# THE ORGANIC CHEMISTRY
# OF DRUG SYNTHESIS

VOLUME 2

# The Organic Chemistry of Drug Synthesis

**VOLUME 2**

**DANIEL LEDNICER**

Mead Johnson and Company

Evansville, Indiana

**LESTER A. MITSCHER**

The University of Kansas School of Pharmacy
Department of Medicinal Chemistry
Lawrence, Kansas

A WILEY-INTERSCIENCE PUBLICATION

JOHN WILEY AND SONS, New York · Chichester · Brisbane · Toronto

*Library of Congress Cataloging in Publication Data:*

Lednicer, Daniel, 1929-
   The organic chemistry of drug synthesis.

  "A Wiley-Interscience publication."
  1. Chemistry, Medical and pharmaceutical.
2. Drugs.  3. Chemistry, Organic.  I. Mitscher,
Lester A., joint author.  II. Title.

RS421.L423    615'.191    76-28387
ISBN 0-471-04392-3

Printed in the United States of America

10 9 8 7 6

It is our pleasure again to dedicate
a book to our helpmeets: Beryle and Betty.

"Has it ever occurred to you that medicinal chemists are just like compulsive gamblers: the next compound will be the real winner."[*]

[*]R. L. Clark at the 16th National Medicinal Chemistry Symposium, June, 1978.

# Preface

The reception accorded "Organic Chemistry of Drug
Synthesis" seems to us to indicate widespread interest
in the organic chemistry involved in the search for
new pharmaceutical agents. We are only too aware of
the fact that the book deals with a limited segment
of the field; the earlier volume cannot be considered
either comprehensive or completely up to date.
Because the earlier book did, however, lay the
groundwork for many of the structural classes or
organic compounds that have proven useful in the
clinic, it forms a natural base for a series that
will, in fact, be comprehensive and up to date.
This second volume fills some of the gaps left by
the earlier work and describes developments in the
field up to the end of 1976. More specifically, we
have included literature and patent preparations for

those compounds granted a USAN* generic name prior to and including 1976 that did not appear in Volume I.

In assembling the first volume, we faced an apparently staggering mass of material. It seemed at the time that attempts to be inclusive would lead to an undigestible compendium. In order to keep the reader's interest, we chose instead to be selective about material to be included. Specifically, the first volume deals predominantly with organic compounds actually used in the clinic. It is, of course, well known that many compounds die in various stages of clinical trials, either from lack of effect, lack of superiority over existing drugs, or the presence of disqualifying side effects. Particularly since 1962, sponsoring companies have become much more demanding in the standards to be met by a drug before undertaking the cost involved in the clinical work leading to an NDA.[†] For that reason, this period has seen a large increase in the number of compounds that have been granted generic names but have failed to achieve clinical use. Many such failed analogues were omitted from the previous volume. Since we now intend to make the series comprehensive, and since those analogues do have heuristic value, we have chosen to violate chronology and include them in the present volume. Volume 2 thus goes beyond simple updating.

[*]United States Adopted Name
[†]New Drug Application

The organization of the material by chemical classes used earlier has been retained since it provided a convenient method for lending coherence to the subject matter. However, changes in emphasis of research in medicinal chemistry have led us to change the organization of the individual chapters. The small amount of new work devoted to some structural types (e.g., phenothiazines) that formed large units in the earlier book failed to provide sufficient material to constitute a chapter here; what material was available has simply been included under some broader new heading. As was the case previously, syntheses have been taken back to commonly available starting materials as far as possible. An exception to this rule will be found in the section on steroids. Many of the compounds described are corticoids, that are the products of intricate multistep syntheses. In the earlier volume, we described the preparation of some quite highly elaborated corticoids using plant sterols as start-ing materials. Many of these corticoids are used for preparation of compounds in this volume. Since there seems little point in simply reiterating those sections, a starting material is judged to be readily available if its preparation is described in the first volume. The reference will be to that book rather than to the original literature.

We have endeavored, too, to approach biological activity in the same fashion as we did earlier. The first time some therapeutic indication occurs will be the occasion for a concise simplified discussion of the disease state and the rationale for the specific method of drug therapy. Biological activities are noted for each generic compound at the same time as its preparation. It will be emphasized again that the activities quoted are those given by the authors; this book is not intended as a critical text in pharmacology.

"Organic Chemistry of Drug Synthesis, Volume 2" is addressed to the same audience as was Volume 1: graduate students in medicinal and organic chemistry, as well as practitioners in the two fields. This book also assumes that the reader will have a good understanding of synthetic organic chemistry and at least a rudimentary knowledge of biology.

Finally, we express our sincere appreciation to several individuals who contributed time and talent to this project. Ms. Carolyn Kelly patiently typed the many versions of the manuscript, including the final camera-ready copy, in the midst of the press of her daily responsibilities. Sheila Newland drew the structural formulae, and John Swayze read the entire manuscript and made several useful suggestions to help clarify the text and reduce the number of typos. Ken McCracken and Peggy Williams were extremely helpful in guiding us through the intricacies of the IBM "Office System 6".


Daniel Lednicer                    Evansville, Indiana
Lester A. Mitscher                  Lawrence, Kansas
                                    January, 1980

# Contents

Chapter 1.  Monocyclic and Acyclic Aliphatic
Compounds                                          1
1. Cyclopentanes                                   1
    a.  Prostaglandins                             1
    b.  Other Cyclopentanoids                      7
2. Cyclohexanes                                    8
    a.  Cyclohexane and Cyclohexene
        Carboxylic Acids                           8
    b.  Cyclohexylamines                          12
    c.  Miscellaneous                             17
3. Adamantanes                                    18
4. Noncyclic Aliphatics                           20
References                                        23

Chapter 2.  Derivatives of Benzyl and Benzhydryl
Alcohols and Amines                               26
1. Derivatives of Benzylamine                     27
2. Benzhydrylamine Derivatives                    30
3. Benzhydrol Derivatives                         31
References                                        34

Chapter 3.  Phenylethyl and Phenylpropylamines    36
            1.  Phenylethyl and Phenyl-
                propylamines                       36
                a.  Those With a Free ArOH
                    Group                          36
                b.  Those Agents With an
                    Acylated or Alkylated ArOH
                    Group                          44
            2.  1-Phenyl-2-Aminopropanediols       45
            3.  Phenylethylamines                  47
            4.  Phenylpropylamines                 55
            References                             59

Chapter 4.  Arylalkanoic Acids and Their
            Derivatives                            63
            1.  Antiinflammatory Arylacetic
                Acids                              63
            2.  Diaryl and Arylalkyl Acetic
                Acids: Anticholinergic Agents      71
            3.  Miscellaneous Arylalkanoic
                Acids                              78
            References                             82

Chapter 5.  Monocyclic Aromatic Compounds         85
            1.  Derivatives of Benzoic Acid        85
                a.  Acids                          85
                b.  Anthranilic Acid and
                    Derivatives                    88
                c.  Amides                         92
            2.  Derivatives of Aniline             95
            3.  Derivatives of Phenol              98
                a.  Basic Ethers                   98
                b.  Phenoxyacetic Acids            101
                c.  Ethers of 1-Aminopropane-
                    2,3-diol                       105
            4.  Arylsulfones and Sulfonamides      111
                a.  Sulfones                       111
                b.  Sulfonamides                   112
            5.  Functionalized Benzene
                Derivatives                        119
                a.  Alkyl Analogues                119
                b.  Miscellaneous Derivatives      126
            References                             127

Chapter 6.  Steroids                                    135
            1.  Estranes                                136
            2.  Androstanes                             153
            3.  Pregnanes                               164
                a.  11-Desoxy Derivatives              164
                b.  11-Oxygenated Pregnanes            176
            References                                  200

Chapter 7.  Polycyclic Aromatic and Hydro-
            aromatic Compounds                          207
            1.  Indanes and Indenes                     208
            2.  Naphthalenes                            211
            3.  Fluorenes                               217
            4.  Anthracenes                             219
            5.  Dibenzocycloheptanes and
                Dibenzycycloheptenes                    221
            6.  Tetracyclines                           226
            References                                  228

Chapter 8.  Five-Membered Heterocycles                  232
            1.  Derivatives of Pyrrole                  233
            2.  Derivatives of Furan                    238
            3.  Derivatives of Imidazole               242
            4.  Derivatives of Pyrazole                261
            5.  Derivatives of Oxazole and
                Isoxazole                               262
            6.  Derivatives of Thiazole                267
            7.  Miscellaneous Five-Membered
                Heterocycles                            270
            References                                  273

Chapter 9.  Six-Membered Heterocycles                   278
            1.  Pyridines                               278
            2.  Piperidines                             284
            3.  Piperazines and Pyrazines              298
            4.  Pyrimidines                             302
            5.  Miscellaneous Structures                304
            References                                  308

Chapter 10. Morphinoids                                 314
            1.  Compounds Derived from
                Morphine                                315
            2.  Morphinans                              323
            3.  Benzomorphans                           325

|  | 4. Phenylpiperidines | 328 |
|  | References | 337 |

| Chapter 11. | Five-Membered Heterocycles Fused to One Benzene Ring | 340 |
|  | 1. Indoles | 340 |
|  | 2. Reduced Indoles | 348 |
|  | 3. Indazoles | 350 |
|  | 4. Benzimidazoles | 352 |
|  | 5. Miscellaneous | 354 |
|  | References | 358 |

| Chapter 12. | Six-Membered Heterocycles Fused to One Benzene Ring | 361 |
|  | 1. Quinolines | 362 |
|  | 2. Isoquinolines | 373 |
|  | 3. Quinazolines | 379 |
|  | 4. Cinnolines and Quinoxalines | 387 |
|  | 5. Miscellaneous Benzohetero-cycles | 390 |
|  | References | 396 |

| Chapter 13. | Benzodiazepines | 401 |
|  | References | 407 |

| Chapter 14. | Heterocycles Fused to Two Benzene Rings | 409 |
|  | 1. Central Rings Containing One Heteroatom | 410 |
|  | 2. Benzoheterocycloheptadienes | 420 |
|  | 3. Derivatives of Dibenzolactams | 424 |
|  | 4. Other Dibenzoheterocycles | 430 |
|  | References | 432 |

| Chapter 15. | β-Lactam Antibiotics | 435 |
|  | 1. Penicillins | 437 |
|  | 2. Cephalosporins | 439 |
|  | 3. Cephamycins | 442 |
|  | References | 443 |

| Chapter 16. | Miscellaneous Fused Heterocycles | 445 |
|  | 1. Compounds with Two Fused Rings | 446 |
|  | 2. Compounds with Three or More Fused Rings | 451 |

    3.  Purines and Related Hetero-
        cycles                              463
    4.  Polyaza Fused Heterocycles         469
    5.  Ergolines                          475
    References                             480

Indexes                                    483

Cross Index of Drugs                       485

Index                                      501

Errata for VOLUME 1 of ORGANIC CHEMISTRY OF
DRUG SYNTHESIS                             513

# 1

# Monocyclic and Acyclic Aliphatic Compounds

1.  CYCLOPENTANES

a.  Prostaglandins

When realistic quantities of the natural prostaglandins became available, their extreme potency and wide-ranging biological activities were discovered and visions of therapeutic application in the regulation of fertility, control of ulcers, blood pressure, bronchial asthma, and many other conditions led to a torrent of chemical and biological studies which currently measures about four papers daily, and at least one a week dealing with synthesis alone. Initial chemical emphasis lay in developing efficient syntheses of the natural substances to solve the supply problem. Presently, the emphasis has shifted to preparation of analogues which are intended to be less expensive, more selective in their action, and longer lasting. The five drug candidates in this

1

section are significant representatives of the
hundreds of such analogues available.

The naturally occurring prostaglandins, $E_1$, $E_2$
and $A_1$, have potent antisecretory activity when
given parenterally and have been suggested for use
in treatment of gastric ulcers.  Unfortunately,
these natural compounds have relatively poor oral
activity and rapid metabolism makes their action
short-lived.  Molecular manipulation proved that an
oxygen atom at $C_{11}$ was not necessary for bioactivity
but these compounds also lacked the desired oral
activity. This problem was solved by a study of the
metabolizing enzymes and by borrowing an artifice
from steroid chemistry (*viz*-methyl testosterone,
Volume I).  The most rapid metabolic deactivating
reaction is oxidation to the bioinert $C_{15}$-oxo prostaglandins.  Converting the latter to a tertiary
methyl carbinol led to the desired orally active
gastric antisecretory agents.

Starting with 2-carbomethoxycyclopentanone *(1)*,
t-BuOK catalyzed alkylation of methyl ω-bromohepta-
noate gave diester *2* which was then hydrolyzed and
decarboxylated.  The conjugated double bond was then
introduced by a bromination-dehydrobromination
sequence to give versatile prostaglandin synthon *3*.
Esterification to *4* was followed by conjugate addition
of sodio nitromethane to give *5*.  Nitroketone *5* was
converted to the sodium salt of the corresponding
nitronic acid with sodium in methanol and this was
hydrolyzed with icecold dilute $H_2SO_4$ to ketoaldehyde
*6*.  This sequence is the Nef reaction.  Wittig

reaction of this sodio dimethyl-2-ketoheptyl phosphonate gave 7.[1,2]   Ester hydrolysis to 8 followed by
careful reaction with methyl magnesium bromide
produced the orally active bronchiodilator, *doxaprost*
(9).[2]   Doxaprost, at least as originally prepared,
is conformationally undefined at $C_{15}$ and is probably
a mixture of R and S isomers.

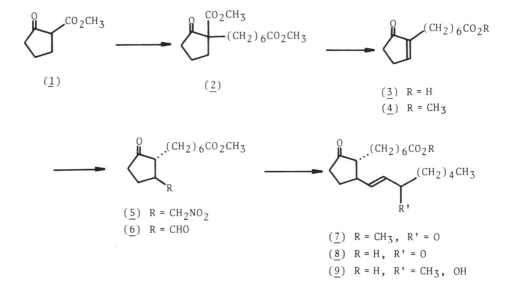

(1)

(2)

(3) R = H
(4) R = $CH_3$

(5) R = $CH_2NO_2$
(6) R = CHO

(7) R = $CH_3$, R' = O
(8) R = H, R' = O
(9) R = H, R' = $CH_3$, OH

Enzymic studies demonstrated that the 15-
dehydrogenase was also inhibited by saturation of
the $C_{13}$ double bond and *deprostil (12)* embodies this
chemical feature as well.[3]  Catalytic hydrogenation
of 7 produced 10 which was hydrolyzed to 11 and
reacted with methyl magnesium bromide in ether. As
above, careful control of conditions allowed the
organometallic reagent to add selectively to the

less hindered side chain carbonyl to produce the
orally active potent gastric antisecretory agent,
*deprostil (12).* Interestingly, studies with resolved
*12* showed that the unnatural epimer at $C_{15}$ was more
potent.

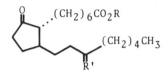

(<u>10</u>)  R = CH$_3$,  R' = O
(<u>11</u>)  R = H,  R' = O
(<u>12</u>)  R = H,  R' = CH$_3$, OH

Introduction of an allene function in place of
an olefinic double bond is not commonly employed by
medicinal chemists, although such derivatives are
occasionally used as progestational steroids.  It is
interesting, therefore, that the presence of this
synthetic feature is consistent with typical prostaglandin biopotency.[4]  In this case, the well-known
Corey-lactol synthon, *13*, was reacted with dilithio
pent-4-yn-1-ol to give acetylenic carbinol *14* which
was protected by esterification with acetyl chloride
to give *15*. Treatment of *15* with LiMe$_2$Cu led to
allene *16*.  The mechanism of this curious reaction
is not clear.  Possibly the reagent forms an organometallic derivative of the acetylene moiety with
expulsion of the acetate group and double bond
migration as a consequence.  When this sequence was
applied in earlier papers to terminal acetylenes
(*e.g.*, *J. Am. Chem. Soc.*, *91*, 3289 (1969)), terminal

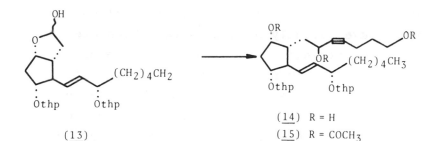

(13)

(14) R = H
(15) R = COCH₃

(16)

(17)

methylation accompanied allene formation and loss of the acetoxy group. Careful alkaline hydrolysis of allene *16* preferentially cleaved the terminal primary ester. The resulting alcohol was then oxidized to the carboxylic acid with Jones' reagent. Saponification under more strenuous conditions removed the remaining acetate group and acid treatment removed the thp ethers. There is thus obtained *prostalene* *(17)*, which has been described as a bronchodilator and hypotensive agent.

Animal husbandry requires the careful selection and management of breeding stock and a prize stud is an economically valuable asset. The expensive service fee makes it very important that the female be in estrus at the time of mating. In order to

optimize the breeding process, two prostaglandin
analogues have recently been marketed which are
potent luteolytic agents used to regularize or
synchronize estrus in horses. The inclusion of an
aryloxy residue in place of the last three carbons
of the aliphatic moiety at the methyl terminus of
the prostaglandins greatly increases activity and
apparently decreases metabolic deactivation.

The synthesis begins with *18*, a well-known
prostaglandin synthon first developed by Corey.[5]
This is condensed with the appropriate phosphonate
ylide reagents (*19* or *20*) which are themselves
prepared by reaction of the appropriate ester or
acid chloride of an aryloxyacetic acid with the
anion of the dimethyl methylphosphonate. The resulting *trans*-eneone (*21* or *22*) is reduced with zinc
borohydride, the p-phenylphenylester serving to give
preferential reduction to the 15α-ols. The ester is
then hydrolyzed with $K_2CO_3$/MeOH and the two alcoholic
functions are protected as the tetrahydropyranyl
ethers. Reduction with diisobutylaluminum hydride
at -78°C produces lactols *23* and *24* and their $C_{15}$
epimers. Reaction with the Wittig reagent from 5-
triphenylphosphonopentanoic acid and acid catalyzed
removal of the protecting groups followed by chromatography gives *fluprostenol (25)* and *cloprostenol
(26)*,[6] respectively. These compounds are several
hundred times more potent by injection than prostaglandin $F_{2\alpha}$ as luteolytic agents, although striking
species differences are observed.

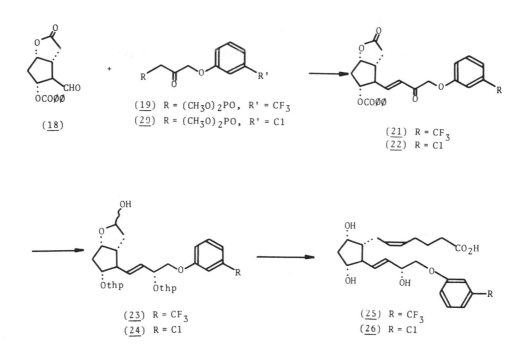

(18)

(19) R = $(CH_3O)_2PO$, R' = $CF_3$
(20) R = $(CH_3O)_2PO$, R' = Cl

(21) R = $CF_3$
(22) R = Cl

(23) R = $CF_3$
(24) R = Cl

(25) R = $CF_3$
(26) R = Cl

b.   Other Cyclopentanoids

Clinical success with the monoamine oxidase inhibitor
and amphetamine analogue *tranylcypromine (27)* led to
an exploration of the effect of ring size on activity.[7]  It was found that an interesting dissociation
of properties could be achieved and the best of the
series, *cypenamine (30)*, is an antidepressant without
significant MAO inhibitory activity.  One of the
more convenient syntheses[8] makes use of the finding
that hydroxylamine-O-sulfonic acid is soluble in
diglyme and therefore is suitable for conversion of
organoboranes from hindered and unhindered olefins
into the corresponding amines.  1-Phenylcyclopentene

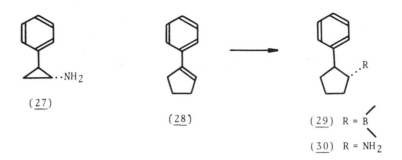

(27)

(28)

(29) R = B

(30) R = NH$_2$

*(28)* is hydroborated to *29* in the usual way with
borohydride and BF$_3$.  Addition of H$_2$NOSO$_3$H followed
by acid hydrolysis completes the synthesis of *cypenamine (30)* with excellent regio and stereospecificity.
The reaction sequence is a net *cis* anti-Markownikoff
addition of the elements of NH$_3$ to *28*.

    2.   CYCLOHEXANES

    a.   Cyclohexane and Cyclohexene Carboxylic
Acids This subgroup is classified strictly for
chemical convenience because their pharmacological
properties are unrelated to one another.

    Clotting of blood is, of course, one of the
more significant ways in which the body protects
itself from excessive blood loss after injury.
After the healing takes place, the clot, which is a
three-dimensional polypeptide, is broken down by
proteolytic enzymes such as fibrinolysin or plasmin.
In some pathological states, fibrinolysis is hyper-
active and inhibitors have a hemostatic value.

    Plasmin does not occur in free form but is
generated as needed from an inactive precursor,
plasminogen.  The active of plasminogen to plasmin
is a proteolytic event and can be inhibited by ω-

aminocarboxylic acids having a structural or spatial
resemblance to lysine. One such agent is *p-amino-
methylbenzoic acid (33)* and its reduction product
*tranexamic acid (34).*[9] First p-cyanotoluene *(31)* is
oxidized to the carboxylic acid *(32)* with $CrO_3$; then
reduction of the nitrile group with Raney cobalt in
the presence of liquid ammonia produces p-aminomethyl-
benzoic acid *(33)*. Reduction of the aromatic ring of

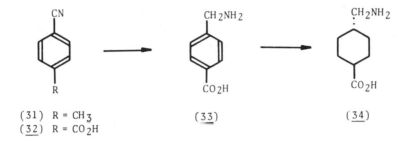

(31) R = CH_3
(32) R = CO_2H                    (33)                    (34)

33 with a platinum catalyst produces mainly the *cis*
isomer. Upon heating under nitrogen at 315-325°,
isomerization occurs to the *trans*-analogue *(34)*
which possesses all of the hemostatic activity.

Many substances other than estrone possess
estrogenic activity and some of these bear only
little formal resemblance to the natural hormone.
Many years ago, doisynolic acid *(39)*, a steroid
degradation product, was shown to have such activity.
Over the years many simple compounds have been
synthesized following the idea of molecular dissection. One of these is *fenestrel (38)*.[10] Hageman's
ester *(35)* is alkylated to *36* by t-BuOK and ethyl-
bromide. The regioselectivity observed is generally

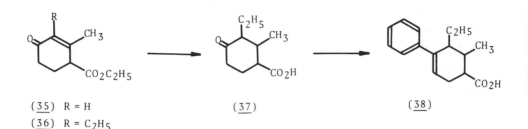

(35) R = H
(36) R = C$_2$H$_5$

(37)

(38)

(39)

(40)

(41) R = CN
(42) R = CO$_2$H

(43)

regarded to be a consequence of the greater reactivity of the enolate at C$_2$ over the other possible
enolates (at C$_4$ and C$_6$).  The double bond is reduced
with hydrogen and a palladium catalyst and saponification produces *37* of unspecified stereochemistry.
Treatment with phenyl magnesium bromide followed by
dehydration with tosic acid in acetic acid leads to
the estrogen, *fenestrel (38)*.  Presumably, the
double bond remains tri- rather than tetrasubstituted
in this case because of the steric interactions this
latter case would engender between the ethyl and
phenyl groups.  The stereochemistry of *fenestrel* is
complex so formula *38* implies no stereochemical
meaning.

A smooth muscle relaxant apparently of the
antimuscarinic type whose actions, therefore, are
somewhat reminiscent of atropine, is *isomylamine*
*(43)*.[11]  Its synthesis begins with the sodamide
catalyzed alkylation of cyclohexyl nitrile *(40)* with
1-bromo-3-methylbutane and the resulting nitrile
*(41)* is hydrolyzed to the acid *(42)* with HBr in
acetic acid. Alkylation of the sodium salt of this
acid using β-chloroethyldiethylamine leads to the
desired *43*.

Coughing is a useful physiologic device utilized
to clear the respiratory tract of foreign substances
and excessive secretions.  Coughing, however, does
not always serve a useful purpose but can rob the
patient of sleep.  A number of agents are available
to suppress this.  Many of these are narcotic and
have an undesirable abuse potential. One of the
agents available which is claimed to be nonnarcotic
is *amicibone (45)*.[12]  The synthesis involves
base-catalyzed alkylation of benzyl cyclohexan-
ecarboxylate *(44)* with β-hexamethyleneiminoethyl
chloride  a reaction which may go through an
aziridinium intermediate.

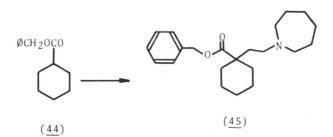

ØCH₂OCO

(44)                                              (45)

b.  Cyclohexylamines

Although substantial strides have been made toward
the chemotherapeutic control of cancer, much remains
to be accomplished with respect to broadening of
activity spectrum, decreasing host toxicity, increasing remission time, etc., of the various chemotherapeutic agents available.  Lacking an all-encompassing
rationale upon which to build a drug design program,
many potentially useful leads have emerged from
directed screening efforts.  The nitrosoureas *carmustine (BCNU, 48)*, *lomustine (CCNU, 58)* and *semustine
(MeCCNU, 56)* are cases in point belonging to the
group of cytotoxic alkylating agents.

Cell multiplication requires the rapid synthesis
of functional DNA.  Those cells which are dividing
most rapidly, for example, cancer cells, are particularly sensitive to agents which disrupt this
process.  The alkylating agents alkylate the purine
and pyrimidine bases and so convert them to unnatural
compounds.  This has the consequence of stopping DNA
synthesis and/or inhibiting transcription of the
genetic code from DNA.  Normal host cells generally
spend time in a resting stage where they are less
damaged by these cytotoxic agents.  Tumor cells, by
contrast, are almost always in an active phase of
the cell cycle.  Following up a lead discovered at
the Cancer Chemotherapy National Service Center, it
was ultimately shown that unsymmetrical N-nitro-
soureas are quite potent alkylating agents and
several are now in clinical trial.

BCNU is synthesized[13,14] by treating phosgene
with ethyleneimine without the addition of a base to
take up the HCl liberated.  Reaction of the intermediate urea (46) in situ with hydrogen chloride
serves to open the aziridine rings to afford sym-
bis-2-chlorethylurea (47).  This is nitrosated with
sodium nitrite in formic acid to give BCNU (48).

$$2\ \big[\!\!\big>\!NH\ +\ COCl_2 \longrightarrow \big[\!\!\big>\!N\overset{O}{\overset{\|}{C}}N\!\!<\!\!\big] \longrightarrow (Cl(CH_2)_2N)_2\overset{H}{\overset{|}{C}}\overset{O}{\overset{\|}{}} \longrightarrow ClCH_2CH_2\overset{N=O}{\overset{|}{N}}CONHCH_2CH_2Cl$$

$$(\underline{46}) \qquad\qquad (\underline{47}) \qquad\qquad\qquad (\underline{48})$$

On standing in water under various conditions,
two main modes of degradation occur and these are
rationalized as follows.

The nonnitrosated nitrogen of 49 supplies
electrons for an intromolecular displacement of Cl
to give intermediate imino ether 50 which collapses
to isocyanate 51 and highly reactive 52 which latter
fragments, ejecting nitrogen and capturing OH to
produce acetaldehyde, after enolization.  In the
second mode, a cyclic fragmentation process (53)
leads to isocyanate 51 and N-hydroxy-2-chloroethyl-
azine (54) which undergoes fragmentation, losing
nitrogen and capturing OH (to give 2-chloroethanol)
or $NH_3$ (to give 2-chloroethylamine). As 2-chloroethyl-
amine is a known source of aziridine, this substance
has potential alkylating activity.  Also, ejection

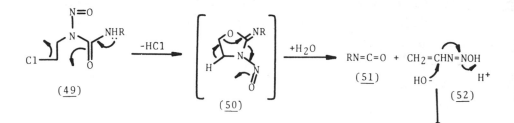

(49) → (50) → (51) + (52) → CH$_3$CHO + N$_2$ + H$_2$O

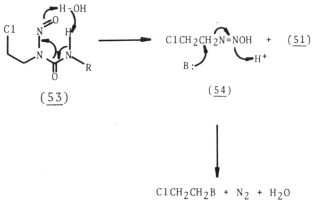

(53) → ClCH$_2$CH$_2$N=NOH (54) + (51)

ClCH$_2$CH$_2$B + N$_2$ + H$_2$O
B=OH; NH$_2$

of nitrogen from *52* to *54* leads to electron deficient
species which react with nucleophiles.  The isocyanate *(51)* also adds nucleophiles.  Thus, it is
not certain at this stage which of these is the most
responsible agent for the bioactivity or whether the
antitumor properties are a blend of these.

The reader has noted that unsymmetrical ureas can nitrosate on either nitrogen and that these decomposition modes enable one to assign structure to the products.  This, in fact, also has preparative significance and both *lomustine (CCNU, 58)* and its methyl analogue *semustine (MeCCNU, 56)* are made in this way.[14]  In the *semustine* synthesis, *BCNU (48)* is decomposed in the presence of two equivalents of *trans*-4-methylcyclohexylamine to give an 84% yield of unsymmetrical urea *55*--probably *via* the trapping of intermediate isocyanate *51* (R = $CH_2CH_2Cl$). Nitrosation with $NaNO_2/HCO_2H$ produces *semustine (56)* contaminated with some of the alternate nitroso analogue.  Use of cyclohexylamine in this reaction sequence leads to *lomustine (58)* instead.  There is some evidence to suggest that *in vivo* 4-hydroxylation to *59* may be of great importance in the activity of *lomustine*.

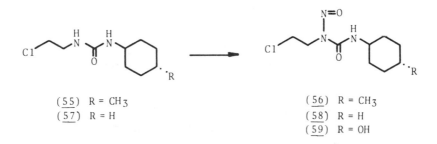

(55) R = CH₃          (56) R = CH₃
(57) R = H            (58) R = H
                      (59) R = OH

A more complex cyclohexylamine, *tiletamine* *(65)*, is a useful anesthetic in that injection leads to loss of consciousness without an untoward decrease in blood pressure or heart rate and without undue respiratory depression.  Its synthesis[15] begins with

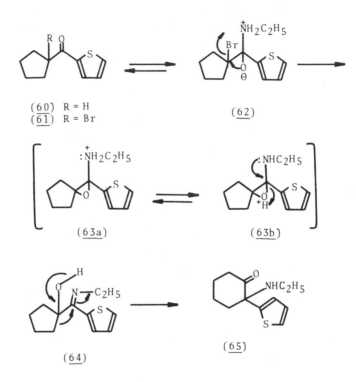

(60) R = H
(61) R = Br

(62)

(63a)          (63b)

(64)

(65)

bromination of α-thienylcyclopentylketone *(60)* to
give *61*.  Reaction with ethylamine appears to involve
carbonyl addition to *62* followed by epoxy formation
*(63ab)* and then rearrangement to ethylimine *64* after
proton loss.  It is, of course, apparent that bromide
*61* could not undergo a Favorskii rearrangement.
Thermolysis of *64* results in a ring expansion and
formation of *tiletamine (65)*.  The close structural
relationship between *tiletamine* and *ketamine*[16] is
probably not coincidental.

c.   Miscellaneous

The molecular dissection embodied in the morphine rule (66) has served as a useful empirical guide for the synthesis of analgesic agents even though a number of significant agents fit the rule poorly. Briefly, the morphine rule suggests that substances containing an aromatic ring attached to a quaternary carbon which is in turn separated from a tertiary amine by two carbons might be active.   One such is tramadol (69).   It is synthesized[17] by reacting the Grignard reagent prepared from m-methoxybromobenzene (67) with 2-dimethylaminomethylenecyclohexanone (68), itself obtained by Mannich reaction on cyclohexanone, to give tramadol (69).   The isomers are separated by fractional crystallization of the HCl salts.

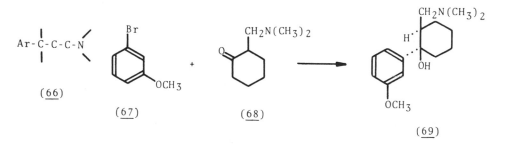

A closely related analgesic which does not fit into the morphine rule is nexeridine (73).   In this case,[18] 2-phenylcyclohexanone (70) is reacted with the lithium salt of N,N-dimethylpropionamide (71) to give tertiary alcohol 72.   Reduction of the latter with lithium aluminum hydride gives nexeridine (73).

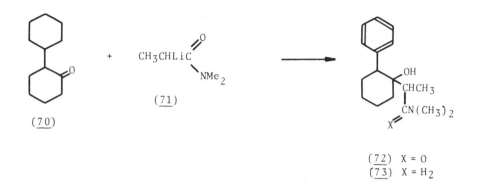

$$CH_3CHLiC \overset{O}{\underset{NMe_2}{}}$$

(71)

(70)

(72) X = O
(73) X = H₂

### 3.  ADAMANTANES

The adamantane moiety is of medicinal chemical
interest because of its inertness, compactness
relative to lipid solubilizing character, and symmetry.  Considerable interest, therefore, was en-
gendered by the finding that *amantadine* (78) was
active for the chemoprophylaxis of influenza A in
man.  There are not many useful chemotherapeutic
agents available for the treatment of communicable
viral infections, so this finding led to considerable
molecular manipulation. The recent abrupt end of the
National Influenza Immunization program of 1976
prompted a new look at the nonvaccine means for
prophylaxis or treatment of respiratory tract infections due to influenza A, especially in that the
well-known antigenic shift or drift of the virus
obviates usefulness of the vaccine but not *amantadine*.
The synthesis[19] begins with the halogenation of
adamantane (74) with bromine to give 76 or chlorine
and AlCl₃ to give 75.  The four bridgehead positions

are identical and surprisingly reactive. Reaction

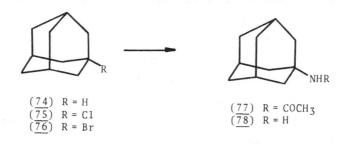

(74) R = H
(75) R = Cl
(76) R = Br

(77) R = COCH₃
(78) R = H

of 76 with acetonitrile in sulfuric acid leads
through an apparent SN₁ reaction to amide 77 which
is hydrolyzed by base to give *amantadine (78)*. A
similar antiviral agent, *rimantadine (83)*, is also
useful for treatment of respiratory diseases due to
type A influenza virus. It is synthesized[20] from

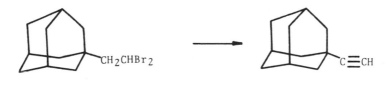

(79)

(80)

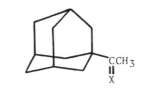

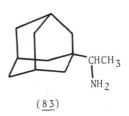

(81) X = O
(82) X = NOH

(83)

adamantyl bromide (76) by $AlBr_3$ catalyzed addition
of vinylbromide to give 79 which is then dehydro-
halogenated by heating with KOH to give acetylene
80.   Hydration to methyl ketone 81 is achieved by
HgO-catalyzed reaction with sulfuric acid.   After
oxime formation (82) lithium aluminum hydride reduction leads to *rimantidine (83)*.

The high lipophilicity of adamantyl moieties
suggests that drugs containing them might pass into
tissues of high lipid content or cross the blood-
brain barrier.   Indeed *carmantadine (85)* is active
against the spasms associated with Parkinson's
disease.   *Amantadine (78)* reacts[21] with methyl 2,4-
dibromobutyrate to give ester 84 which can be hydrolyzed with aqueous barium hydroxide to complete the
synthesis of *carmantidine (85)*.

(78) ⟶

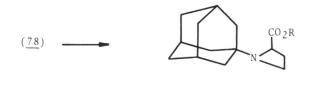

(84)  R = $CH_3$
(85)  R = H

### 4.   NONCYCLIC ALIPHATICS

Many of the biguanides have oral hypoglycemic
activity, and *metformin (87)* is such an antidiabetic
agent.   Cyanamide has a highly reactive nitrile
function because of the electropositive $NH_2$ group

attached and at pH 8-9 self-adds to form "dicyanamide"
(86, for which cyanoguanidine would be a better
name).  Fusion with dimethylamine[22] leads efficiently
to metformin (87) by addition to the nitrile function.
Metformin is closely related to buformin.[23]

The discovery and clinical acceptance of
meprobamate, and the relative chemical accessibility
of this group of compounds has led to intensive
exploration of 1,3-biscarbamates.  It was found that

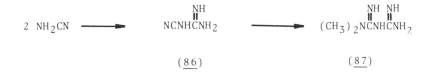

$$2 \ NH_2CN \longrightarrow \overset{\overset{NH}{\|}}{NCNHCNH_2} \longrightarrow \overset{\overset{NH}{\|} \ \overset{NH}{\|}}{(CH_3)_2NCNHCNH_2}$$

(86)                              (87)

substitution of one of the NH hydrogens by an alkyl
group changed the emphasis of the biological response
from muscle relaxant and anticonvulsant to centrally
acting muscle relaxant whose action differs somewhat
from meprobamate.  Carisoprodol was the best member
of one of these series and lorbamate (92) is its
cyclopropyl analogue. The chief synthetic problem to
be overcome was the differentiation of the two
primary alcohol groups of 89, readily accessible by
lithium aluminum hydride reduction of the appropriate
di-substituted malonate (88).  This was solved[24] by
an ester exchange reaction with diethylcarbonate to
give 90 which produced carbamate 91 on reaction with

cyclopropylamine.  Ester exchange of *91* with ethyl
carbamate led efficiently to *lorbamate* (*92*), a
useful muscle relaxant.

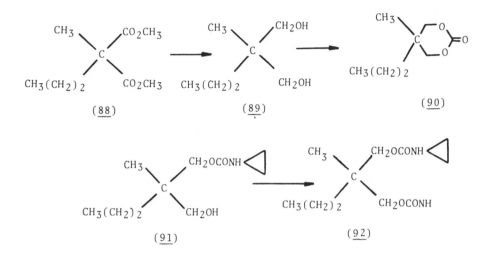

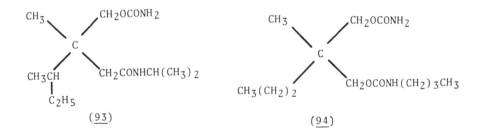

Relatively simple variants of this basic scheme
led to the minor tranquilizers *nisobamate* (*93*)[25] and
*tybamate* (*94*).[26]

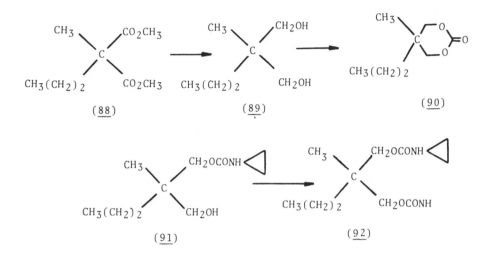

REFERENCES

1. J. F. Bagli and T. Bogri, *Tetrahedron Lett.*, 3815 (1972); for a photochemically-based alternate synthesis, see J. F. Bagli and T. Bogri, *J. Org. Chem.*, *37*, 2132 (1972).

2. M. Baumgarth, J. Hartin, K. Irmscher, J. Kraemer, D. Orth, H. E. Radunz and H. J. Schliep, Ger. Patent 2,305,437 (1974); W. Lippmann, *Prostaglandins*, *7*, 1 (1974).

3. J. F. Bagli, T. Bogri and S. N. Sehgal, *Tetrahedron Lett.*, 3329 (1973).

4. P. Crabbe and H. Carpio, *J. Chem. Soc.*, *Chem. Commun.*, 904 (1972).

5. E. J. Corey, N. M. Weinshenker, T. F. Schaaf and W. Huber, *J. Am. Chem. Soc.*, *91*, 5675 (1969).

6. D. Binder, J. Bowler, E. D. Brown, N. S. Crossley, J. Hutton, M. Senior, L. Slater, P. Wilkinson and N. C. A. Wright, *Prostaglandins*, *6*, 87 (1974).

7. W. R. McGrath and W. L. Kuhn, *Arch. Int. Pharmacodyn. Ther.*, *172*, 405 (1968).

8. M. W. Rathke, N. Inoue, K. R. Varma and H. C. Brown, *J. Am. Chem. Soc.*, *88*, 2870 (1966).

9. M. Levine and R. Sedlecky, *J. Org. Chem.*, *24*, 115 (1959); Anon., Spanish Patent 358,367 (1970).

10. A. Mebane, U. S. Patent 3,344,147 (1967); A. H. Nathan and J. A. Hogg, *J. Am. Chem. Soc.*, *78*, 6163 (1956).

11.  C. H. Tilford, L. A. Doerle, M. G. VanCampen,
     Jr., and R. S. Shelton, *J. Am. Chem. Soc.*, *71*,
     1705 (1949).

12.  A. Frank, A. Kraushaar, H. Margreiter and R.
     Schunk, Austrian Patent 237,593 (1964).

13.  H. Bestian, *Ann. Chem.*, *566*, 210 (1950).

14.  T. P. Johnson, G. S. McCaleb and J. A.
     Montgomery, *J. Med. Chem.*, *6*, 669 (1963); T. P.
     Johnson, G. S. McCaleb, P. S. Opliger and J. A.
     Montgomery, *Ibid.*, *9*, 892 (1966).

15.  Anon., Netherlands Patent 6,603,587 (1966); C.
     L. Stevens, A. B. Ash, A. Thuillier, J. H.
     Amin, A. Balys, W. E. Dennis, J. P. Dickerson,
     R. P. Galinski, H. T. Hanson, M. D. Pillai and
     J. W. Stoddard, *J. Org. Chem.*, *31*, 2593 (1966).

16.  D. Lednicer and L. Mitscher, *Organic Chemistry
     of Drug Synthesis*, *1*, 59 (1977).

17.  Anon., British Patent 997,399 (1965); *Chem.
     Abstr.*, *63:* 9871f (1965).

18.  B. V. Shetty and T. L. Thomas, Ger. Patent
     2,509,053 (1975).

19.  K. Gerzon, E. V. Krumkalus, R. L. Brindle, F.
     J. Marshall and M. A. Root, *J. Med. Chem.*, *6*,
     760 (1963); H. Stetter, J. Mayer, M. Schwarz
     and K. Wulff, *Chem. Ber.*, *93*, 226 (1970).

20.  P. E. Aldrich, E. C. Hermann, W. E. Meier, M.
     Paulshock, W. W. Prichard, J. A. Snyder and J.
     C. Watts, *J. Med. Chem.*, *14*, 535 (1971); H.
     Stetter and P. Goebel, *Chem. Ber.*, *95*, 1039
     (1962).

21.   E. H. Gold, U. S. Patent 3,917,840; *Chem.*
      *Abstr.*, *84:* 59221k (1976).
22.   S. L. Shapiro, V. A. Parrino and L. Freedman,
      *J. Am. Chem. Soc.*, *81*, 3728 (1959).
23.   D. Lednicer and L. Mitscher, *Organic Chemistry*
      *of Drug Synthesis*, *1*, 221 (1977).
24.   B. L. Ludwig, L. S. Powell and F. M. Berger, *J.*
      *Med. Chem.*, *12*, 462 (1969).
25.   F. M. Berger and B. L. Ludwig, U. S. Patent
      2,937,119 (1960); G. Schneider, M. Halmos, P.
      Meszaros and O. Kovaks, *Monatsh.*, *94*, 426
      (1963).

# 2

# Derivatives of Benzyl and Benzhydryl Alcohols and Amines

As will become apparent in a perusal of this book, organic molecules owe their biological activity to a variety of structural features. Sometimes a set of activities is associated with the structural backbone of a molecule. For example, most prostanoids share certain biological properties despite some changes in functionality; the same will be noted later for steroids. Some biological activities are associated with a specific arrangement of structural subunits; e.g., β-adrenergic blocking agents tend to be derivatives of aryloxypropanolamines. Some activities are quite directly associated with a specific functionality; no better example of this exists than the host of guanidine-containing sympathetic blocking agents. Sometimes, however, no such discernable

relationship can be detected between activity and
structure.  Such classes are often marked by widely
divergent activities.  Derivatives of benzyl- and
benzhydrylamines and alcohols fall into this latter
category.

1.  Derivatives of Benzylamine

In the course of some work aimed at delineation of
the structure-activity relationships of the antidepressant monoamine oxidase (MAO) inhibiting drug
*pargyline (1)*, it was noted that activity was consistent with quite wide modification of the substitution on nitrogen.  One of the best drugs to emerge
from this study is *encyprate (4)*. Hydrogenation of
the Shiff base from benzaldehyde and cyclopropylamine
*(2)* gave the secondary amine *(3)*.  Treatment of this
with ethyl chloroformate afforded the MAO inhibitor
*encyprate (4)*.[1,2]

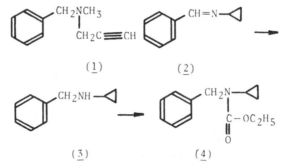

A derivative of benzylhydrazine, *procarbazine
(8)*, exhibits antineoplastic activity.  In an interesting insertion-type sequence, reaction of the p-
toluamide *(5)* with ethyl azodicarboxylate leads
directly to the substituted hydrazine *(6)*.  It is
not unlikely that the first mole of the diazo compound

oxidizes the benzylic methyl group to an anion or
radical anion; addition of that to a second mole of
diazo compound would give the observed product (6).
Methylation by means of sodium hydride and methyl
iodide proceeded at the less hindered amide to give
(7).    Acid hydrolysis of the carbethoxy groups leads
finally to (8).[3]

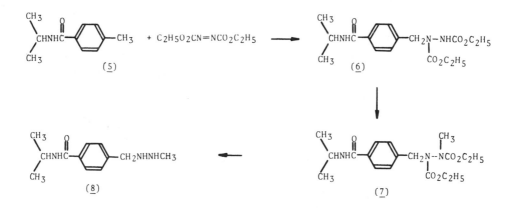

An important feature of the antibiotic *chloramphenicol (9)* is the presence of the dichloroacetamide
function. Inclusion of this amide in a simpler
molecule, *teclozan (15)*, leads to a compound with
antiamebic activity.  Whether this is cause and
effect or fortuitous is unclear.  The synthesis
begins with alkylation of the alkoxide derived from
ethanolamine *(10)* with ethyl iodide to give the
aminoether *(11)*.   Reaction of α,α'-dibromo-p-xylene
*(12)* with 2-nitropropane in the presence of base
leads to dialdehyde *(13)*. The reaction probably
proceeds by O-alkylation on the nitropropyl anion

followed by bond reorganization and subsequent
hydrolysis of the resulting enol ether. Reductive
alkylation of the dialdehyde with aminoether *(11)*
gives diamine *(14)*. Acylation by means of dichloroacetyl chloride affords *teclozan (15)*.[4]

The presence of the dichloroacetamide grouping
is apparently not an absolute requirement for anti-

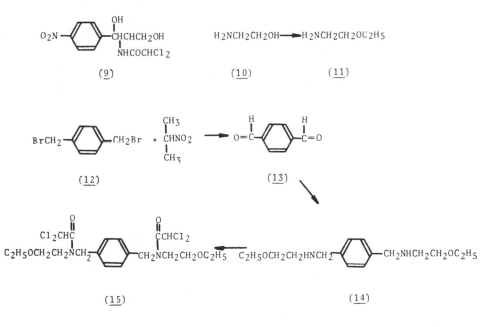

amebic activity. In one pertinent example, reductive
alkylation of dialdehyde *(16)* with n-hexylamine
affords *17a* and Eschweiler-Clark methylation of *17a*
by heating with formaldehyde in formic acid then
leads to the antiamebic drug *symetine (17b)*.[5]

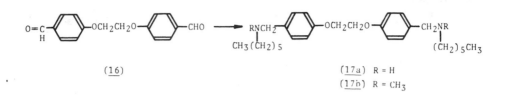

(16)                              (17a)  R = H
                                  (17b)  R = CH₃

## 2. Benzhydrylamine Derivatives

Attachment of piperazine nitrogen directly to a
benzhydryl carbon leads to a pair of compounds which
show vasodilator activity, and which should be
useful in disease states marked by impaired blood
circulation. Reaction of piperonyl chloride (18)
with a mixture of piperazine and piperazine dihydro-
chloride leads to the monoalkylation product (19).
(It may be supposed that the mixture of free base
and salt equilibrates to the monobasic salt, thus
making the second amine less nucleophilic.) Alkylation of 19 by means of benzhydryl chloride then
affords the coronary vasodilator medibazine (20).[6]

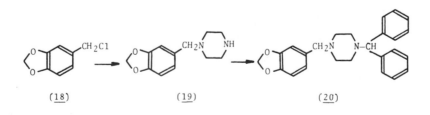

(18)                    (19)                    (20)

In an analogous sequence, condensation of piperazine with 4,4'-difluorobenzhydryl chloride gives the monoalkylation product *(22)*. Reaction of *22* with cinnamyl bromide affords *flunarizine (23)*.[7] *Flunarizine* is also a coronary vasodilator.

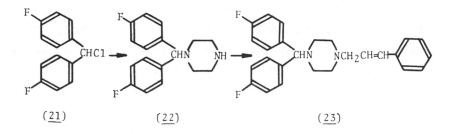

(21)                  (22)                       (23)

3.  Benzyhydrol Derivatives
*Cyprolidol (26)*, a highly modified benzhydrol derivative, is reported to exhibit antidepressant activity; it is of note that this agent bears little structural relation to either the MAO inhibitors or tricyclic antidepressants.  Addition of the carbene from

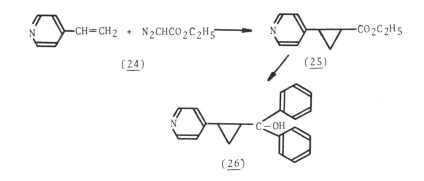

(24)

(25)

(26)

decomposition of ethyl diazoacetate to 4-vinyl-
pyridine gives the cyclopropane (25) (stereochemistry
unspecified).  Condensation of the ester with phenylmagnesium bromide affords cyprolidol (26).[8]

Basic ethers of benzhydrols are among some of
the better known antihistaminic compounds.  The
earlier volume describes well over a dozen of these
drugs.  However, research in the area of allergy has
recently shifted away from compounds which antagonize
the action of histamine to drugs that intervene in
earlier stages of the allergic reaction.  The basic
ethers are therefore represented here by but a few
entries.  In the preparation of rotoxamine (28),
reaction of pyridine-2-carboxaldehyde with the
Grignard reagent formed from p-bromochlorobenzene
gives the carbinol (27); alkylation with N,N-dimethyl-
chloroethylamine and optical resolution gives rotoxamine (28), the levorotatory form of carbinoxamine.[9]

A slightly more complex scheme is required for
preparation of an antihistaminic agent bearing a
secondary amine, e.g., tofenacin (32).  In the
synthesis of tofenacin, alkylation of the benzhydrol
(29) with ethyl bromoacetate affords the alkoxy
ester (30); saponification followed by conversion to
the methylamide gives (31), which is reduced with
lithium aluminum hydride to complete the synthesis
of 32.[10]

Antihistaminic properties are well known to be
preserved even when nitrogen is included in a ring,
such as in clemastine (36).  Synthesis of 36 is
begun by reaction of 4-chlorobenzophenone (33) with

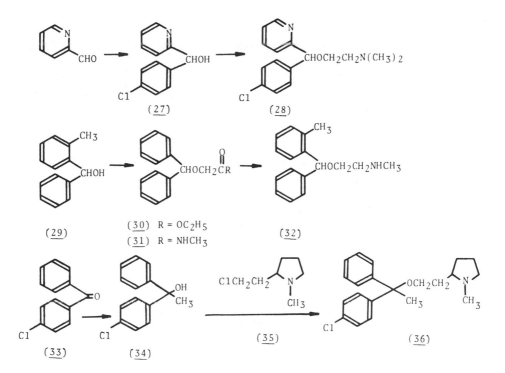

(27)  (28)

(29)  (30) R = OC₂H₅
(31) R = NHCH₃  (32)

(33)  (34)  (35)  (36)

methyl magnesium bromide to give the carbinol (34).
Alkylation of 34 with the chloroethyl pyrrolidine
(35) then yields *clemastine* (36).[11]

    Arrhythmias, that is, disturbances in the
regular timed beating of the heart, often result in
life-threatening situations, since the pumping
efficiency of the heart is directly related to its
rhythmic synchronous contractions. Much activity has
thus been expended in searching for drugs which
abolish irregularities of the beat without compromis-
ing other aspects of cardiac function.  One apparently

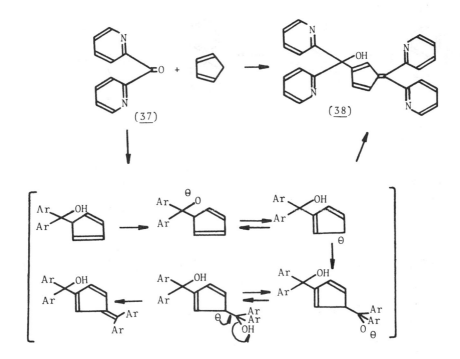

quite complex compound which exhibits such activity
is, in fact, the product of a relatively simple
reaction: condensation of cyclopentadiene with
bis(2-pyridyl)ketone *(37)* in the presence of base
affords directly *pyrinoline (38)*.[12] The condensation
can be rationalized by a scheme such as that shown.

REFERENCES
1.  B. W. Horrom and W. B. Martin, U. S. Patent
    3,088,226 (1963); *Chem. Abstr.*, *59:* 9888e
    (1963).
2.  L. R. Swett, W. B. Martin, J. D. Taylor, G. M.
    Everett, A. A. Wykes and Y. C. Gladish, *Ann. N.*

Y. Acad. Sci., 107, 891 (1963).

3.  Anon., Belgian Patent 618,638 (1962); *Chem. Abstr.*, *59:* 6313c (1963).

4.  A. R. Surrey and J. R. Mayer, *J. Med. Chem.*, *3*, 409 (1961).

5.  K. Gerzon and E. R. Shepard, U. S. Patent 2,759,977 (1956); *Chem. Abstr.*, *51:* 3664a (1956).

6.  Anon., Belgian Patent 616,371; *Chem. Abstr.*, *60: 1767e (1964).*

7.  *P. A. J. Janssen, Ger. Offen., 1,929,330 (1972).*

8.  *Anon., Belgian Patent 649,145 (1964); Chem. Abstr., 64:* 8151c (1966).

9.  A. O. Swain, U. S. Patent 2,800,485 (1957).

10. Anon., Belgian Patent 628,167 (1964); *Chem. Abstr.*, *60:* 11942h (1964).

11. Anon., British Patent 942,152 (1963); *Chem. Abstr.*, *60:* 9250g (1963).

12. Anon., British Patent 1,009,012 (1965); *Chem. Abstr.*, *64:* 3503g (1966).

# 3

# Phenylethyl and Phenylpropylamines

1. PHENYLETHYL AND PHENYLPROPYLAMINES

    a. Those With a Free ArOH Group

The autonomic nervous system controls tissues and
organs whose functions are largely automatic, *i.e.*,
not requiring conscious effort for activation.
Norepinephrine is the accepted neurotransmitter at
the nerve endings and the motor endplate in the
sympathetic branch of the autonomic nervous system.
Administration of norepinephrine *(1)* mimics the
effect of stimulation of these nerves, causing
responses such as vasoconstriction, increased heart
rate, relaxation of the ileum, contraction of the
uterus in pregnant animals, and relaxation of the
lung and bronchial muscles.  Synthetic substances
eliciting some of these responses are called sympathomimetic agents, and a wide variety are known.  More
recently, adrenergic agents (another synonym for

sympathomimetic agents) have been functionally
divided into those acting at α-receptors--  those
mainly associated with excitatory processes such as
vasoconstriction--and at β-receptors--those mainly
associated with inhibitory processes such as vaso-
dilatation.  Pharmacological agents which block each
of these receptor groups (antagonists) are predominantly used in classifying the drugs.  A finer
subdivision of the β-receptors into $\beta_1$--which are
involved in certain heart muscle and intestinal
smooth muscle responses--and $\beta_2$--which are involved
in certain other smooth muscles such as bronchi,
uterus and blood vessels--has been found extremely
useful.  *Isoproterenol (2)* is the archetypal β-
agonist, having strong activity against both $\beta_1$ and
$\beta_2$ receptors.  Generally, the R-configuration at the
benzylic carbon is required for maximal potency
amongst the agonists and antagonists of this type.

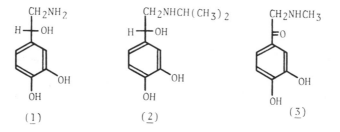

One can infer correctly from the foregoing that
increased bulk on the nitrogen generally increases
selectivity toward the β-receptors.  Further, a

catechol ring or a system electronically equivalent
to it is needed for optimum activity, especially at
the β-receptors, while alkyl branching in the ethanolamine side chain generally decreases potency.

The chemistry of most of the drugs in this
family is quite simple, accounting in part for the
very large number of analogues which have been made.
The foundation for the chemistry in this series was
laid long ago by Stolz[1] in his classic synthesis of
the ophthalmic agent *adrenalone (3)* in which he
reacted catechol with chloroacetyl chloride and then
displaced the reactive chlorine atom with methylamine
to complete the synthesis.   Borohydride reduction
would have given epinephrine (adrenaline).

This process, or simple variants of it, is used
to prepare many drugs.   For example, one method for
the synthesis of *fenoterol (6)*, a bronchodilator,
starts with sidechain bromination of m-diacetoxy-

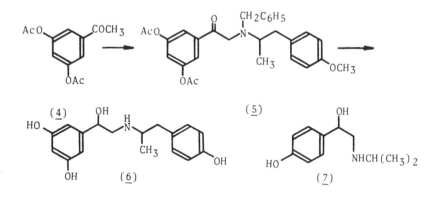

acetophenone *(4)* and then displacement of halogen by
1-(p-methoxyphenyl)-2-N-benzylaminopropane to give
5.[2] Hydrogenation removes the benzyl group, whose
function was to prevent overalkylation. Next, HBr
cleaves the ether and ester groups, and either
catalytic or hydride reduction completes the synthesis of 6. Separation of diastereoisomers was
achieved by fractional crystallization.

Analogous methods are used to prepare the
ophthalmic agent *deterenol (7)*;[3] the bronchodilators
*clorprenaline (8)*[4] and *isoetharine (9)*;[5] the vasodilators *bamethan (10)*[6] and *ifenprodil (11)*;[7] and
the smooth muscle relaxant *ritodrine (12)*.[8]

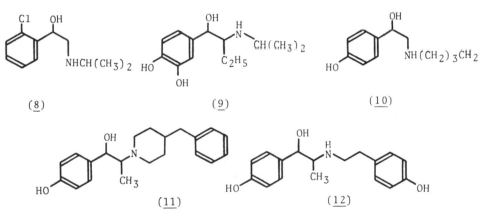

Direct alkylation of the appropriate aryl-
ethanolamine is, of course, widely used as, for
example, in treatment of *ephedrine (13a)* with ethyl
iodide to give the adrenergic agent, *etafedrine
(13b)*,[9] or with cinnamyl chloride to give the muscle
relaxant, *cinnamedrine (14)*.[10] Likewise, alkylation

of β-hydroxyphenethylamine with 2-chloropyrimidine
gives *fenyripol (15)*, also a muscle relaxant.[11]
   The Mannich reaction can also be used to add an
alkyl group in the condensation of ℓ-norephedrine
*(16)* with formaldehyde and m̲-methoxyacetophenone to
give *oxyfedrine (17)*, a coronary vasodilator.[12]

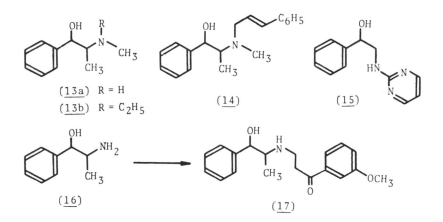

(13a)  R = H
(13b)  R = C$_2$H$_5$

(14)

(15)

(16)

(17)

   A departure from the catechol pattern of the
natural neurotransmitters was achieved following
application of the fact that arylsulfonamido hydrogens
are nearly as acidic as phenolic OH groups.  Nitration
of p̲-benzyloxyacetophenone gave *18* which was reduced
to *19* with Raney nickel and hydrazine, and in turn
reacted with mesyl chloride to give sulfonamide *20*.
Methanesulfonate *20* was then transformed to *soterenol
(21)*, a clinically useful bronchodilator, in the

usual way.[13]  The analogue *mesuprine (22)* was made
by a slight variation in this scheme.[13]  The β-
blockers *sotalol (23)* and *metalol (24)*[14] are made in
essentially the same fashion.  These agents *(23* and
*24)* owe their activity to their capacity to occupy
β-adrenergic receptors without triggering the normal

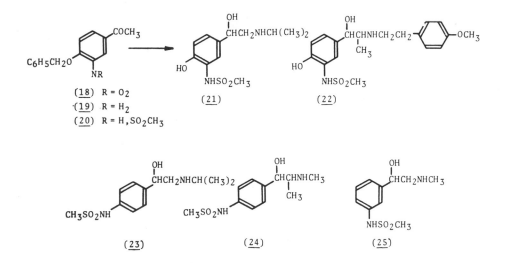

physiological response.  The resemblance of *23* and
*24* to the normal agonist helps them serve as antagonists.  Greater coverage of β-blockers will be
found in Chapter 5.

Amidephrine *(25)*, an adrenergic agent very
closely related to *metalol*, finds use as a bronchodilator.[15]  *Carbuterol (27)*, another bronchodilator,
is made by reacting 3-amino-4-benzyloxyacetophenone
with phosgene to give isocyanate *26*.  Subsequent

treatment of *26* with ammonia produces a urea derivative, which is converted to *carbuterol* by the
familiar bromination, amine displacement and reduction sequence.

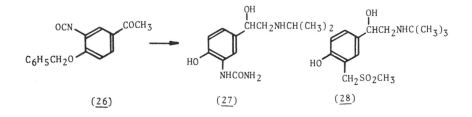

<table>
<tr><td>(26)</td><td>(27)</td><td>(28)</td></tr>
</table>

It is evident that some leeway is available in
the substituents tolerable in the m-position.  The
bronchodilator *sulfonterol (28)* is descended from
this observation.[16]  Chloromethylanisole *(29)* is
reacted with methylmercaptan to give *30*, and the
newly introduced group is oxidized to the methyl-
sulfonyl moiety of *31* with hydrogen peroxide.  Ether
cleavage, acetylation and Fries rearrangement of the
phenolic acetate produces *32*, which is next brominated
with pyrrolidinone hydrobromide tribromide and then
oxidized to the glyoxal *(33)* with dimethyl sulfoxide.

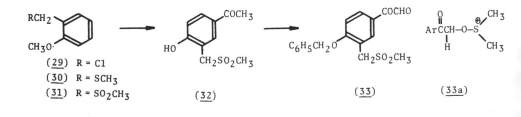

(29) R = Cl
(30) R = SCH₃
(31) R = SO₂CH₃          (32)          (33)          (33a)

The last reaction perhaps involves an intermediate
such as *33a* which expells a proton and dimethyl
sulfide.  Formation of the Schiff's base with t-
butylamine, reduction with sodium borohydride and
hydrogenolysis of the benzyl ether produces
*sulfonterol (28)*.  Despite the fact that the methylene
hydrogen of *sulfonterol* must be much less acidic
than of the corresponding urea proton on *carbuterol*
or the sulfonamide proton on *soterenol*, good bioactivity is retained.

That even further leeway is possible is shown
by the utility of the saligenin analogue *albuterol
(36)* as a bronchodilator.[17]  One of the several
syntheses starts by Fries rearrangement of aspirin
followed by esterification to *34* which is then
brominated and reacted with benzyl t-butylamine to
give *35*.  Hydride reduction reduces both carbonyls,
and hydrogenolysis of the benzyl group completes the
synthesis. Presumably, chelation, believed to be
significant in the molecular mode of action of the
catecholamines, can still take place with *albuterol*.

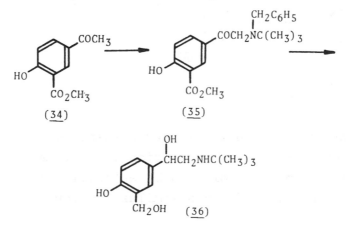

b.   Those Agents With An Acylated or Alkylated
     ArOH Group

Once again we come upon a chemical classification
that has no pharmacological significance.   The three
drugs in this small group cause widely different
biological responses.

Reaction of the Grignard reagent prepared from
m-trifluoromethylbromobenzene *(37)* with methyl-
1,2-dibromoethylether leads to alkoxy bromide *38*,
which is then reacted with methylamine to give the
anorexic agent *fludorex (39)*.[18]

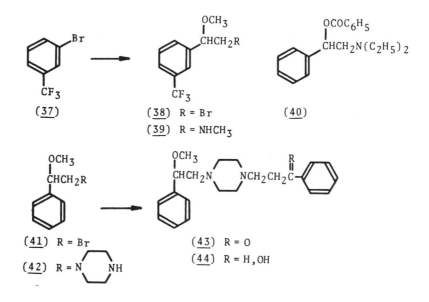

(37)

(38) R = Br

(39) R = NHCH₃

(40)

(41) R = Br

(42) R = N◯NH

(43) R = O

(44) R = H,OH

The gastric anticholinergic agent, *elucaine*
*(40)*, is synthesized by reaction of styrene oxide
with diethylamine, followed by esterification with
benzoyl chloride.[19]   In a similar fashion, *eprozinol*

(44), a bronchodilator, is synthesized by adding the
elements of $CH_3OBr$ to styrene, by reaction with
t-butylhypobromite in methanol, to give *41*. This is
next reacted with piperazine to give *42*. A Mannich
reaction with formaldehyde and acetophenone leads to
ketone *43*, and reduction with borohydride completes
the synthesis of *eprozinol*.[20]

### 2. 1-PHENYL-2-AMINOPROPANEDIOLS

*Chloramphenicol* was the first orally active, broad-
spectrum antibiotic to be used in the clinic, and
remains the only antibiotic which is marketed in
totally synthetic form. Its initial popularity was
dampened, and its utilization plummeted when it was
found that some patients developed an irreversible
aplastic anemia from use of the drug. Of the hundreds
of analogues synthesized, none are significantly
more potent or certain to be safer than *chloramphenicol* itself. Two analogues have been given
generic names and fall into this chemical classification. It was found early in the game that
activity was retained with p-substituents, and that
electron withdrawing substituents were best. The
synthesis of *thiamphenicol*[21] *(50)* begins with p-
thiomethylacetophenone *(45)*, which is brominated and
then reacted with hexamethylenetetramine to give *46*,
which is in turn converted to amide *47* by reaction
with dichloroacetyl chloride. Reaction with formaldehyde and bicarbonate introduces the hydroxymethyl
function of *48*, and subsequent Meerwein-Pondorff-
Verley reduction with aluminum isopropoxide gives

*49.* The p-SCH$_3$ function was oxidized to the methyl-
sulfonyl group of racemic *thiamphenicol (50)* with
peracetic acid. The drug has been resolved by
saponification of *49,* treatment with an optically
active acid, reamidation and oxidation. Closely
related *cetophenicol (52)* is synthesized from the
p-cyano analogue *51* by reaction with methyl lithium
followed by amide exchange to give *52.*[22]

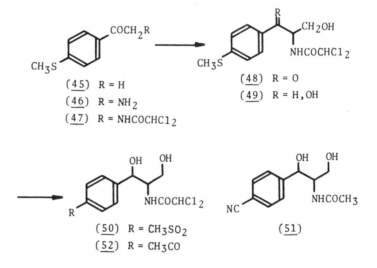

(45) R = H

(46) R = NH$_2$

(47) R = NHCOCHCl$_2$

(48) R = O

(49) R = H,OH

(50) R = CH$_3$SO$_2$

(52) R = CH$_3$CO

(51)

### 3.  PHENYLETHYLAMINES

Phenylethylamines lacking the β-hydroxy group of
norepinephrine *(1)* and related neurotransmitters are
much more lipophilic.  They exert a much more pronounced central--as opposed to peripheral--sympatho-
mimetic effect.  Their action is, however, not
direct.  It is generally accepted that these agents
function at least in part by liberating endogenous
catecholamines from storage sites.  These, then,
exert their characteristic actions.  It will be
recalled that amphetamine is used clinically for
appetite suppression, as an euphoriant-antidepressant,
as a nasal decongestant, to improve psychomotor
performance, to treat drug depression, in treating
children with minimal brain dysfunction (hyper-
kinesis) and so on.  Insomnia, anxiety and, especially with large doses, occasionally psychotomimetic
activity are undesirable side effects.  Removal of
side effects or greater selectivity of action is, as
usual, the objective of molecular manipulation in
this drug class.

*Amphetamine (53)* is the prototype drug in this
group. One significant objective of molecular manipulation in this group is to retain the appetite
depressant activity without significant central
stimulation.  This is as yet unrealized. Some of the
drugs prepared with this purpose in mind are discussed
in this section.  Reductive alkylation of the nitrogen
atom of amphetamine with β-chloropropionaldehyde
produces the anorexic agent *mefenorex (54)*.[23]  The

Schiff's base of amphetamine with chloral, *amphecloral*
(55), is a single molecule combination of a stimulant
-anorexic and a sedative.[24]  Presumably, *in vivo*
hydrolysis releases the sedative, chloral, to combat
the excitant action of amphetamine with the intended
retention of the anorexic action.

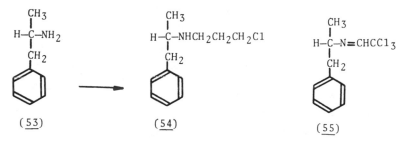

(53)                    (54)                    (55)

   The psychotropic (stimulant) action of
*amphetaminil* (57) may be intrinsic or due to *in vivo*
hydrolysis of the α-aminonitrile function--akin to a
cyanohydrin--to liberate amphetamine itself.  It is
synthesized by forming the Schiff's base of amphetamine with benzaldehyde to give 56, and then nucleophilic attack on the latter with cyanide anion to
form *amphetaminil* (57).[25]

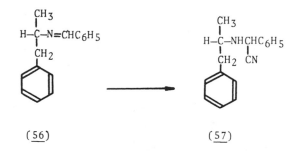

    (56)                    (57)

   The alkyl terminus of the side chain need not
be methyl for retention of activity.  *Aletamine* (59)

is such an agent. It is prepared by the Hofmann
rearrangement of α-allyl-β-phenylpropionamide (58).[26]

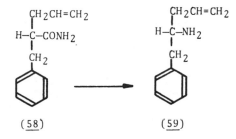

(58)                    (59)

The action of monoamine oxidase in terminating
the bioactivity of primary amines in this class is
inhibited by their conversion to secondary amines,
which are not substrates for this enzyme. Greater
selectivity of action, for reasons that are obscure,
is often seen when a trimethoxyphenyl moiety is
present in the drug. Such considerations may have
played a role in the design of *trimoxamine (66)*, an
antihypertensive agent.[27] The synthesis starts with
trimethoxybenzyl chloride *(60)*, which is alkylated
with the anion from ethyl allylacetoacetate and NaH
to give *61*, which is cleaved to ester *62* with sodium
ethoxide *via* a retro-Claisen reaction. Saponification
to acid *63* is followed by conversion to a mixed
anhydride by means of ethyl chlorocarbonate. Treatment with ammonia gives amide *64*. Hoffman rearrangement with NaOBr gives *65*, which is converted to the
secondary amine *66* by reaction with ethyl chlorocarbonate, followed by lithium aluminum hydride
reduction.

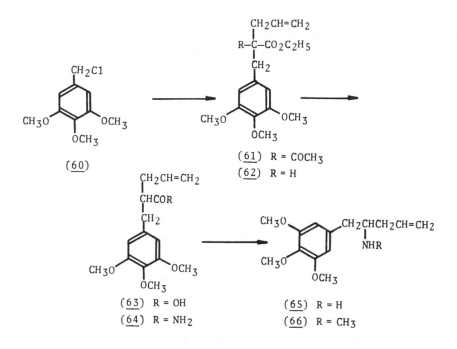

Drugs most often react with biopolymers called receptors in order to exert their pharmacological effects and the receptors are optically asymmetric and should therefore require a most favorable configuration and conformation for maximal activity. Thus, there has been much interest in preparation of rigid analogues both for their utility in mapping receptors and because it was felt that an intrinsically correct fit would maximize intrinsic potency. One drug designed with these considerations in mind is *rolicyprine (68)*, an antidepressant.[28] This drug is most probably a latentiated form (prodrug) of the free amine, *tranylcypromine (67)*. Restriction of the primary amino group into a rigid ring system decreases its conformational possibilities enormously.

Use of the relatively small cyclopropane ring drastic-
ally reduces the potential for deleterious steric
bulk effects and adds only a relatively small lipophilic increment to the partition coefficient of the
drug.  One of the clever elements of the *rolicyprine*
synthesis itself is the reaction of d,l-*tranylcypromine (67)* with L-5-pyrrolidone-2-carboxylic
acid (derived from glutamic acid) to form a highly
crystalline diastereomeric salt, thereby effecting
resolution.  Addition of dicyclohexylcarbodiimide
activates the carboxyl group to nucleophilic attack
by the primary amine thus forming the amide *rolicyprine (68)*.

Dopamine (69) is a well-known neurotransmitter
which interacts with many receptors in the central

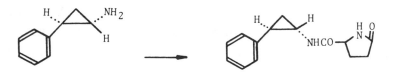

(67)                                    (68)

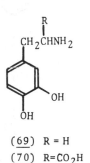

(69)  R = H
(70)  R=CO$_2$H

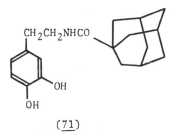

(71)

nervous system. In Parkinsonism, a fine tremor and
muscular rigidity is present which finds its biochemical basis in low levels of dopamine in certain
regions of the CNS. Administration of dopamine
itself is insufficient to overcome this defect, as
it cannot efficiently penetrate the blood-brain
barrier. Before the discovery that the corresponding amino
acid, *DOPA (70)*, which efficiently entered the
brain, was converted enzymatically to *dopamine*, and
thereby constituted effective therapy, various means
were employed to attempt such central delivery.    One
of these used the lipophilicity of adamantoyl
analogues.    *Dopamine* was reacted with the acid
chloride of adamantane-1-carboxylic acid to give
*dopamantine (71)*, an anti-Parkinsonian agent.[29]
     A relatively old compound, p-*chlorophenylalanine*
*(74)*, is able to penetrate the blood-brain barrier
into the CNS and serves as a serotonin inhibitor.
Interestingly, it increases copulatory behavior in

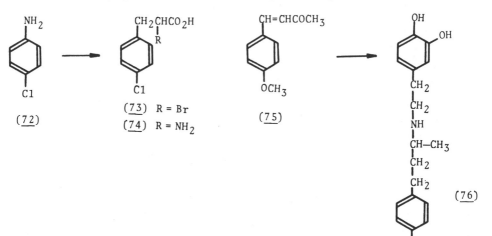

experimental animals, as does testosterone, and has
achieved some notoriety on this ground.  One of the
syntheses begins by diazotization of p-chloroaniline
(72), followed by Meerwein reaction with cuprous
bromide and acrylic acid to give 2-bromopchloro-
hydrocinnamic acid (73); which is then reacted with
ammonia to give p-*chlorophenylalanine* (74).[30]

Dobutamine (76), on the other hand, is a *dopamine*
derivative which does not act centrally, but is of
interest because of its coronary vasodilator
properties.  Such drugs are potentially of value in
treatment of angina pectoralis. Further, it is now
undergoing extensive clinical trials as an inotropic
agent for use in heart failure.  Its synthesis is
effected by Raney nickel catalyzed reduction of
methyl p-methoxyvinylphenylketone (75) to its dihydro
analog followed by reductive alkylation with β-
(3,4-dimethoxyphenyl)ethylamine.  The ether groups
are cleaved with HBr to complete the synthesis of
76.[31]

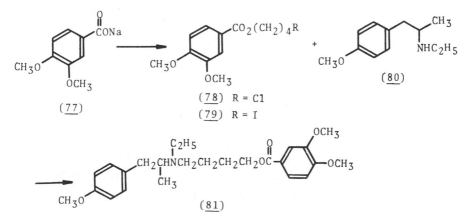

*Mebeverine (81)*, a smooth muscle relaxant, is
prepared, *i.a.*, by reacting sodium 3,4-dimethoxy-
benzoate *(77)* with 1,4-dichlorobutane to form chloro-
ester *78* which is in turn transformed to the corresponding iodide *(79)* on heating with NaI in methylethyl ketone.  Alkylation of 2-ethylamino-3-p-methoxy-
phenylpropane *(80)* with *79* leads to *mebeverine*
*(81)*.[32]

*Mixidine (84)*, an amidine related to *dopamine*
*(84)*, has coronary vasodilator properties.  It is
prepared by reaction of β-(3,4-dimethoxy)phenethyl-
amine *(82)* with the ethylimino derivative of N-
methyl-2-pyrrolidone *(83)* in an apparent addition-
elimination sequence.[33]

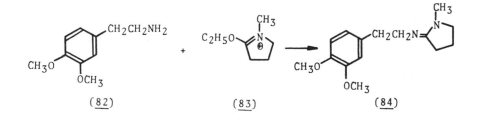

b.  Miscellaneous

*Xylamidine (87)* is an amidine which serves as a
serotonin inhibitor.  This agent is prepared by
alkylation of m-methoxyphenol with α-chloropropio-
nitrile, KI and potassium carbonate in methylethyl
ketone to give *85*, which is in turn reduced with

lithium aluminum hydride to give the primary amine
86.    When 86 is treated with m-tolylacetonitrile in
the presence of anhydrous HCl, the synthesis is
completed.[34]    Alternately, one can react primary
amine 86 with m-tolylacetamidine under acid catalysis
to produce *xylamidine*.

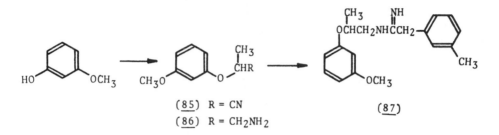

(85)  R = CN
(86)  R = CH₂NH₂

(87)

#### 4.    PHENYLPROPYLAMINES
The drugs of this group also have widely different
pharmacological properties, indicating the general
absence of a common pharmacophoric moiety in the
group.

Alverine (88) is an anticholinergic agent
prepared by reductive alkylation of ethylamine with
two equivalents of phenylpropionaldehyde.[35]

Alkylation of cyclohexylidinephenylacetonitrile
(89) with 2-chloroethyldimethylamine, using NaH as
base, gives nitrile 90.    Note that the product
results from alkylation of the enolate which results
in a double bond shift.    This product (90) is transformed to unsaturated amine 91 on heating with HCl.

Catalytic hydrogenation of the double bond then
produces *gamfexine (92)*, an antidepressant.[36]

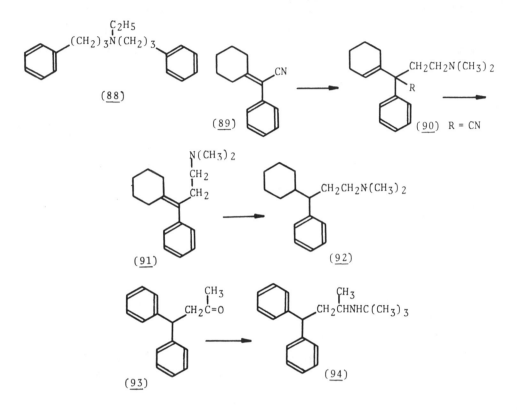

(88)

(89)

(90)  R = CN

(91)

(92)

(93)

(94)

Reductive amination of methyl 2,2-diphenylethyl
ketone *(93)* with t-butylamine in formic acid leads
to *terodiline (94)*, a coronary vasodilator.[37]

The relationship between serum cholesterol
levels and cardiovascular disease remains suggestive,
despite intensive research into the subject.  In any
case, agents which can lower serum cholesterol
levels are of therapeutic interest. *Beloxamide (98)*,

an N-benzyloxyacetamido derivative, is such an hypocholesterolemic agent.   It is synthesized by alkylating N-carbethoxyhydroxylamine with benzyl bromide,
using sodium ethoxide.   The resulting carbamoyl
ester (95) is alkylated again, this time with 3-
phenylpropyl bromide and sodium ethoxide to give 96,
which is then cleaved to the alkylated O-benzyl-
hydroxylamine derivative 97.   Reaction with acetyl
chloride completes the synthesis of beloxamide.[38]

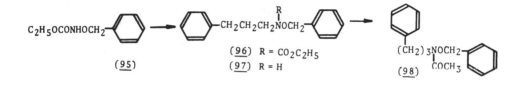

(95)   (96) R = $CO_2C_2H_5$   (97) R = H   (98)

A propoxyphene-like analgesic which obeys the
empirical morphine rule is pyrroliphene (101).   A
Mannich reaction involving pyrrolidine, formaldehyde
and propiophenone gave amino ketone 99, which was
converted to tertiary carbinol 100 by reaction with
benzyl magnesium chloride; reaction with acetyl

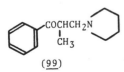

(99)

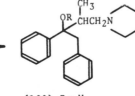

(100) R = H
(101) R = COCH₃

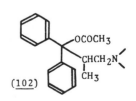

(102)

chloride completed the synthesis.[34] It is gratifying
that *pyrroliphene (101)* retained the desired bioactivity as its synthesis was apparently impelled by
the observation that the initial target compounds
(*e.g., 102*) were not very stable chemically.

A somewhat related analgesic, *noracymethadol*
*(108)*, is an active metabolite of *acetylmethadol*.

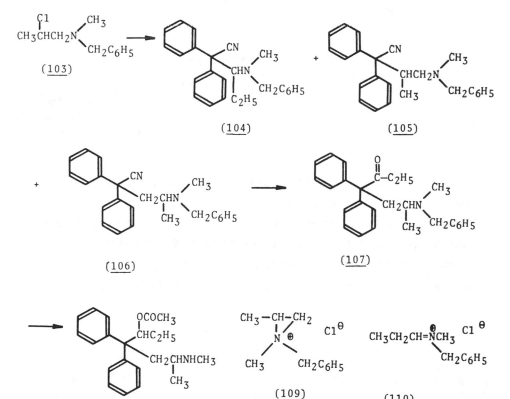

It can be synthesized from methyl benzyl 2-chloro-
propylamine *(103)* by sodium amide induced alkylation
of 2,2-diphenylacetonitrile to give a mixture of
amines *104*, *105* and *106*.  Amines *105* and *106* are the
expected products of nucleophilic attack on the
presumed intermediate asymmetric aziridinium *109*.
Amine *104* can be rationalized by assuming dehydrohalogenation and rearrangement of the resulting
enamine to the charged iminium ion *(110)* which would
rapidly add the nucleophile to give the observed
product.  In any event, treatment of nitrile *106*
with ethyl magnesium bromide, followed by hydrolysis,
produced intermediate ketone *107*.  This was reduced
to the secondary carbinol with lithium aluminum
hydride and acetylated before catalytic debenzylation
of the amine using palladium on carbon catalyst.[40]
Given the nature of the initial alkylation reaction,
it is doubtful that this is a practical synthesis.

REFERENCES

1.  F. Stolz, *Chem. Ber.*, *37*, 4149 (1904).

2.  Anon., Belgian Patent 640,433 (1967); *Chem.
    Abstr.*, *62:* 16124e (1964).

3.  R. J. Adamski, P. E. Hartje, S. Namajiri, L. J.
    Spears and E. H. Yen, *Synthesis*, *2*, 478 (1970);
    J. R. Corrigan, *J. Am. Chem. Soc.*, *67*, 1894
    (1945).

4.  J. F. Nash, U. S. Patent 2,887,509 (1959).

5.  M. Bochmuehl, G. Ehrhart and L. Stein, German
    Patent 638,650 (1936); *Chem. Abstr.*, *31:* 3209[4]
    (1937).

6.   J. R. Corrigan, M. Langerman and M. L. Moore,
     *J. Am. Chem. Soc.*, *67*, 1894 (1945).

7.   C. Carron, A. Jullien and B. Bucher,
     *Arzneimittelforsch.*, *21*, 1992 (1971).

8.   P. Claassen, U. S. Patent 3,410,944 (1965);
     *Chem. Abstr.*, *63:* 17965n (1965).

9.   T. Ueda, S. Toyoshima, K. Takahashi and M.
     Muraoka, *Chem. Pharm. Bull.*, *3*, 465 (1955).

10.  L. H. Welsh and G. L. Keenan, *J. Amer. Pharm.*
     *Assn.*, *Sci. Ed.*, *30*, 123 (1941).

11.  A. P. Gray and D. E. Heitmeier, U. S. Patent
     3,274,190 (1966); *Chem. Abstr.*, *66:* P18725u
     (1967).

12.  K. Thiele, Belgian Patent 630,296 (1963); *Chem.*
     *Abstr.*, *61:* 1800f (1964).

13.  A. A. Larsen, W. A. Gould, H. R. Roth, W. T.
     Comer, R. H. Uloth, K. W. Dungan and P. M.
     Lish, *J. Med. Chem.*, *10*, 462 (1967).

14.  R. H. Uloth, J. R. Kirk, W. A. Gould and A. A.
     Larsen, *J. Med. Chem.*, *9*, 88 (1966).

15.  C. Kaiser, D. F. Colella, M. S. Schwartz, E.
     Garvey and J. R. Wardell, Jr., *J. Med. Chem.*,
     *17*, 49 (1974).

16.  C. Kaiser, M. S. Schwartz, D. F. Colella and J.
     R. Wardell, Jr., *J. Med. Chem.*, *18*, 674 (1975).

17.  D. T. Collin, D. Hartley, D. Jack, L. H. C.
     Lunts, J. C. Press, A. C. Ritchie and P. Toon,
     *J. Med. Chem.*, *13*, 674 (1970); Y. Kawamatsu, H.
     Asagawa, E. Imamiya and H. Hirano, Japanese
     Patent 74 70,939 (1974).

18.  M. Sahyun, Netherlands Patent 6,608,794 (1966);
     *Chem. Abstr.*, *67:* 64023a (1967).

19.  S. L. Shapiro, H. Soloway, E. Chodos and L.
     Freedman, *J. Am. Chem. Soc.*, *81*, 203 (1959).

20.  H. E. Saunders, British Patent 1,188,505 (1970);
     *Chem. Abstr.*, *72:* 90466v (1970).

21.  R. A. Cutler, R. J. Stenger and C. M. Suter, *J.
     Am. Chem. Soc.*, *74*, 5475 (1952); C. M. Suter,
     S. Shalit and R. A. Cutler, *J. Am. Chem. Soc.*,
     *75*, 4330 (1953).

22.  M. Von Strandtmann, J. Shavel, Jr., and G.
     Bobowski, Belgian Patent 638,755 (1964); *Chem.
     Abstr.*, *62:* 11740bc
            (1965).

23.  H. Beschke, K. H. Klingler, A. von Schlictegroll
     and W. A. Schaler, German Patent 1,210,873
     (1966); *Chem. Abstr.*, *64:* 19486c (1966).

24.  C. Cavallito, U. S. Patent 2,923,661 (1960);
     *Chem. Abstr.*, *54:* 9846c (1966).

25.  J. Klosa, German Patent 1,112,987 (1959); *Chem.
     Abstr.*, *56:* 3409d (1962).

26.  D. D. Micucci, U. S. Patent 3,210,424 (1965);
     *Chem. Abstr.*, *63:* 17897f (1965).

27.  F. J. McCarty, P. D. Rosenstock, J. P. Palolini,
     D. D. Micucci, L. Ashton, W. W. Bennetts and F.
     P. Palopoli, *J. Med. Chem.*, *11*, 534 (1968); F.
     P. Palopoli, D. D. Micucci and P. D. Rosenstock,
     U. S. Patent 3,440,274 (1969); *Chem. Abstr.*,
     *75:* 140487n (1971).

28.  J. H. Biel, U. S. Patent 3,192,229 (1965);
     *Chem. Abstr.*, *66:* 104,804u (1967).

29.  H. P. Faro and S. Symchowicz, German Patent
     2,254,566 (1973); *Chem. Abstr.*, *79:* 104963
     (1973).

30.  J. H. Burckhalter and V. C. Stephens, *J. Am.
     Chem. Soc.*, *73*, 56 (1961); G. H. Cleland, *J.
     Org. Chem.*, *26*, 3362 (1961).

31.  R. Tuttle and J. Mills, German Patent 2,317,710
     (1973); *Chem. Abstr.*, *80:* 14721z (1974).

32.  Anon., Belgian Patent 609,490 (1962); T. Kralt,
     H. O. Moes, A. Lindner and W. J. Asma, German
     Patent 1,126,889 (1962); *Chem. Abstr.*, *59:* 517b
     (1963).

33.  G. I. Poos, French Patent 1,576,111 (1969);
     *Chem. Abstr.*, *72:* 132,511p (1970).

34.  Anon., Netherlands Patent 6,508,754 (1966);
     *Chem. Abstr.*, *65:* 2181e (1962).

35.  W. Steuhmer and E. A. Elbraechter, *Arch. Pharm.*,
     *287*, 139 (1954).

36.  M. D. Aceto, L. S. Harris, A. M. Lands and E.
     J. Alexander, U. S. Patent 3,328,249 (1967);
     *Chem. Abstr.*, *67:* 99834t (1967).

37.  Anon., British Patent 923,942 (1963).

38.  B. J. Ludwig, F. Duersch, M. Auerbach, K.
     Tomeczek and F. M. Berger, *J. Med. Chem.*, *10*,
     556 (1967).

39.  A. Pohland and H. R. Sullivan, *J. Am. Chem.
     Soc.*, *75*, 4458 (1953).

40.  A. Pohland, U. S. Patent 3,021,360 (1962);
     *Chem. Abstr.*, *56:* 3568c (1962).

# 4
# Arylalkanoic Acids and Their Derivatives

1. ANTIINFLAMMATORY ARYLACETIC ACIDS

Inflammation is an intimate part of every organism's
apparatus for dealing with injuries imposed by the
environment.  Under normal circumstances, the complex
sequence of events characterizing inflammation
ceases soon after the environmental challenge stops.
Not infrequently, however, the inflammatory process,
once started, continues despite the fact that the
original triggering event has passed.  The incident
swelling and pain is familiar to all.  Treatment of
chronic or persistant inflammation has gone through
some clearly recognizable cycles.  From about the
turn of the century, the standard drug therapy for
treatment of this syndrome has consisted of *aspirin*
or another of the simpler aromatics, such as
*antipyrine* and *acetaminophen*.  The layman chooses
these materials for self-administration.  Use of

these drugs for severe conditions is, however,
limited by their relatively low activity--particularly
in treatment of the inflammation due to arthritis--and
the incidence of side effects when used at higher
doses.  The discovery of the antiinflammatory activity
of *cortisone* and related corticosteroids quickly led
to common prescription of these potent drugs for a
wide variety of inflammatory conditions.  This
widespread use uncovered the host of endocrine
effects the corticoids elicit upon chronic administration.  This phenomenon required the more selective
use of these compounds.

Quite recently, a series of arylacetic acid
derivatives has come into clinical use as potent
antiinflammatory agents. In general, these compounds
show profiles of activity quite similar to *aspirin*,
and though as a rule they are more active and are
less likely to cause or exacerbate gastric ulcers.
Many of these compounds have been shown to be effective in the treatment of arthritis.  Since they
apparently work by a mechanism different from that
of the corticosteroids and are structurally unrelated,
they have no corresponding endocrine effects.

An interesting example of this class of nonsteroidal antiinflammatory agents is *ketoprofen (5)*.
It is synthesized by reaction of the diazonium salt
from amine *1* with potassium ethyl xanthate, followed
by alkaline hydrolysis to afford thiophenol *2*.
Reaction of the sodium salt of *2* with 2-iodobenzoic
acid results in formation of the corresponding bis-
arylsulfide *via* nucleophilic aromatic substitution.

Friedel-Crafts cyclization of the dibasic acid gives
thiaxanthone *4*. Note that the symmetry of this
intermediate assures formation of a single product.
Desulfurization by means of Raney nickel leads,
finally, to the antiinflammatory agent, *ketoprofen*
*(5)*.[1]

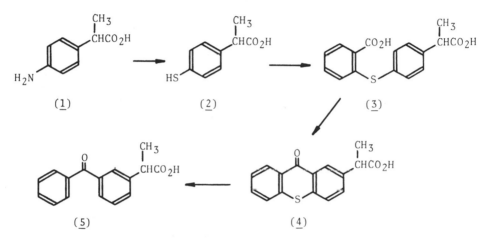

Quite a different route is employed to prepare
heterocyclic analogues of *5*.  For example, acylation
of thiophene with p-fluorobenzoyl chloride *(6)*
affords ketone *7*.  Nucleophilic aromatic substitution
with the enolate from diethyl methylmalonate gives
the diester *8*.  Saponification, followed by decarboxylation, gives *suprofen* *(9)*.[2,3]  A similar sequence
starting with the more highly substituted acid
chloride *(10)* affords *cliprofen* *(13)*.[2,3]

Structure-activity studies in the phenylacetic
acid antiinflammatory series have shown that inclusion
of a methyl group on the benzylic carbon usually
leads to maximal activity. It is of note that this

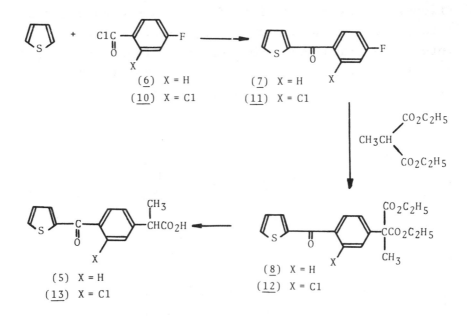

(6) X = H           (7) X = H     X
(10) X = Cl         (11) X = Cl

(5) X = H
(13) X = Cl

(8) X = H
(12) X = Cl

group can be replaced, in at least one case, by
chlorine.  Acylation of phenylcyclohexane with ethyl
oxalyl chloride affords the glyoxylic ester *14*.
Chlorination proceeds *meta* to the carbonyl group to
give *15*.[4]  Reduction of the keto moiety gives the
corresponding mandelate *16*, which reacts in turn
with thionyl chloride to replace the hydroxyl group
by chlorine to give *17*; ester hydrolysis affords
*fenclorac (18)*.[5]

    In a similar vein, the keto bridge in 5 can be
replaced by oxygen with retention of activity.
Reduction of acetophenone derivative *19* by means of
sodium borohydride leads to the corresponding alcohol
*(20)*.  Reaction with phosphorus tribromide gives *21*.
Displacement of the halide with cyanide gives

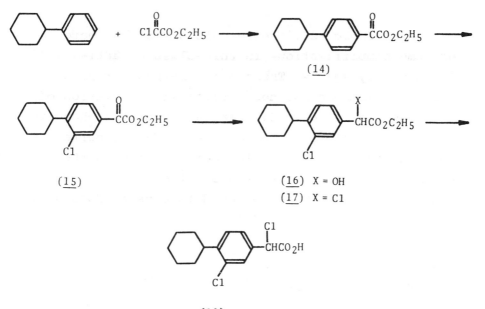

(14)

(15)                              (16) X = OH
                                 (17) X = Cl

(18)

substituted acetonitrile *22*, whose saponification
affords the antiinflammatory acid, *fenoprofen (23)*.[6]

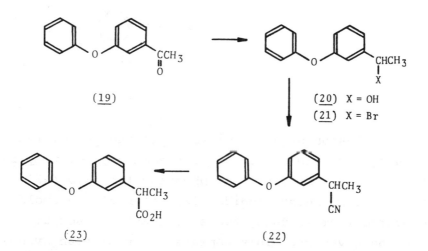

(19)                              (20) X = OH
                                 (21) X = Br

(23)                              (22)

Alclofenac (26)[7] represents one of the more
extreme simplifications in this class of antiinflammatory agents. The general method for preparation of related compounds[8] starts with acylation of
ochlorophenol to give 24. Alkylation of the phenolic
group of 24 with allyl bromide affords the corresponding ether (25). Willgerodt reaction on the
acetophenone results in transposition of the side
chain and oxidation to the acid to give alclofenac
(26).

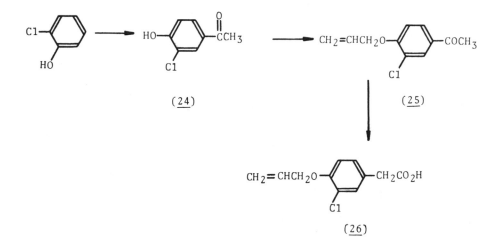

(24)                                            (25)

(26)

Inclusion of basic nitrogen in the p-position
is also compatible with antiinflammatory activity in
this series. Nitration of phenylacetic acid (27)
affords 28. Methyl iodide alkylation of the enolate
prepared from 28 using two equivalents of sodium
hydride gives 29. This appears to involve an Ivanov
intermediate (28a). Catalytic reduction of the

nitro group leads to the corresponding aniline *(30)*.
Acetylation to *31*, followed by reaction with chlorine,
serves to introduce the desired aryl halogen atom.
Removal of the acetyl group, followed by cyclo-
alkylation of the primary aniline *(33)* with
1,4-dibromo-2-butene affords *pirprofen (34)*.[9]

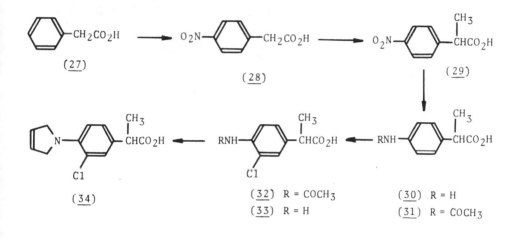

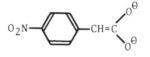

Anthranilic acid derivatives, such as *flufenamic
acid (35)*, constitute another effective series of
non-steroidal antiinflammatory agents.  Homologation

of the acid function in that series would of course
lead to the arylacetic acid series.   It is of note
that one such hybrid compound, *diclofenac (40)*, does
in fact exhibit antiinflammatory activity.   In an
interesting synthesis, the diphenylamine *36* is first
condensed with oxalyl chloride to give the oxanilic
acid chloride *37*.   Friedel-Crafts cyclization under
quite mild conditions gives the isatin *38*.   Reduction
of the keto group by means of the Wolff-Kishner
reaction gives lactam *39*, whose hydrolysis affords
*diclofenac (40).*[10]

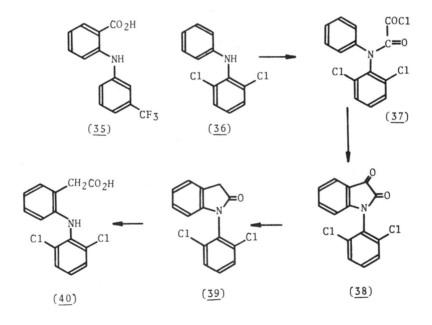

2.   DIARYL AND ARYLALKYL ACETIC ACIDS: ANTI-
     CHOLINERGIC AGENTS

Acetylcholine is the neurotransmitter amine of the
parasympathetic autonomic nervous system.  A host of
bodily responses, such as gastric secretion, intestinal motility, and constriction of the bronchi,
depend on cholinergic transmission.  Quite some time
ago it was discovered that responses due to activation
of the cholinergic system can be antagonized by
*atropine (41)*.  Experience with this natural product
foreshadowed the shortcomings of most subsequent
anticholinergic drugs.  That is, these agents, as a
class, show little selectivity for a given organ
system.  They tend to ablate all responses mediated
by the parasympathetic nervous system.  This lack of
selectivity leads to a set of side effects, such as
dryness of the mouth, blurred vision, and CNS effects,
which are quite predictable as extensions of the
pharmacology.  As has been detailed elsewhere,
numerous SAR studies have reduced the requirements
for anticholinergic activity to an ester of a benzilic
acid with an alcohol related to ethanolamine; esters
of cyclic aminoalcohols tend to be more active than
the acyclic counterparts.

     Clinical trials of some of the more potent
tertiary amines revealed these to exhibit marked
psychotomimetic activity.[11]  Much subsequent work
thus dealt with the quaternary salts which do not
reach the central nervous system. Many of the uses
of anticholinergic drugs involve "topical" application
(*e.g.*, interior of the stomach, intestine or bronchi);

the drugs could thus in principle show a clinically
useful effect without first being absorbed parenterally. In addition, quaternization, while greatly
inhibiting absorption, should assure that the drug
will not cross the blood-brain barrier.

Preparation of the quaternary anticholinergic
agent *benzilonium bromide (47)* is begun by conjugate
addition of ethylamine to methylacrylate, giving
aminoester *42*. Alkylation of *42* with methyl bromoacetate leads to diester *43*, which is transformed
into pyrrolidone *44* by Dieckmann cyclization, followed by decarboxylation. Reduction of *44* by lithium
aluminum hydride leads to the corresponding aminoalcohol *(45)*. Transesterification of alcohol *45*
with methyl benzilate leads to *46*. *Benzilonium
bromide (47)* is obtained by alkylation of ester *46*
with ethyl bromide.[12]

In a similar sequence, reaction of ketoester *52*
with 2-thienylmagnesium bromide gives a modest yield
of the benzilic ester *53*. Transesterification of
this with aminoalcohol *51*, prepared analogously to
*45* by starting with methylamine, gives, after quaternization with methyl bromide, *heteronium bromide
(54).*[12]

Similarly, lactam formation of diethyl glutamate
*(55)* leads to ethyl pyroglutamate *(56)*. Reduction
by means of lithium aluminum hydride gives the
aminoalcohol *57*, which is then N-methylated to give
*58*. Treatment with thionyl chloride leads to the
chloroamine *59* and displacement of halogen (possibly
*via* an aziridinium intermediate) with sodium benzilate

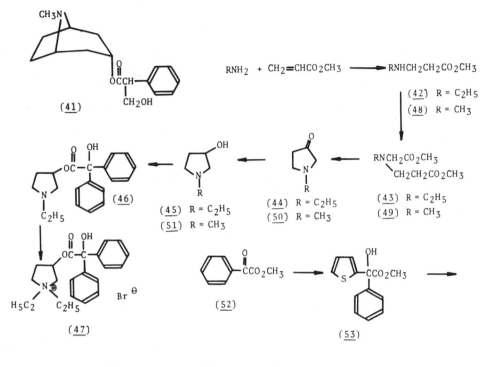

RNH$_2$ + CH$_2$=CHCO$_2$CH$_3$ ⟶ RNHCH$_2$CH$_2$CO$_2$CH$_3$

(42) R = C$_2$H$_5$
(48) R = CH$_3$

RNCH$_2$CO$_2$CH$_3$
CH$_2$CH$_2$CO$_2$CH$_3$

(43) R = C$_2$H$_5$
(49) R = CH$_3$

(44) R = C$_2$H$_5$
(50) R = CH$_3$

(45) R = C$_2$H$_5$
(51) R = CH$_3$

(46)

(47)

(41)

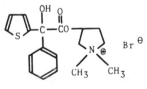

(52)

(53)

(54)

73

affords *poldine (60).*[13] Alkylation of *60* with
dimethyl sulfate gives *poldine methylsulfate (61),*
in which the two-carbon bridge between quaternary N
and O is preserved by placing a methylene in the -
position of the pyrrolidine nucleus.

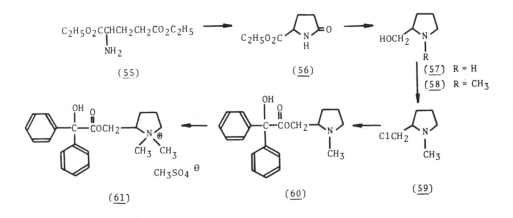

Benzilate esters of piperidinols, as well as
those of acyclic aminoalcohols, show similar anticholinergic activity. For example, ester interchange
between methyl benzilate and N-methyl-4-piperidinol,
followed by quaternization of the resulting ester
with methyl bromide, gives *parapenzolate bromide*
*(62).*[14] In analogous fashion, ester interchange
between methyl benzilate and N-ethyl-N-n-propyl-
ethanolamine yields *benapryzine (63).*[15]

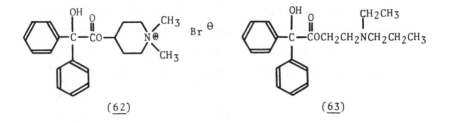

(62)                                              (63)

Biological activity in this series shows considerable tolerance for modification in the ester
moiety as well.   Esters in which one of the aromatic
rings is fully reduced still show good anticholinergic
activity.   One such agent, *propenzolate (66)*, is
prepared by displacement of halogen from N-methyl-
3-chloropiperidine *(64)* by the sodium salt of acid
65. [16]

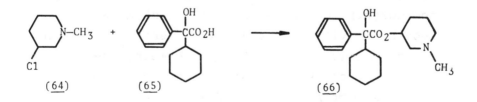

(64)              (65)                             (66)

In yet a further variation on this scheme, the
basic center in the molecule can be present as an

amidine.   In the synthesis of *oxyphencyclimine (69)*,
reaction of chloroacetonitrile with methanol and
hydrogen chloride leads to the corresponding iminoether *67*.   Condensation of *67* with N-methyl propyle-
nediamine gives the corresponding tetrahydropyrimidine *(68)*.   Displacement of the halogen with the
sodium salt of *65* affords *oxyphencyclimine (69).*[17]

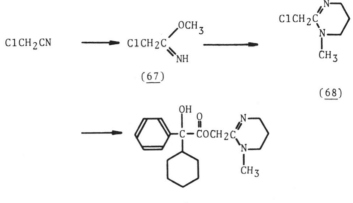

(67)

(68)

(69)

Omission of the hydroxyl group and one of the
cyclic hydrocarbons from the acid moiety is apparently not inconsistent with biological activity.   Thus,
the ester from 2-phenylbutyryl chloride and diethyl-
aminoethoxyethanol, *butamirate (71)*, shows anti-
spasmodic activity.   In analogous fashion, reaction
of the acid chloride from *72* with N-methyl-4-
piperidinol, followed by quaternization, gives
*pentapiperium methylsulfate (73).*[18]

Apparently, minor chemical modifications of the
benzilcarboxylic acid containing molecules led to a
compound which shows surprising analgesic activity.
Condensation of N-methylphenethylamine *74* with

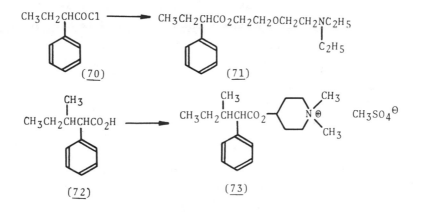

(70)          (71)

(72)          (73)

ethylene oxide gives aminoalcohol 75; which is then

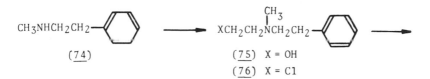

(74)          (75) X = OH
              (76) X = Cl

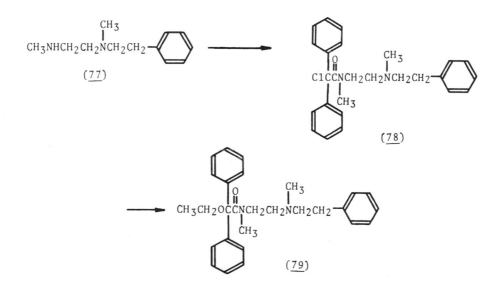

(77)

(78)

(79)

converted to the halide *(76)* by means of thionyl
chloride.   Reaction with methylamine leads to the
key diamine *77*.   Acylation of the diamine with
chlorodiphenylacetyl chloride (to *78*), followed by
displacement of the benzylic halogen by sodium
ethoxide, affords the analgesic agent *carbiphene*
*(79)*.[19]


### 3.   MISCELLANEOUS ARYLALKANOIC ACIDS

It has been known for some time that *thyroxine*, and
related compounds such as *liothyronine (88)* are
effective in lowering serum cholesterol.   The normal
metabolic activity of this class of thyroid active
compounds has precluded their use as hypocholesterolemic agents.

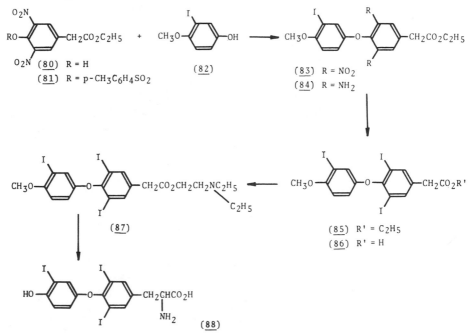

A program aimed at preparation of analogues of
thyroxine which would maximize their effect on
lipids resulted in the preparation of *thyromedan*
(*87*).  This agent, interestingly, proves also to
have good thyromimetic activity.  In the synthesis
of *87*, reaction of the substituted phenylacetate *80*
with tosyl chloride leads to the corresponding
tosylate (*81*).  Reaction of that intermediate with
the salt from phenol *82* results in aromatic nucleophilic displacement of the highly activated tosylate
to afford the diphenyl ether *83*.  The nitro groups
are then reduced catalytically to give diamine *84*.
Diazotization, followed by Sandmeyer reaction with
sodium iodide, affords the desired triiodo intermediate *85*.  Saponification affords the acid (*86*),
and reaction of the sodium salt of the acid with
2-chlorotriethylamine gives *thyromedan* (*87*).[20]

A highly-substituted phenylacetic acid derivative shows activity as a shortacting narcotic
and as an injectable general anesthetic.  This
agent, *propanidid* (*90*), is obtained by alkylation of
phenol *89* with N,N-diethylchloroacetamide.[21]

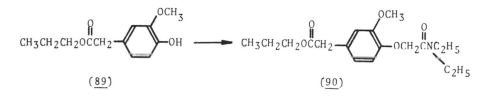

(89)                                                  (90)

*Clofibrate* (*91*) has been in clinical use for
several years as a serum triglyceride lowering
agent.  This drug is an important hypocholesteremic

agent also, blocking cholesterol biosynthesis.
Appearance of this agent on the market occasioned
intensive work in many laboratories aimed at discover-
ing additional compounds with this activity.  A
distantly related analogue, *halofenate (98)*, was, in
fact, found to be effective.  In addition, however,
clinical trials revealed this analogue to have
marked concomitant uricosuric activity; that is, the
drug promotes excretion of uric acid. In order to
synthesize *halofenate*, acid *92* is first converted to
the acid chloride by means of thionyl chloride;
bromination affords the α-halo derivative *93*.  This
is then allowed to react with methanol to give the
corresponding methyl ester *(94)*.  Displacement of
bromine with the anion from *meta*-trifluoromethylphenol
leads to ester *95*.  The ester is then hydrolyzed and

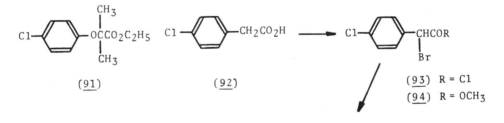

(91)                              (92)                              (93) R = Cl
                                                                    (94) R = OCH₃

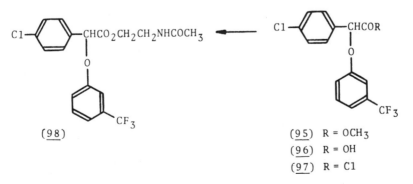

(98)                                                (95) R = OCH₃
                                                    (96) R = OH
                                                    (97) R = Cl

the product *(96)* is converted to the acid chloride
*(97).*   Acylation of N-acetylethanolamine with *97*
yields *halofenate (98).*[22]

   A disubstituted butyramide, *disopyramide*,
distantly related to some acyclic narcotics interestingly shows good antiarrhythmic activity.  Alkylation of the anion from phenylacetonitrile with 2-
bromopyridine yields *99.*   Alkylation of the anion
from the latter with N,N-diisopropyl-2-chloroethyl-
amine leads to the amine *100.*   Hydration of the
nitrile in sulfuric acid affords *disopyramide (101).*[23]

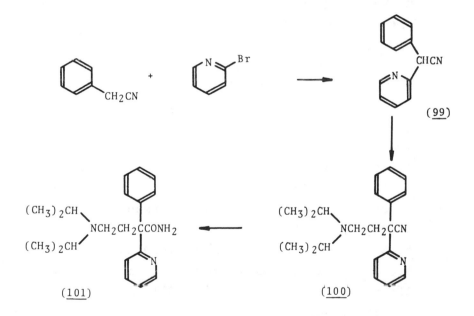

   Finally, reaction of the half acid chloride of
malonate *102* with N,N-diethylethylenediamine gives
the muscle relaxant *fenalamide (103).*[24]

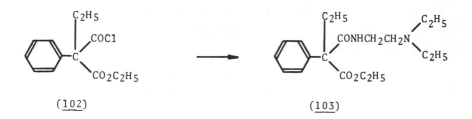

(102)                                      (103)


REFERENCES

1.  D. Farge, M. N. Messer and C. Moutonnier, U. S.
    Patent 3,641,127 (1972); *Chem. Abstr.*, *68:* 524
    (1968).

2.  P. A. J. Janssen, G. H. P. Van Daele and J. M.
    Boey, German Patent 2,353,375 (1974).

3.  P. G. H. Van Daele, J. M. Boey, V. K. Sipido,
    M. F. L. De Bruyn and P. A. J. Janssen,
    *Arzneimittelforsch.*, *25*, 1495 (1975).

4.  D. Julius and N. J. Santora, U. S. Patent
    3,321,267 (1971).

5.  D. Julius and N. J. Santora, German Patent
    2,122,273 (1972).

6.  M. S. Winston, U. S. Patent 3,600,437 (1971).

7.  N. P. BuuHoi, G. Lambelin and C. Gillet, South
    African Patent 68 05,495 (1969); *Chem. Abstr.*,
    *71:* 101,554e (1971).

8.  G. Gariraghi, S. Banfi, U. Cornelli, M. Pinza
    and G. Pifferi, *Il Farmaco, Ed. Sci.*, *32*, 286
    (1977).

9.  R. W. J. Carney and G. DeStevens, German Patent
    2,012,237 (1970).

10. A. Sallman and R. Pfister, German Patent
    1,815,802 (1969).

11. R. W. Brimbelcombe, *Advances in Drug Research*,
    7, 165 (1973).

12. W. Ryan and C. Ainsworth, *J. Org. Chem.*, *27*,
    2901 (1962).

13. F. F. Blicke and C.J. Lu, *J. Am. Chem. Soc.*,
    *77*, 29 (1955).

14. J. Klosa and G. Delmar, *J. Prakt. Chem.*, *16*, 71
    (1962).

15. M. D. Mehta and J. G. Bainbridge, U. S. Patent
    3,746,743 (1973).

16. J. H. Biel, U. S. Patent 2,995,492 (1957).

17. J. A. Faust, A. Mori and M. Sanyun, *J. Am.
    Chem. Soc.*, *81*, 2214 (1959).

18. H. Martin and E. Habicht, U. S. Patent
    2,987,517 (1961).

19. J. Krapcho and C. F. Turk, *J. Med. Chem.*, *6*,
    547 (1963).

20. B. Blank, F. R. Pfeiffer, C. M. Greenberg and
    J. F. Kerwin, *J. Med. Chem.*, *6*, 560 (1963).

21. R. Hiltmann, H. Wollweber, F. Hoffmeister and
    W. Wirth, German Patent 1,134,981 (1962); *Chem.
    Abstr.*, *58*: 4480f (1963).

22. W. A. Bolhofer, U. S. Patent 3,517,050 (1970).

23. J. W. Cusic and H. W. Sause, U. S. Patent
    3,225,054 (1965).

24.  P. Galimberti, V. Gerosa and M. Melandri, U. S.
     Patent 3,025,317 (1962); *Chem. Abstr.*, *56:* 550c
     (1962).

# 5

# Monocyclic Aromatic Compounds

The benzene ring per se does not impart any particular
pharmacological response to a drug.  It is widely
held that its planarity, its ability to bind to
tissue receptors by Van der Waals and charge transfer
mechanisms, and, particularly, its ability to serve
as a conductor of electrons within a substance serve
as modulators, enhancing or diminishing the intensity
of response to a molecule that is otherwise inherently
bioactive.

    1.  DERIVATIVES OF BENZOIC ACID
    a.  Acids
Salicylic acid analogues are often active as nonsteroidal antiinflammatory agents because they interfere with biosynthesis of prostaglandins.  *Diflunisal*
*(3)* appears to be such an agent.  It is synthesized
from the nitrobiphenyl *1* by catalytic reduction to

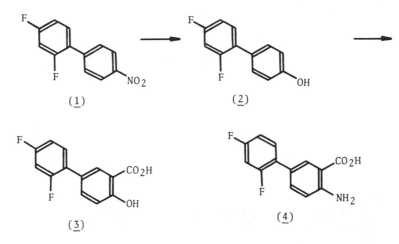

the aniline, diazotization, and heating in aqueous
acid to give phenol *2*. This is carboxylated using
$K_2CO_3$ and carbon dioxide to give *diflunisal*.[1]
Alternatively, the corresponding anthranilic acid
derivative *4* is diazotized, then hydroxylated by
heating in dilute sulfuric acid to give *diflunisal*.[2]

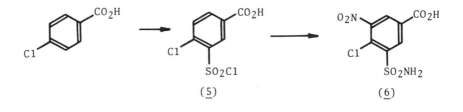

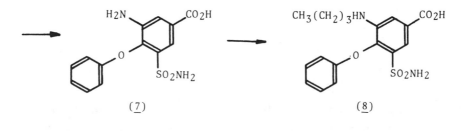

Many benzenesulfonamides have diuretic properties, particularly those having two such functions situated meta to one another. To some extent a carboxyl group can serve in place of one of the sulfonamido groups. *Bumetanide (8)* is such a substance. Chlorosulfonation of p-chlorobenzoic acid leads to 5, which is nitrated, and then converted to sulfonamide 6 with ammonia. The chloro group of 6 is now highly activated toward nucleophilic aromatic substitution, facilitating reaction with phenoxide. Subsequent catalytic reduction in the presence of LiOH produces amino acid 7. Next, treatment with butanol and sulfuric acid not only forms the butyl ester but monoalkylates the amino function. Saponification of the ester group leads to *bumetanide (8)*, a diuretic agent possessing 40-fold greater activity in healthy adults than *furosemide.*[3]

*Tibric acid (10)*, interestingly, has the m-carboxysulfonamido functionality but its activity is expressed, instead, as suppression of serum triglyceride levels. In its reported preparation, chlorosulfonic acid treatment converts 2-chlorobenzoic acid to chlorosulfonate 9, which readily forms the hypolipidemic agent *tibric acid (10)* on reaction with 3,5-dimethylpiperidine.[4]

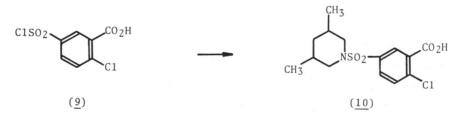

(9)                                  (10)

   b.   Anthranilic Acid and Derivatives
N-Aryl anthranilic acids are frequently found to have
antiinflammatory activity and have been studied
extensively to maximize potency and decrease side
effects (gastric irritation, ulcers, etc.).   These
compounds are often synthesized by reacting an ortho-
halobenzoate salt with a suitably substituted aniline.
This procedure failed, perhaps because of steric
hindrance, in attempting to synthesize *meclofenamic
acid (16)*.[5]   The successful synthesis begins by

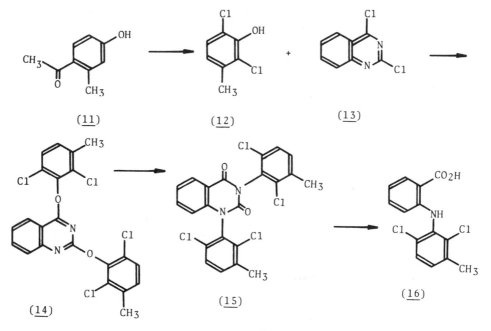

treating 2-methyl-4-hydroxy acetophenone *(11)* with
NaOCl, which both ortho-chlorinates adjacent to the
phenolic OH and effects a haloform reaction. Decarboxylation leads to the chlorinated meta cresol *12*.   When
*12* is converted to its sodium salt with NaH in DMF

and then treated with 2,4-dichloroquinazoline (*13*),
two molecules of the phenol react with the heterocycle
to give the nucleophilic aromatic substitution product
*14*.   When heated, *14* undergoes an O to N-aryl rearrangement (Chapman Rearrangement) to give *15*. Upon saponification, carbon dioxide and 2,5-dichloro-3-methylaniline
are lost and *meclofenamic acid (16)* results.   Reaction
of sodium meclofenamate with ethylchloromethyl ether
in acetone gives *etoclofene (17)*, which is also
active as an antiinflammatory agent.   *Etoclofene*
reportedly causes less gastrointestinal irritation
than *meclofenamic* acid to which it is presumably
converted after passage through the stomach.[6]

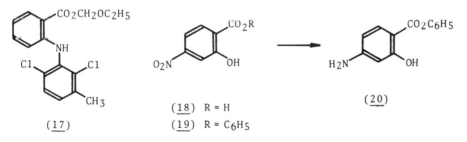

$(\underline{17})$      $(\underline{18})$ R = H    $(\underline{19})$ R = $C_6H_5$      $(\underline{20})$

One of the mainstays in the treatment of tuber-
culosis is *paraaminosalicylic acid (PAS)*.   It is not,
however, a pleasant drug to take.   *Phenyl amino-*
*salicylate (20)* was synthesized from 4-nitrosalicylic
acid *(18)* by esterification of its acid chloride with
phenol to give *19*, which is converted to the desired
product *(20)* by reduction with Raney nickel catalyst.[7]
*Phenyl aminosalicylate* was intended to be more accept-
able to patients than *PAS*.

Unquestionably, the most frequently used analgesic
is *aspirin*.   The reader will recall that *aspirin* is

regarded as a latentiated form of salicylic acid and
is intended to minimize as far as possible the irritation of the gastrointestinal tract that salicylic
acid would otherwise cause.  *Salsalate (24)* represents
another approach to this problem in which self-
esterification has been used to serve the same purpose.
Direct self-condensation is difficult to control,
although low temperature treatment of salicylic acid
with PCl$_3$ does work.  A more stepwise procedure
involves the condensation of benzyl salicylate *(21)*
with the acid chloride of salicylate benzyl ether *22*
to produce protected dimer *23*.  Catalytic hydrogenolysis removes the benzyl groups and completes the
preparation of *salsalate (24)*.[8]

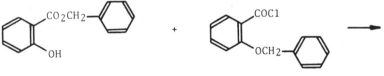

(21)                          (22)

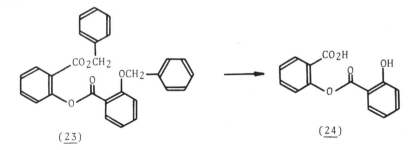

(23)                          (24)

Esterification of certain aromatic acids with
β-aminoethanol and propanol derivatives frequently
results in molecules that show local anesthetic

activity; and some of these derivatives also have an
antiarrythmic action on the heart. *Amoproxan (27)* is
such an agent. It can be synthesized by reacting
epichlorohydrin with 3-methylbutanol and $BF_3$ to give
epoxide *25*. This, then, is reacted with morpholine
to give alcohol *26*, which is then reacted with 3,4,5-
trimethoxybenzoyl chloride to complete the synthesis
of *amoproxan (27)*.[9]

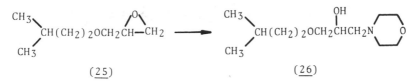

(25)                                      (26)

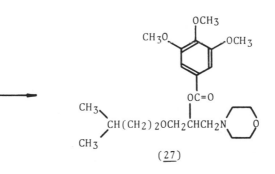

(27)

*Risocaine (28)* manages to retain local anesthetic
activity even without having a "basic ester" moiety.[10]
Its synthesis follows classic lines involving esterification of p-nitrobenzoic acid with thionyl chloride
followed by reaction with propanol, and then catalytic
reduction to complete the scheme.

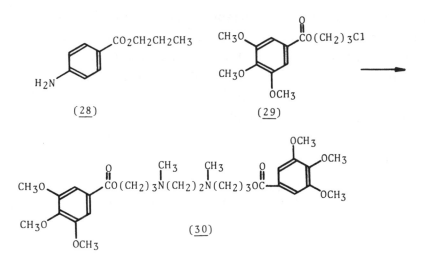

(28)          (29)

(30)

Vasodilators may be of value in the treatment of
conditions resulting from insufficient blood flow
through tissues.  One such agent incorporating a bis-
basic ester moiety is prepared by reacting 3,4,5-tri-
methoxybenzoyl chloride with 3-chloropropanol to give
*29*, and condensing two molar equivalents of this with
N,N'-dimethylethanediamine to give *hexobendine (30)*.[11]

c.  Amides

As one would anticipate, the time honored Schotten-
Baumann reaction and its variants are the key steps
in putting this group of substances together.  Their
intrinsic interest to the medicinal chemist depends
upon their pharmacological properties and, in some
cases, preparation of some of the less common benzoic
acid analogues.

Anticholinergic agents play a role in management
of ulcers by decreasing the secretion of gastric acid

mediated by the neurohormone acetyl choline.  *Prog-*
*lumide (32)* is synthesized from the benzoyl amide of
glutamic anhydride derivative *31* by reaction of the
more activated carbonyl with dipropylamine.[12]

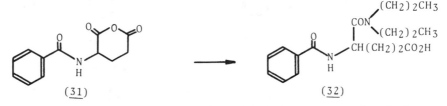

(31)                                    (32)

The diuretic *clopamide (35)* is synthesized from
p-chlorobenzoic acid *(33)* by chlorosulfonation and
subsequent ammonia treatment to give *34*.  This is
converted to its acid chloride with thionyl chloride
and reacted with the desired hydrazine derivative

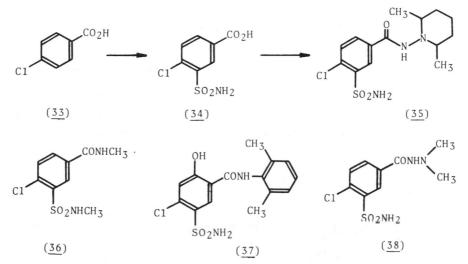

(itself prepared by lithium aluminum hydride reduction
of N-nitroso-2,6-dimethyl piperidine) in a
Schotten-Baumann reaction to give *clopamide*.[13]  The
related diuretics *diapamide (36)*,[14] *xipamide (37)*,[15]

and *alipamide (38)*[16] are made by simple variants on this scheme.

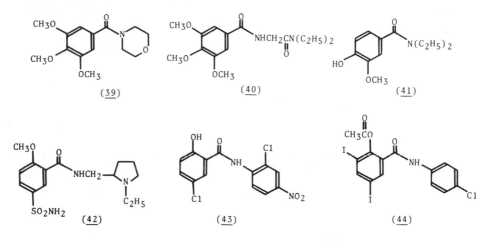

(39)          (40)          (41)

(42)          (43)          (44)

The sedatives *trimetozine (39)*,[17] and *tricetamide (40)*,[18] the CNS stimulants *ethamivan (41)*,[19] and *sulpiride (42)*,[20] the antihelmintic agents *niclosamide (43)*,[21] *clioxanide (44)*,[22] and *bromoxanide (45)*,[23] the coccidiostat *alkomide (46)*,[24] and the antiarrhythmic agent *capobenic acid (47)*[25] are all made from the corresponding benzoic acids in obvious ways.

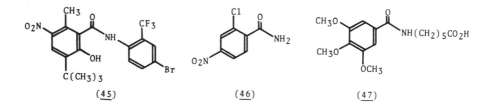

(45)          (46)          (47)

## 2. DERIVATIVES OF ANILINE

The clinical success of hindered acetanilide derivatives, such as *lidocaine*, of course, resulted in the
synthesis of many analogues.  Branching in the acid
moiety is consistent with activity as demonstrated by
the local anesthetic properties of *etidocaine (48)*[26]
and a formally cyclized analogue, *dexivacaine (49).*[27]
*Etidocaine* is prepared from 2,6-dimethylaniline by
sequential reactions with 2-bromobutyryl chloride and
ethylpropylamine.  The preparation of *dexivacaine*
follows the same pattern.  However, in this case,
resolution by crystallization of its quinic acid salt
was carried out, whereupon it was found that the S-
enantiomer was the longer acting.

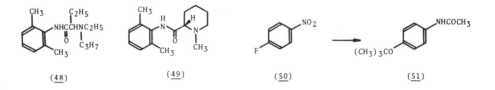

(48)          (49)          (50)          (51)

*Acetanilide* is a well-established analgesic
agent.  It is perhaps not suprising then that *butacetin
(51)* has such activity; however, it appears to have
been synthesized while searching for antitubercular
agents.  The synthesis proceeds from 4-fluoronitro-
benzene *(50)* <u>via</u> a nucleophilic aromatic displacement
reaction with potassium <u>tert</u>-butoxide, followed by
Raney nickel reduction and acetylation.[28]

A molecular dissection of the alkaloid *vasicine*
*(52)* ultimately resulted in the expectorant and
mucolytic agent *bromhexine (54).*[29] The synthesis
starts with displacement of halogen on 2-nitrobenzyl-
bromide *(53)* by N-methyl cyclohexylamine, followed by
Raney nickel and hydrazine reduction of the nitro
group.   Bromination in acetic acid then affords
*bromhexine.*

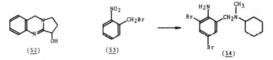

Serotonin *(55)* is a putative neurotransmitter,
especially in the central nervous system, and has a
number of peripheral effects as well.   There have
been numerous attempts to associate disturbances in
serotonin catabolism and anabolism with mental disease,
and antagonists have been prepared as an aid to
investigation of these theories and as potential
therapeutic agents.   BAS *(56)* is one such inhibitor
and its structural similarity to *55* makes it under-
standable that it should be such.   On the other hand,
*cinanserin (58)* is 157 times more potent as a serotonin
inhibitor than *56*, and its structural relationship to
either *55* or *56* is much less obvious.   This under-
scores one of the more frustrating features of deli-
berate drug design--that the best analogues occasionally differ strikingly in structure from the lead
molecule so that success requires an unsatisfying
amount of semirandom molecular manipulation and a
very close liason with the pharmacologist into whose
hands the drugs are placed for evaluation.   In any

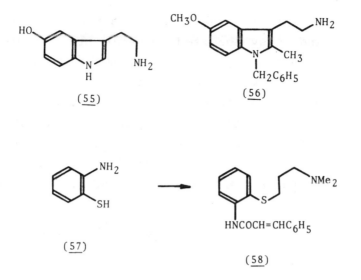

(55)

(56)

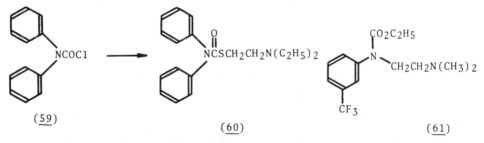

(57)

(58)

event, *cinanserin* is synthesized from 2-aminothio-
benzene *(57)* by S-alkylation using N,N-dimethyl-3-
chloropropylamine and $NaOCH_3$, followed by reaction
with cinnamoyl chloride to give *58*.[30]

(59)

(60)

(61)

*Phencarbamide (60)*[31] is a structural analogue of
acetylcholine which acts as an anticholinergic agent,
possibly by serving as a false agonist.  It is made
by reacting N,N-diphenylcarbamoyl chloride *(59)* with
2-mercapto-N,N-diethylethamine.

Flubanilate (61) has central nervous stimulating
activity and is synthesized conveniently from N-
(2-dimethylamino)ethyl-3-trifluoromethylaniline by
reaction with ethylchlorocarbonate.[32]

A number of aminobenzophenone derivatives possess
nonsteroidal antiinflammatory activity.   Illustrative
is diflumidone (63).   Its synthesis involves treatment
of 3-aminobenzophenone (62) with difluoromethane-
sulfonic anhydride in the presence of triethylamine.[33]

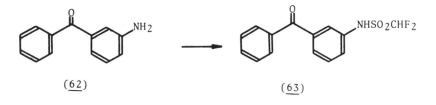

(62)                              (63)

(64)

The closely related antiinflammatory agent triflumidate
(64) can be prepared by abstracting the now acidic NH
proton of the trifluoromethyl analogue of 63 with
sodium hydroxide and reacting the resulting anion
with ethyl chlorocarbonate to give 64.[34]

    3.   DERIVATIVES OF PHENOL
    a.   Basic Ethers
The chemical fragment, OCCN=, occurs very frequently
in drugs, perhaps deriving some inspiration from

acetyl choline. The fact that drugs containing this
unit do not possess some common pharmacological
property suggests that the function is involved in
transport rather than being a pharmacophore. Several
agents containing this moiety are described in this
section.  *Boxidine (69)* has hypolipidemic properties.[35]

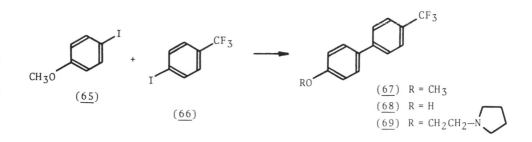

It was synthesized from p-iodoanisole *(65)* by copper-
catalyzed coupling with p-trifluoromethyliodobenzene
*(66)* to give the expected statistical mixture from
which unsymmetrical product *67* could be separated.
Ether cleavage with HBr and HOAc gave *68;* this was
then alkylated with the aziridinium ion derived from
N-(2-chloroethyl)pyrrolidine, using NaH as base, to
complete the synthesis of *boxidine (69)*.

The quaternary ammonium salt *73, thenium
closylate*, is an anthelmintic agent.  Many substances
of this general type are effective by interfering
with nervous conduction, and thereby muscle tone, of
intestinal worms.  This allows their expulsion, not
always in the dead state.  The synthesis[36] proceeds
from 2-thienylamine *(70)* by monoalkylation with 2-
phenoxyethyl bromide *(71)* to give secondary amine *72*.

This is converted by methyl iodide to the quaternary
salt which is converted to the p-chlorobenzene sulfonate salt (73) for pharmacological purposes.

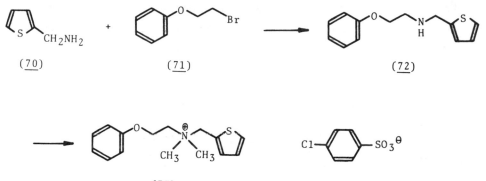

(70)                    (71)                        (72)

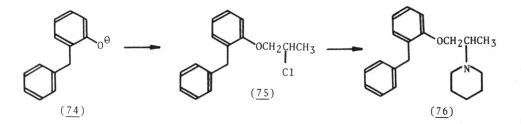

(73)

When 1,2-dichloropropane is reacted with o-benzyl-
phenoxide ion (74), halide 75 results, which is then
converted to the antitussive agent *benproperine* (76)
on treatment with piperidine.[37]

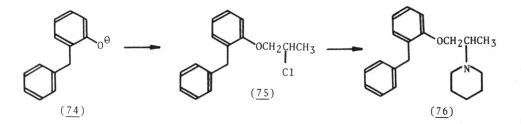

(74)              (75)                    (76)

*Guanethidine* (77) was the first of a series of
antihypertensive agents which act by interfering with
adrenergic transmission.  It was subsequently found
that simple substitution of the guanidine function
onto a nucleus with appropriate lipophilicity almost
invariably affords such sympathetic inhibitors.

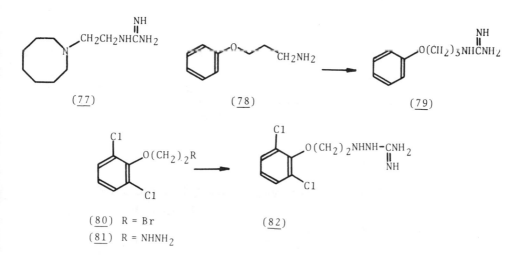

(77)   (78)   (79)

(80) R = Br   (82)
(81) R = NHNH₂

Thus, for example, guanidine analogues *guanoxyfen*
*(79)* and *guanochlor (82)* also possess antihypertensive
activity. *Guanoxyfen* is synthesized[38] by base-
catalyzed condensation of phenol with chloroacetonitrile, followed by hydride reduction to amine *78*.
The guanido function is introduced by reaction with
S-methylthiourea to give *guanoxyfen (79)*.  When 2-
(2,6-dichlorophenoxy)ethyl bromide *(80)* is reacted
with hydrazine to give *81*, and this is reacted with
S-methylthiourea, *guanochlor (82)* results.[39]


  b.   Phenoxyacetic Acids
The clinical success of *clofibrate* has naturally led
to the synthesis of numerous analogues intended for
use as hypocholesterolemic agents.  One of these,
*clofenpyride (84)*, is synthesized readily from p-
chlorophenoxy-2,2-dimethylacetic acid *(83)* by conversion to the acid chloride and reaction with 3-hydroxy-
methylpyridine.[40]  Substitution of a single aromatic

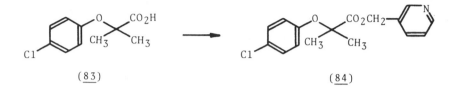

(83)                                    (84)

ring in the place of the gem-dimethyl groups of *84* is
compatible with activity.  Interestingly, the resulting
molecule, *halofenate (90)* is also reported to show
uricosuric activity.  Conversion of p-chlorophenyl-
acetic acid *(85)* to its acid chloride *(86)* activates
the benzylic methylene group to bromination with
molecular bromine, and the resulting mixed dihalide
*(87)* is reacted with methanol to give ester *88*.
Nucleophilic halide displacement with the sodium salt
of m-trifluoromethylphenol gives intermediate *89*,
which is saponified with KOH, converted to the acid

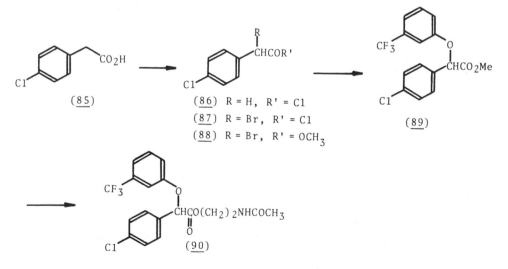

(85)

(86) R = H, R' = Cl
(87) R = Br, R' = Cl
(88) R = Br, R' = OCH$_3$

(89)

(90)

chloride with thionyl chloride, and then esterified
with N-acetylethanolamine to give *halofenate (90)*.[41]

Insertion of a second aryl ether oxygen function
is also consistent with hypocholesterolemic activity.
Burger et al. have published an early and apparently
general synthesis of such compounds.[42]   In the specific
case of *lifibrate (92)*, bis-(4-chlorophenoxy) acetic
acid *(91)* is converted to the acid chloride with
thionyl chloride, and then reacted with N-methyl
piperidine-4-ol to give the desired basic ester *92*.

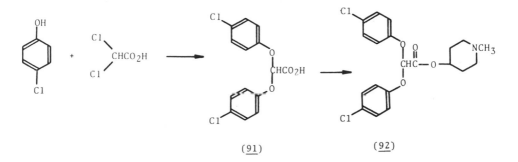

(91)                    (92)

A seemingly simple variation on these structures
results in central stimulant activity instead.
p-Methoxyphenyloxyacetic acid *(93)* is reacted with
N,N-diethylethanolamine via the acid chloride to give
*mefexamide (94)*.[43]

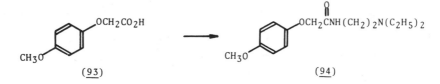

(93)                    (94)

The diuretic properties of *ethacrynic acid (95)*
were at one time attributed to its role as a Michael

acceptor.  The enone was believed to react with SH
groups on enzymes in the kidney.  This interesting
view was weakened by the discovery that some related
molecules which do not possess this structural feature

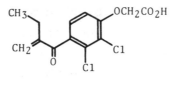

(95)

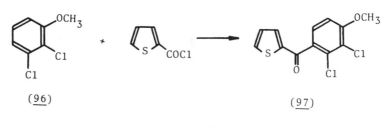

(96)                                              (97)

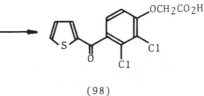

(98)

still possess marked diuretic activity.  An analogue
of *ethacrynic acid* is synthesized by condensing 2,3-
dichloromethoxybenzene *(96)* with the acid chloride of
thiophene α-carboxylic acid to give *97*.  Ether cleavage
with $AlCl_3$, followed by sodium salt formation, etheri-
fication with ethyl chloroacetate, and then saponification gives *ticrynafen (98)*.[44]

c.  Ethers of 1-Aminopropane-2,3-diol

There has been enormous interest recently in the
pharmacological properties of selective β-adrenergic
blocking agents following the clinical success of
*propranolol*.  That the many pharmacological responses
elicited by norepinephrine and epinephrine in various
tissues are the consequence of macromolecular receptor substances of slightly different specificities
has been known for some time.  Such differences are
often most conveniently demonstrated through use of
selective inhibitors, and functional classifications
of such receptors are usually made on that basis.
Ahlquist devised a system of receptor classification
based largely upon whether excitatory or inhibitory
responses followed administration of adrenergic
agents.[45]  The α-receptor was associated generally
with excitatory responses (vasoconstriction, uterine
and nictating membrane stimulation) while the
β-receptor was associated with inhibitory responses
(vasodilation, inhibition of uterine muscle).

While the physiological responses following
β-receptor stimulation are many, those most prominent
are those on the cardiovascular system and on the
smooth muscles of the bronchial tree.  Subsequently,
a lack of faithful parallelism between the cardiac
and bronchial effects led Lands et al.[46] to propose a
further subdivision of the β-receptors into $\beta_1$, which
stimulates cardiac muscle and lipolysis, and $\beta_2$,
which relaxes bronchioles and influences the vasculature and shows metabolic effects.  Epinephrine *(99)*

is an archetypal adrenergic agent stimulating α, $\beta_1$, and $\beta_2$ receptors.

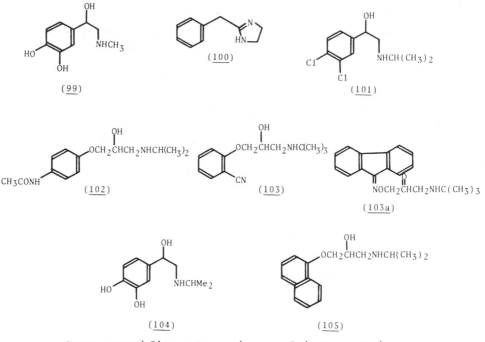

(99)

(100)

(101)

(102)

(103)

(103a)

(104)

(105)

Some specific antagonists of interest in classifying receptors are *tolazoline (100*, α-receptor antagonist), *dichloroisoproterenol (101*, β-receptor antagonist), *practolol (102*, $\beta_1$receptor antagonist), and *bunitrolol (103*, $\beta_2$receptor antagonist). Recently described compound *103a* departs from the previous structural norm and possesses strong $\beta_2$receptor blocking selectivity. These classifications are rendered somewhat difficult because few of these agents are completely selective and may have additional pharmacological properties, such as varying degrees of intrinsic sympathomimetic agonist action.

*Isoproterenol (104)* is an important agent for classification because of its selective β-receptor agonist
activity.  It is of special interest that its chrono-
tropic (increase in heart rate) and inotropic (increase
in force of contraction) effects exceed that of
epinephrine; it is also used in the management of
mild to moderate asthma due to its bronchodilating
effect, resulting in increased vital capacity of the
lungs.

It is in this context that *propranolol (105)* and
its myriad analogues need to be judged.  Administration
of *105* leads to a decrease in heart rate, cardiac
contractile force and myocardial oxygen consumption.
These drugs often have some intrinsic adrenergic
sympathomimetic activity which leads, i.a., to an
increase in airway resistance of little consequence
to most patients but of potential danger to asthmatics.
Another factor of interest is a direct action on cell
membranes, affecting their responsiveness to electrical
stimulation and, in isolated atria, decreasing spontaneous frequency, maximal driving frequency,
contractility and increasing the electrical threshold.
In contrast to the β-blocking action, these "local
anesthetic" actions are nonstereospecific.  Whether
these local anesthetic actions are important in
antiarrhythmic action is being debated.

The therapeutic use of these agents is in control
of cardiac arrhythmias, angina pectoris, and in
essential and renovascular hypertension.  The various
ancillary activities lead to side effects and much

effort has been expended to refine out these extra-
neous responses.  It is not universally agreed whether
some intrinsic sympathetic activity (I.S.A.) is
desirable or not and, if so, how much a drug should
have.

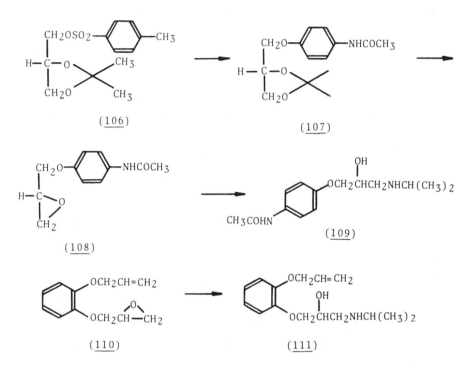

(106)                          (107)

(108)                          (109)

(110)                          (111)

The means used to prepare these agents can be
illustrated by the following examples.  *Practolol*
*(109)*[47] gives less clinical bronchoconstriction in
some patients than propranolol because its receptor
action is more selective.  Serious occasional toxicity
not related to β-blockade has led to its withdrawal
from clinical use.  A synthesis is available which
relates the absolute configuration of the more potent

optical isomer to (+)-lactic acid.  The glycerol
derivative *106* is available from D-mannitol and
retains the optical activity as the two primary
alcohol functions are differentially protected.
Displacement with sodium p-acetamidophenoxide gives
*107* which is deblocked with dilute acid, selectively
reacts at the primary alcohol function with one molar
equivalent of tosyl chloride and pyridine, then
treated with NaOH in dimethylsulfoxide to yield
epoxide *108*.  Epoxide opening with isopropylamine
leads to optically active *practolol (109)*, showing
that the 1-compounds are related to R-(-)-epinephrine.
    The synthesis of *oxprenolol (111)* follows a
similar course.[49]  Epoxide *110*, readily synthesized
by reaction of the sodium salt of pyrocatechol mono-
allylether with epichlorohydrin, is reacted either
with isopropylamine or with HCl (to form the intermediate halohydrin) followed by isopropylamine.

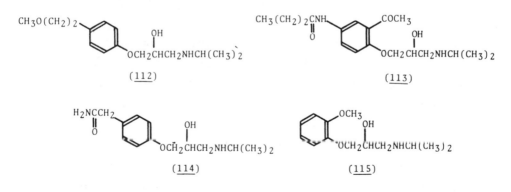

Metoprolol *(112)*,[50] *acebutolol (113)*,[51] *atenolol*
*(114)*,[52] and *moprolol (115)*[23] are all closely related

and made by this basic route or simple variations of
it.

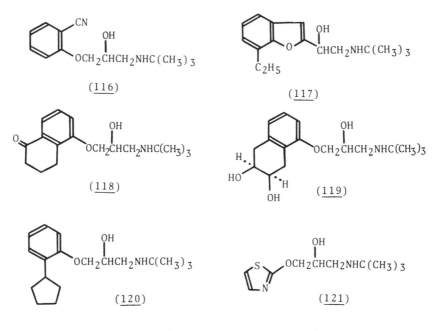

(116)

(117)

(118)

(119)

(120)

(121)

Replacement of isopropylamine by tert-butyl
amino often results in an increase in potency.  This
substitution is used in the β-blockers *bunitrolol*
*(116),*[54] *bufuralol (117),*[55] *bunolol (118),*[56] *nadolol*
*(119),*[57] and *phenbutalol (120).*[58] *Tazolol (121)*[59]
whose structure is similar, is not a good β-blocker,
possessing substantial ISA.[59]

Substitution of groups other than i-propyl or
t-butyl on nitrogen also leads to active compounds.
Primary amine *122* is reacted with p-(β-chloroethoxy)-
benzamide *(123)* to give the β-blocker, *tolamolol*
*(124).*[60]

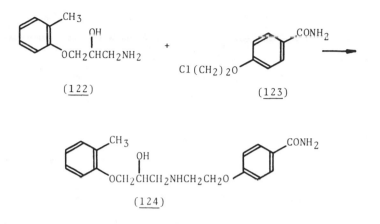

(122)                        (123)

(124)

### 4.  ARYLSULFONES AND SULFONAMIDES

### a.  Sulfones

Until the development of the antibacterial sulfones, Hanson's Disease (leprosy) remained a potentially horrible affliction, treated with largely ineffective ancient remedies.  The antibacterial sulfonamides do not do well against this disease and, interestingly, the sulfones which are effective, are not very useful

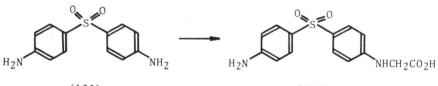

(125)                        (126)

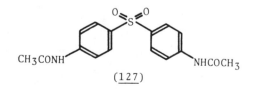

(127)

against most other bacterial infections.  *Dapsone*
*(125)* is such an agent.  It is somewhat inconvenient
to administer to patients because of its rather low
water solubility.  In the search for more easily
administered drugs, *125* was reacted with bromoacetic
acid to give *acediasulfone (126)* which can be
administered as a water soluble salt.[61]

Acedapsone *(127)*, which is conveniently prepared
by acetylation of *dapsone*, was intended to be a
prodrug.[62]  Leprous patients being treated with
*dapsone* were observed to have a lower incidence of
malaria and *acedapsone* was made to capitalize on this
observation.  It, indeed, has both antileprotic and
antimalarial activity.

b.   Sulfonamides

Because of bacterial resistance and unacceptable side
effects in some patients, the antibacterial sulfonamides no longer enjoy the clinical vogue they once
had.  Still, their cheapness, undeniable efficacy in
susceptible infections, and the hope of overcoming
their deficiencies leads to a continuing interest
despite thousands having been synthesized to date.
Some of the more significant agents not included in
Volume I of this work follow.

Generally, $N_1$-acylsulfonamides are less effective
than those having a single $N_1$-aryl group.  One such
acyl analogue, *sulfabenzamide (130)* is prepared
simply from *sulfanilamide (128)* by bisbenzamide
formation (to *129*) using benzoyl chloride and pyridine,
followed by partial saponification.[63]

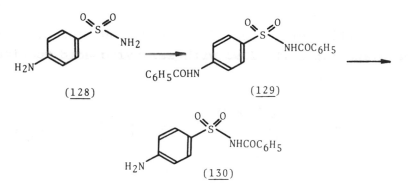

(128)          (129)

(130)

The classic syntheses of the antibacterial
sulfonamides involve reaction of the appropriate
arylamine with an acid addition salt of p-amino-
benzenesulfonyl chloride, or p-nitrobenzenesulfonyl
chloride followed by reduction.  Chemical interest
largely resides in preparation of the corresponding
arylamines.  For the synthesis of *sulfacytine (134)*,
N-ethyl uracil *(131)* was converted to its thioamide
*(132)* by reaction with phosphorous pentasulfide.  The
newly introduced sulfur is then displaced with ammonia
in methanol to give *133*.  Standard reactions complete

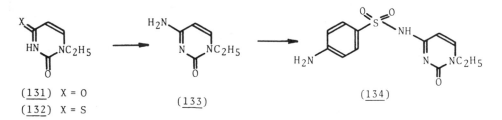

(131) X = O          (133)                    (134)
(132) X = S

the synthesis of *134*.[64]  Reaction of cyanoacetone
*(135)* with phenylhydrazine gives the corresponding
*pyrazole (136)*, which is then converted to *sulfazamet*
*(137)* in the usual way.[65]  An antibacterial agent
promoted for use in ulcerative colitis is made by

diazotization of *sulfapyridine (138)* and coupling of
the diazonium salt *(139)* with salicylic acid to give
*sulfasalazine (140).*[66]

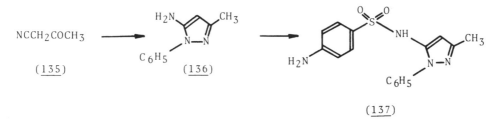

NCCH$_2$COCH$_3$

(135)               (136)

(137)

*Mafenide (142)* was synthesized in part to see
whether the p-amino group of the classical sulfonamides
had to be attached directly to the ring for efficacy
as an antibacterial agent.  The answer is apparently
yes.[67]  Reduction of p-cyanobenzenesulfonamide *(141)*
produces *mafenide*, which is not a clinically useful
antibacterial agent.

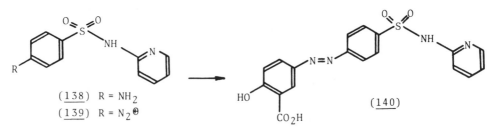

(138)  R = NH$_2$
(139)  R = N$_2$$^\oplus$

(140)

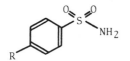

(141)  R = CN
(142)  R = CH$_2$NH$_2$

Coccidiosis is an economically significant respiratory disease of fowl. During the course of studies directed toward antimalarial agents, *sulfanitran (143)* was prepared and found to be a coccidiostat. It is prepared conveniently by reaction of p-acetoamidobenzenesulfonyl chloride with p-nitroaniline in acetic acid.[68]

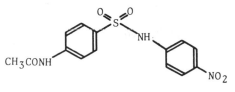

(143)

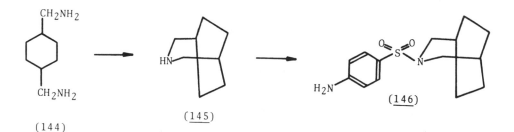

(144)          (145)          (146)

Benzenesulfonamides having two substituents on $N_1$ usually have poor antibacterial potency. Such is the case with *azabon (146)*. This central stimulant is prepared in the usual fashion from 3-azabicyclo-[2.2.2]nonane *(145)*, which is itself prepared by pyrolysis of aliphatic diamine *144*.[69]

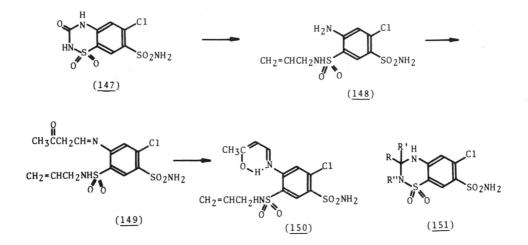

(147)     (148)

(149)     (150)     (151)

*Ambuside (149)*, a diuretic, is prepared from
cyclic urea derivative *147* by allylation of the more
acidic NH group with allyl bromide by means of NaH,
followed by hydrolytic ring opening to give 2-allyl-
sulfamyl-5-chloro-4-sulfamylaniline *(148)*.   This is
in turn treated in acid with 2-ketopropionaldehyde
dimethylacetal to give the Schiff base *ambuside*
*(149)*.[70] The enolanil form *(150)* of *ambuside* shows
some similarity to the open form of some of the
cyclic thiazide diuretics *(151)* which have been
speculated to be the active form of these molecules.

   c.   Sulfonylureas
Linear descendants of the antimicrobial sulfonamides,
the orally active sulfonylureas continue to be of
interest as alternatives to insulin injections in
patients with adult-onset diabetes.  *Tolpyrramide*
*(153)* is synthesized from unsymmetrical O-methylurea

derivative *152* and tosyl chloride, followed by mild
acid treatment to cleave the O-methyl group.[71]

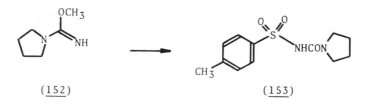

(152)                                (153)

Glyparamide (155) is made by displacement of the
best leaving group of unsymmetrical urea *154* with
sodio p-chlorobenzenesulfonamide.[72]   *Glibornuride*
(*159*) is an **endo-endo** derivative made from camphor-

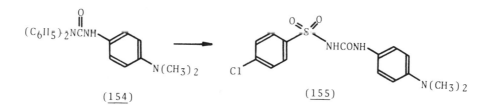

(154)                                (155)

3-carboxamide (*156*) by borohydride reduction (**exo**
approach) (to *157*), followed by a Hoffman reaction to
carbamate *158*, followed by displacement with sodio-
tosylamide to give *glibornuride*.[73]   *Glyoctamide (160)*
is the tosylamide of cyclooctylurea.[74]   *Glipizide*
(*163*) is synthesized from 5-methylpyrazine-2-carboxylic
acid (*161*) and 4-(2-aminoethyl)benzene sulfonamide to
give sulfonamide *162*, which forms *glipizide (163)* on
reaction with cyclohexylisocyanate and base in
acetone.[75]

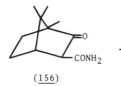  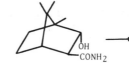 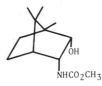

(156) → (157) → (158)

→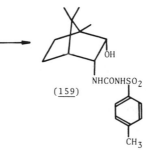

(159)

$CH_3$

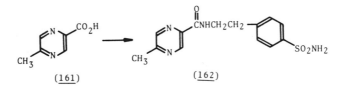

(161) (162)

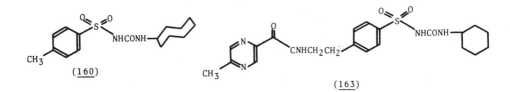

(160) (163)

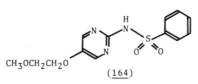

(164)

118

Though *glymidine (164)* does not contain a
sulfonylurea moiety, this function is probably
fulfilled by the aminopyrimidine nucleus, which can
be considered to be the cyclized equivalent. It is
formed simply by reaction of the corresponding
alkoxyaminopyrimidine with benzene sulfonyl chloride.[76]

### 5. FUNCTIONALIZED BENZENE DERIVATIVES
### a. Alkyl Analogues
Parkinson's Disease has been fairly convincingly
demonstrated to be the manifestation of a deficit of
brain dopamine. Administration of this biogenic amine
is ineffective in alleviating the symptoms of this
disease since the drug fails to cross the blood-brain
barrier.  Some success has been achieved by
administering the amino acid precursor of dopamine:
dihydroxyphenylalanine (DOPA).  Though this last
substance does penetrate the brain, its activity is
limited by prior degradation-starting with decarboxylation in the periphery. A compound which would
inhibit the enzyme which catalyzes this first step,
DOPA decarboxylase, should permit more efficient
utilization of DOPA.  A compound very closely related
structurally to the substrate for the enzyme fulfills
this function. *Carbidopa 168* was designed for this
purpose. Carbidopa's synthesis begins with a modified
Strecker reaction using hydrazine and potassium
cyanide on arylacetone *165* to give *166.*  This is then
hydrolyzed with cold HCl to give carboxamide *167.*

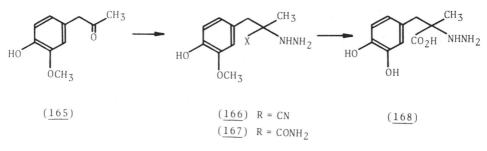

(165)                    (166)  R = CN                    (168)
                         (167)  R = CONH$_2$

More vigorous hydrolysis with 48% HBr cleaves the
amide bond and the arylether group to produce *carbidopa*
*(168)*.[77]  There is some evidence that *carbidopa* has
some anti-Parkinsonian activity in its own right.    If
this is confirmed, then its mode of action will be
different from that for which the drug was designed
and prepared.

Another aminoacid-like drug is the antineoplastic
agent *melphalan (173)*.  Tumor cells spend less time
in resting phases than normal cells so at any given
time, they are more likely to be metabolically active
than most normal host cells.  The rationale behind
incorporating an alkylating function in a molecule
resembling a primary cellular metabolite was to get a
greater safety margin by fooling tumor cells into
taking up the toxin preferentially.  p-Nitrophenyl-
alanine *(169)* was converted to its phthalimide analogue
by heating with phthalic anhydride, and this was
converted to its ethyl ester *(170)*.  Catalytic
reduction produced the aniline *(171)*. Heating in acid
with ethylene oxide led to *172*, which was converted
to the bischloride with phosphorous oxychloride, and
the protecting groups were removed by heating in
hydrochloric acid to give *melphalan (173)*.[78]

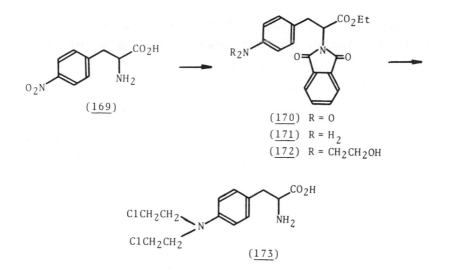

(169)

(170) R = O
(171) R = H$_2$
(172) R = CH$_2$CH$_2$OH

(173)

Baclofen (176), a muscle relaxant and hypnotic, is synthesized from ethyl p-chlorocinnamate (174) via the Triton B catalyzed Michael addition of nitromethane (to 175) followed by Raney nickel reduction and saponification. Baclofen is formally a GABA (gamma-aminobutyric acid) analogue.[79]

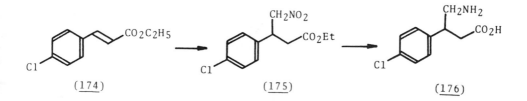

(174)                    (175)                    (176)

Reaction of p-chlorobenzylmagnesium chloride with the Mannich product from 2-butanone (177) produces the antitussive agent, clobutinol (178).[80] The tranquilizer cintriamide (179) is prepared most

conveniently by a simple Shotten-Baumann reaction of
the acid chloride.[81]  For reasons that are not very
clear, the 1,2,3-trimethoxybenzene moiety is frequently
associated with CNS activity.

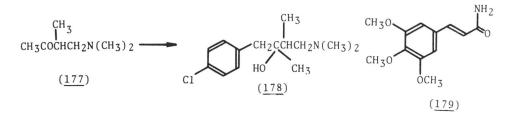

(177)                    (178)                    (179)

Very reactive nitrogen mustards and aziridine-
containing molecules are usually too toxic for general
therapeutic use, but find use in neoplastic disease.
*Benzodepa (182)* is such an agent.  Treatment of ethyl
carbamate with phosphorous pentachloride leads to
cyanate *180* which readily adds benzyl alcohol to
produce carbamate *181*.  Displacement of the active

$H_2N\overset{O}{\overset{\|}{C}}OC_2H_5$ $\longrightarrow$ $Cl_2\overset{O}{\overset{\|}{P}}N=C=O$ $\longrightarrow$ $Cl_2\overset{O}{\overset{\|}{P}}NH\overset{O}{\overset{\|}{C}}OCH_2C_6H_5$ $\longrightarrow$

(180)                    (181)

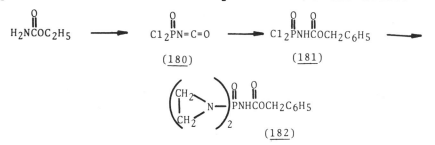

(182)

chlorines with ethyleneimine leads to the very reactive
*benzodepa (182).*[82]  It was previously known that
carbamates and bisaziridininylphosphinyl agents had
antitumor properties, so it was natural to combine
both moieties in a single molecule to see if synergism
would develop.

As noted above, guanido-containing drugs often exhibit antihypertensive activity. Interposition of an additional nitrogen atom is consistent with activity. There is some evidence to suggest that these hydrazines owe their activity to a mechanism different from the guanidines. One such derivative was originally synthesized to be a herbicide.[83] Hydrazone formation

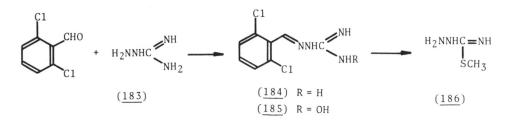

(183)         (184) R = H          (186)
              (185) R = OH

between 2,6-dichlorobenzaldehyde and hydrazinyl guanidine *183* leads efficiently to *guanabenz (184)*. The closely related analogue *guanoxabenz (185)* is prepared in the analogous fashion using the hydrazinyl-oxyguanidine derivative prepared by reacting thiomethyl-imine *186* with hydroxylamine and then with 2,6-dichlorobenzaldehyde.[84]

A group of arylalkylketones containing a basic substituent in the side chain shows CNS activities. *Roletamide (190)* is a hypnotic agent. It is prepared from 3,4,5-trimethoxybenzaldehyde *(187)* by addition of sodium acetylide (to give *188*), followed by Jones oxidation of ethynylarylketone *189*. Michael addition of pyrrolidine-3-ene leads to *roletamide (190)*.[85]

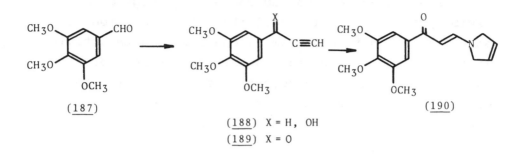

<u>(187)</u>

(<u>188</u>) X = H, OH
(<u>189</u>) X = O

<u>(190)</u>

Reaction of m-chlorobenzonitrile with ethyl
Grignard reagent produces ethylarylketone *191*.
Bromination in methylene chloride followed by displacement of the α-bromoketone moiety with t-butylamine
leads to the antidepressant agent *bupropion (192)*.[86]
While the closely related central stimulant *pyrovalerone (193)* can also be made simply by reacting the
requisite α-haloaralkylketone with pyrrolidine, a

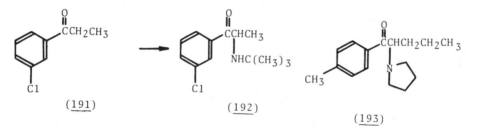

(<u>191</u>)

(<u>192</u>)

(<u>193</u>)

more interesting synthesis goes through quaternary
amine *194* which undergoes a Stevens rearrangement on
treatment with base to provide intermediate *195*,
which is hydrogenated to *pyrovalerone*.[87] This mecha-
nistic interpretation is supported by studies with
unsymmetrical olefins wherein it is seen that the
double bond migrates on conversion of *194* to *195*.

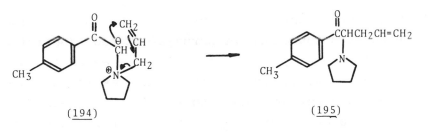

(194)                                (195)

Conversion of a ketone to a highly substituted imine interestingly leads to a compound which shows analgesic activity, *anidoxime (197)*.   Phenyl 2-diethylaminoethyl ketone is converted to its oxime *(196)* in the usual way, and this is converted to *anidoxime* by reaction with p-methoxyphenylisocyanate.[88]

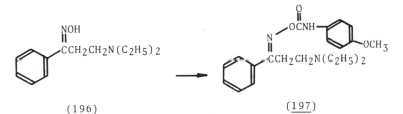

(196)                                (197)

An arylamidine found subsequently to have antiarrythmic activity was actually synthesized in the hope of producing a hypoglycemic agent.   Iminochloride *198* is prepared from the corresponding benzamide and the chlorine iş displaced with n-amylpiperidine to produce *bucainide (199)*.[89]   To posit a similarity to

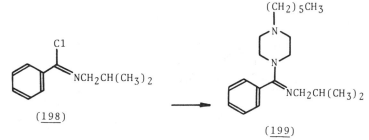

(198)

(199)

the well-established antiarrythmic benzamide procainamide and its congeners is perhaps not too fanciful.
    While some arylaliphatic acids are established
as antiinflammatory agents, it is interesting to note
that some arylketones share this activity. *Fenbufen*
*(200)* is prepared simply by a Friedel-Crafts acylation
of biphenyl with succinic anhydride.[90]  The same
reaction using cyclohexylbenzene leads to *201*.

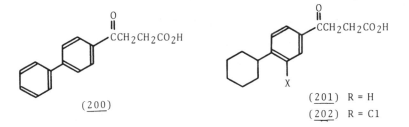

(200)

(201) R = H
(202) R = Cl

Chlorination enhances activity and is accomplished by
treatment of *201* with chlorine in methylene chloride
catalyzed by aluminum chloride.  The nonsteroidal
antiinflammatory agent *bucloxic acid (202)* results.[91]

    b.  Miscellaneous Derivatives
Reaction of 2,6-ditertiarybutyl-4-thiolphenol with
acetone leads to the dithioketal *probucol (203)* which
has hypolipidemic activity.[92]

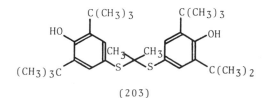

(203)

Some tumors are estrogen-dependent and the use of an antiestrogen has therapeutic value. One such antineoplastic agent appears to be patterned after *clomiphene*. Complex aryl ketone *204* is treated with phenyl magnesium chloride and the resulting tertiary

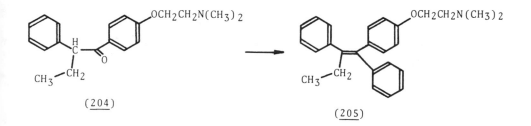

(204)                                          (205)

carbinol is dehydrated. The resulting isomers are separated to give *tamoxifen (205)*. Structural assignment amongst the isomers is performed by pmr measurements.[93]

## REFERENCES

1.  W. Ruyle, L. H. Sarett and A. Matzuk, French Patent 1,522,570 (1968); *Chem. Abstr.*, *71:* P30241u (1969).

2.  W. Ruyle, L. H. Sarett and A. Matzuk, South African Patent 67 01,021 (1968); *Chem. Abstr.*, *70:* P106,209k (1969).

3.  P. W. Fect, *J. Med. Chem.*, *14*, 432 (1971).

4.  G. F. Holland, German Patent 2,145,686 (1972); *Chem. Abstr.*, *77:* P48046m (1972).

5.  P. F. Juby, T. W. Huidyma and M. Brown, *J. Med. Chem.*, *11*, 111 (1968).

6.  G. B. Fregnan, A. Subissi and A. L. Torsello, *Il Farmaco, Ed. Sci.*, *30*, 353 (1975); A. Salimbeni, E. Manghisi and M. J. Magistretti, *Il Farmaco, Ed. Sci.*, *30*, 276 (1975).

7.  S. A. Friere, U. S. Patent 2,604,488 (1952): *Chem. Abstr.*, *48:* 12,807d (1954).

8.  C. Cavallito and J. S. Buck, *J. Am. Chem. Soc.*, *65*, 2140 (1943).

9.  R. Y. Mauvernay, N. Busch, J. Simond and J. Moleyre, U. S. Patent 3,781,432 (1970); *Chem. Abstr.*, *74:* 141,861w (1971).

10. J. Buchit, K. H. Hetterich and X. Pereira, *Arzneimittel forschung*, *18*, 1 (1968).

11. O. Kraupp and K. Schloegl, Austrian Patent 231,432 (1964); *Chem. Abstr.*, *60:* 15786g (1964).

12. Anonymous, Netherlands Patent 6,510,006 (1966); *Chem. Abstr.*, *65:* 3793b (1966).

13. E. Jucker and A. Lindenmann, *Helv. Chem. Acta*, *45*, 2316 (1962).

14. M. L. Hoefle, German Patent 1,158,927 (1963); *Chem. Abstr.*, *60:* 10,608a (1964).

15. Anonymous, Netherlands Patent 6,607,680 (1966); *Chem. Abstr.*, *67:* 21,706h (1967).

16. H. A. DeWald and M. L. Hoefle, U. S. Patent 3,043,874 (1962); *Chem. Abstr.*, *57:* 16,503h (1962).

17. G. R. Pettit, M. F. Baumann and K. H. Rangammal, *J. Med. Chem.*, *5*, 800 (1962).

18.  M. E. Kuehne and B. F. Lambert, *J. Am. Chem. Soc.*, *81*, 4278 (1959).

19.  K. Kratzl and E. Krasnicka, *Monatsh. Chemie*, *83*, 18 (1952).

20.  Anonymous, Netherlands Patent 6,500,326 (1965); *Chem. Abstr.*, *64:* 3,486h (1966).

21.  B. Duhm, W. Maul, H. Medenwald, K. Patzschke and L. A. Wagner, *Z. Naturwissenschaften*, *16b*, 509 (1961).

22.  Anonymous, Netherlands Patent 6,604,303 (1966); *Chem. Abstr.*, *66:* 55,247d (1967).

23.  W. H. Meek, German Patent 2,347,615 (1975); *Chem. Abstr.*, *83:* 58,480m (1975).

24.  D. B. Cosulich, D. R. Seeger, M. J. Fahrenbach, K. H. Collins, B. Roth, M. E. Hultquist and J. M. Smith, Jr., *J. Am. Chem. Soc.*, *75*, 4675 (1953).

25.  A. Garzia, German Patent 2,034,192 (1971); *Chem. Abstr.*, *75:* 5513c (1971).

26.  H. J. F. Adams, G. H. Kronberg and B. H. Takman, German Patent 2,162,744 (1972); *Chem. Abstr.*, *77:* 101,244c (1972).

27.  B. F. Tullar, *Acta Chem. Scand.*, *11*, 1183 (1957); *J. Med. Chem.*, *14*, 891 (1971); *Acta Pharm. Sueica*, *8*, 361 (1971).

28.  K. Bowden and P. N. Green, *J. Chem. Soc.*, 1795 (1954).

29.  J. Keck, *Ann.*, *662*, 171 (1963).

30.  J. Krapcho, B. Rubin, A. M. Drungis, E. R. Spitzmiller, C. F. Turk, J. Williams, B. N. Craver and J. Fried, *J. Med. Chem.*, *6*, 219

(1963).

31.    A. Laurent and J. Vilmer, *Ann. Pharm. Fr.*, *29*,
       569 (1971).

32.    Anon., Netherlands Patent 6,405,529 (1964);
       *Chem. Abstr.*, *62:* 10,368g (1965).

33.    J. K. Harrington and J. E. Robertson, German
       Patent 1,917,821 (1969); *Chem. Abstr.*, *73:*
       14,477e (1970).

34.    J. K. Harrington, J. E. Robertson, D. C. Kvain,
       R. R. Hamilton, K. T. McGurran, R. J. Trancik,
       K. F. Swingle, G. G. I. Moore and J. F. Gerster,
       *J. Med. Chem.*, *13*, 137 (1970).

35.    Anon., Netherlands Patent 6,516,582 (1966);
       *Chem. Abstr.*, *65:* 16,901f (1966).

36.    F. C. Copp, British Patent 864,885 (1961); *Chem.
       Abstr.*, *55:* 24,792a (1961).

37.    Anon., British Patent 914,008 (1962); *Chem.
       Abstr.*, *58:* 12,523a (1963).

38.    D. I. Barron, P. M. G. Bavin, G. J. Durant, I.
       L. Natoff, R. G. W. Spickett and D. K. Vallance,
       *J. Med. Chem.*, *6*, 705 (1963).

39.    G. J. Durant, G. M. Smith, R. G. W. Spickett and
       S. H. B. Wright, *J. Med. Chem.*, *9*, 22 (1966);
       Anon., Belgian Patent 629,613 (1963); *Chem.
       Abstr.*, *60:* 14,437d (1964).

40.    Anon., Netherlands Patent 6,610,738 (1968);
       *Chem. Abstr.*, *68:* 39,487t (1968).

41.    W. A. Bulhofer, South African Patent 67 05,870
       (1967); *Chem. Abstr.*, *71:* 101,563g (1969).

42.    A. Burger, D. G. Markees, W. R. Nes and W. L.
       Yost, *J. Am. Chem. Soc.*, *71*, 3307 (1949).

43. G. Thuillier, P. Rumpf and B. Saville, *Bull. Soc. Chim. Fr.*, 1786 (1960).

44. J. J. Godfroid and J. E. Thuillier, German Patent 2,048,372 (1971); *Chem. Abstr.*, *75:* 93,435s (1971).

45. R. P. Ahlquist, *Am. J. Physiol.*, *153*, 586 (1948).

46. A. M. Lands, A. Arnold, J. P. McAuliff, F. P. Luduena and T. G. Brown, Jr., *Nature*, *214*, 597 (1967).

46a. G. Leclerc, A. Mann, C. Wermuth, N. Bieth and J. Schwartz, *J. Med. Chem.*, *20*, 1657 (1977).

47. J. C. Danilewicz and J. E. G. Kemp, *J. Med. Chem.*, *16*, 168 (1973).

48. M. Dukes and L. H. Smith, *J. Med. Chem.*, *14*, 326 (1971).

49. Anon., Belgian Patent 669,402 (1966); *Chem. Abstr.*, *65:* 5402d (1966).

50. A. E. Brandstrom, P. A. E. Carlsson, S. A. I. Carlsson, H. R. Corrodi, L. Ek and B. A. H. Ablad, German Patent 2,106,209 (1971); *Chem. Abstr.*, *76:* 10,427c (1972).

51. K. R. H. Wooldridge and B. Berkeley, South African Patent 68 08,345 (1969); *Chem. Abstr.*, *72:* 78724v (1970).

52. A. M. Barrett, R. Hull, D. J. LeCount, C. J. Squire and J. Carter, German Patent 2,007,751 (1970); *Chem. Abstr.*, *73:* 120,318p (1970).

53. G. Crocl, *Arzneimittelforsch.*, *20*, 1074 (1970).

54. H. Koeppe, K. Zeile and A. Engelhardt, South African Patent 68 03,783 (1968); *Chem. Abstr.*, *71:* 21,878y (1969).

55.  Anon., Netherlands Patent 6,606,441 (1966);
     *Chem. Abstr.*, *67:* 21,808t (1967).

56.  E. J. Merrill, *J. Pharm. Sci.*, *60*, 1589 (1971).

57.  F. P. Hauck, C. M. Cimarusti and V. L. Narayanan,
     German Patent 2,258,995 (1973); *Chem. Abstr.*,
     *79:* 53,096y (1973).

58.  H. Ruschig, K. Schmitt, H. Lessenich and G.
     Haertfelder, South African Patent 68 07,915
     (1969); *Chem. Abstr.*, *72:* 90,054j (1970).

59.  J. A. Edwards, B. Berkoz, G. S. Lewis, O. Helpern,
     J. H. Fried, A. M. Strosberg, L. M. Miller, S.
     Urich, F. Liu and A. P. Roszkowski, *J. Med.
     Chem.*, *17*, 200 (1974).

60.  J. Augstein, D. A. Cox, A. L. Ham, P. R. Leeming
     and M. Snarey, *J. Med. Chem.*, *16*, 1245 (1973).

61.  E. L. Jackson, *J. Am. Chem. Soc.*, *70*, 680 (1948).

62.  E. F. Elslager, Z. B. Gavrilis, A. A. Phillips
     and D. F. Worth, *J. Med. Chem.*, *12*, 357 (1969).

63.  C. Siebenmann and R. J. Schnitzer, *J. Am. Chem.
     Soc.*, *65*, 2126 (1943).

64.  L. Doub, U. Krolls, J. M. Vandenbelt and M. W.
     Fisher, *J. Med. Chem.*, *13*, 242 (1970).

65.  G. B. Crippa and M. Guarnari, *Gazz. Chim. Ital.*,
     *85*, 199 (1955): J. Seydel and E. Kruger-Thiemer,
     *Arzneimittelforsch.*, *14*, 1294 (1964).

66.  A. Korkuczanski, *Prezemsyl Chem.*, *37*, 162 (1958).

67.  E. Muller, J. M. Sprague, L. W. Kissinger and L.
     F. McBurney, *J. Am. Chem. Soc.*, *62*, 2099 (1940).

68.  R. G. Shepherd, *J. Org. Chem.*, *12*, 275 (1947).

69.  A. W. Pircio and C. S. Krementz, U. S. Patent

3,351,528 (1967); *Chem. Abstr.*, *68:* P38,496v (1968).

70. J. E. Robertson, D. A. Dusterhoft and T. F. Mitchell, Jr., *J. Med. Chem.*, *8*, 90 (1965).

71. E. Walton, British Patent 872,102 (1961); *Chem. Abstr.*, *57:* P785g (1962).

72. G. F. Holland and W. M. McLamore, U. S. Patent 3,033,902 (1962); *Chem. Abstr.*, *57:* P11,109f (1962).

73. K. Hohenlohe-Oehringen, *Monatsh. Chem.*, *101*, 610 (1970); H. Breitschnider, K. Hohenlohe-Oehringen and K. Grassmeyr, *ibid.*, *100*, 2133 (1969).

74. Anon., French Patent 1,558,886 (1969); *Chem. Abstr.*, *72:* P43,231e (1970).

75. V. B. Ambrogi and W. Logemann, German Patent 2,012,138 (1970); *Chem. Abstr.*, *73:* 120,674b (1970).

76. K. Gutsche, A. Harwart, H. Horstmann, H. Priewe, G. Raspe, E. Schraufstatter, S. Wirtz and U. Worfel, *Arzneimittelforsch.*, *14*, 373 (1964).

77. M. Sletzinger, J. M. Chemerda and F. W. Bollinger, *J. Med. Chem.*, *6*, 101 (1963).

78. F. Bergel, V. C. E. Burnop and J. A. Stock, *J. Chem. Soc.*, 1223 (1955); F. A. Bergel and J. A. Stock, *ibid.*, 2409 (1954).

79. F. Uchimaru, M. Sato, E. Kosasayama, M. Shimizu and H. Takashi, Japanese Patent 70 16,692 (1970); *Chem. Abstr.*, *73:* 77,617w (1970).

80. Anon., British Patent 898,010 (1962); *Chem. Abstr.*, *57:* 12381i (1962).

81.  R. B. Moffett, *J. Med. Chem.*, *7*, 319 (1964).

82.  Z. B. Papanastassiou and T. J. Bardos, *J. Med. Chem.*, *5*, 1000 (1962).

83.  J. Yates and E. Haddock, British Patent 1,019,120 (1964); *Chem. Abstr.*, *64:* PC111132h (1966).

84.  W. J. Houlihan and R. E. Manning, German Patent 1,902,449 (1969); *Chem. Abstr.*, *71:* P123963q (1969).

85.  S. Safir and R. P. Williams, Belgian Patent 670,495 (1966); *Chem. Abstr.*, *65:* PC13615c (1966).

86.  D. A. Yeowell, German Patent 2,064,934 (1971); *Chem. Abstr.*, *76:* P33965r (1972).

87.  W. Heffe, *Helv. Chim. Acta*, *47*, 1289 (1964).

88.  M. J. Karten and M. L. Kantor, German Patent 1,805,716 (1969); *Chem. Abstr.*, *71:* 980916g (1969).

89.  J. R. Shroff and V. Bandurco, U. S. Patent 3,793,322 (1974); *Chem. Abstr.*, *80:* P96018n (1974).

90.  A. S. Tomcufcic, R. G. Child and A. E. Sloboda, German Patent 2,147,111 (1972); *Chem. Abstr.*, *76:* P158368e (1972).

91.  F. Krausz, H. Demarne, J. Vaillant, M. Brunaud and J. Navarro, *Arzneimittelforsch.*, *24*, 1360 (1974).

92.  M. B. Neuworth, R. J. Laufer, J. W. Barnhart, J. A. Sefranka and D. D. McIntosh, *J. Med. Chem.*, *13*, 722 (1970).

93.  D. J. Collins, J. J. Hobbs and C. W. Emmens, *J. Med. Chem.*, *14*, 952 (1971).

# 6

# Steroids

Early interest in steroid chemistry centered about
cholesterol, the bile acids, and the cardiotonic
glycosides, but a dramatic expansion took place in
the 1930s with the discovery of steroidal sex
hormones and the adrenal cortical hormones.  As each
of the major steroid structures was elucidated,
efforts were bent toward developing synthetic methods
for their preparation. The impetus for this work was
variously to provide amounts of compound sufficient
for more detailed pharmacology and clinical application, to prepare orally active analogues, to prepare
substances of intrinsic non-hormonal pharmacological
activity, and, in some cases, to provide compounds
that would antagonize the action of endogenous hormones.
    The large number of entries outlined in this
chapter might mislead the casual reader into assuming
that these represent a correspondingly large number

of drugs in actual clinical use. This is in fact not
so:  the majority of commercial steroid drugs are to
be found in the first volume of this work.  The
medicinal chemistry and pharmacology of synthetic
steroids was a field of intensive concentration for
the better part of two decades; numerous compounds
were thus produced which showed enough clinical
promise to be assigned a generic name, but for one
reason or another, most failed to find a place on the
drugstore shelf.  The fact that so many of these
compounds do have generic names indicates that they
have interesting activity in various animal assays,
and have shown sufficient clinical promise to merit
inclusion in this work.

The numbering system and normal stereochemistry
of the steroids of interest to this chapter are as
follows:

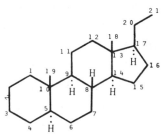

This stereochemical pattern is taken for granted in
the following structures with only departures being
detailed.


1.   ESTRANES
The prototype for the estrane series is the female
sex hormone *estradiol* (<u>1</u>).  Estrogens have important

applications as replacement therapy for hormone-
deficient states found in menopausal and post-
menopausal women for the treatment of menstrual
irregularities, failure of ovarian development, and
in treatment of prostatic carcinoma, etc.  These
compounds also constitute an essential ingredient for
the oral contraceptives.  It is important to recall
that when the synthetic work was done, the Pill was
as yet untainted by any shadow and was regarded as an
unmitigated boon.  There seemed, in fact, to be good
reasons for developing new estrogens of greater
potency and specificity.  It is only fairly recently
that there have been serious questions raised about
the safety of long-term treatment with exogenous
estrogenic compounds, resulting in a lessening
commercial interest in these agents.

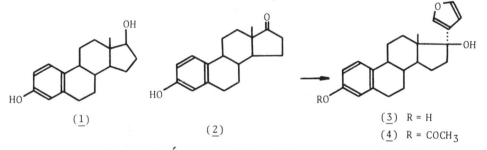

(1)

(2)

(3) R = H

(4) R = COCH$_3$

Reaction of *estrone (2)* with an excess of the
lithium reagent from 3-iodofuran gives intermediate
diol 3.  The stereochemical assignment follows from
the well-known propensity of steroids for attack from
the less-hindered backside ($\alpha$) of the molecule.
Acylation of 3 with acetic anhydride then affords the
estrogen *estrofurate (4)*.[1]

One of the routes for metabolism of the natural estrogens involves oxidation at the 16-position. The resulting compounds (estriols) show paradoxical endocrine activities in animal models. Thus, although these metabolites show estrogenic activity in their own right, they can to some extent block the action of concurrently administered estradiol. The unnatural estriol analogue *epimestrol (8)* shows this kind of activity.

One of the routes to *epimestrol* begins with acylation of estradiol with benzoyl chloride to give the dibenzoate 5. Pyrolysis of the ester leads to formation of the 16,17-olefin. Hydroxylation by means of osmium tetroxide affords the cis-diol 7 due to the intermediacy of the cyclic osmate ester *(6a)*; attack of the reagents from the α side insures formation of the 16,17α-diol.[2] Saponification is followed by alkylation of the phenolic hydroxyl group with dimethyl sulfate in the presence of base to afford *epimestrol (8)*.[3]

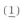 $\longrightarrow$ 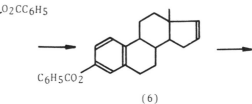 $\longrightarrow$

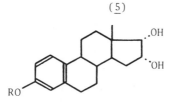

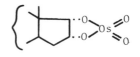

(7) R = H
(8) R = CH$_3$

Replacement of a ring carbon by a heteroatom,
such as nitrogen, has proven a fruitful modification
in many classes of medicinal agents.  The resulting
analogues often possess the same qualitative activity
as the parent compound.  Although this strategy has
been applied extensively to the steroids, it has not
met with overwhelming success.  Two cases of substitution by N in which interesting activity was obtained
both contain the heteroatom at the 8-position.  Such
derivatives are most conveniently prepared by total
synthesis.  For example, condensation of the substituted phenethylamine *9* with 2-cyclopentanonepropionic
acid *(10)* affords directly the bicyclic lactam *12*, as
a mixture of isomeric eneamides.  Though the precise
order of the steps is not clear, the reaction can be
rationalized as proceeding via enamine *11*; enamide
formation will then give the observed products.
Catalytic reduction affords the lactam with the
expected *cis* ring junction *(13)*.  Cyclization by means
of phosphorus oxychloride then gives the tetracyclic
quaternary salt *(14)*.  Treatment with hydrobromic
acid serves both to cleave the methyl ether and to
replace the counterion by bromide.  There is thus
obtained *quinodinium bromide* *(15)*.[4]  This compound
interestingly exhibits antiarrhythmic rather than
hormonal activity, possibly in part because of lack
of D-ring functionality required for estrogen receptor
activation.

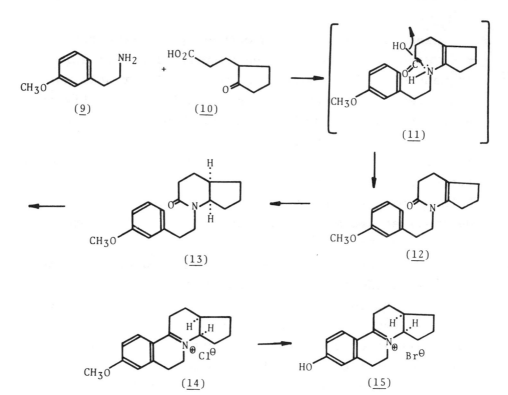

(9)  (10)  (11)

(13)  (12)

(14)  (15)

The scheme used to prepare the direct 8-aza-analogue *21* of estrone bears at least formal simi-larity to the Torgov-Smith steroid total synthesis sequence. Acylation of the phenethylamine *9* with acryloyl chloride gives amide *16*. Michael addition of dimethylamine followed by Bischler-Napieralski cyclo-dehydration gives the dihydroisoquinoline, *17*. Reaction of the heterocycle with 2-methylcyclopentane-1,3-dione in the presence of pyridine leads directly to tetracyclic intermediate *20*.[5] The first step in this transformation probably consists in formation of the olefin *18* by elimination of dimethylamine. Michael addition of the anion from the cyclopentane-

dione gives a transient intermediate such as *19*.
Reaction of the enamine nitrogen with one of the
carbonyl groups leads to the corresponding cyclized
dieneamine *20*. Catalytic reduction leads to stereo-
selective introduction of hydrogen at both C-9 and

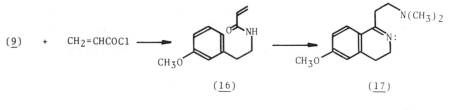

(9)   +   CH₂=CHCOCl ⟶

(16)                    (17)

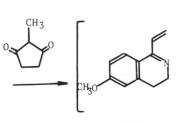

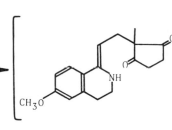

(18)                    (19)

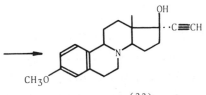

(20)                    (21)

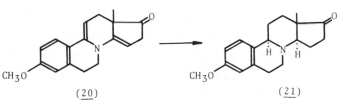

(22)

C-14 from the α face.  It should be noted that except
for the methyl group at C-13, *20* is quite flat; it is
not unreasonable to assume that adsorption to the
catalyst will take place at the face opposite that
substituent, thus leading to the observed stereochemistry.  The product is, of course, racemic.
Reaction of *20* with lithium acetylide completes the
synthesis of *estrazinol (22)*.[6]    It is of note that,
in contrast to *15*, this compound shows activity as an
estrogen.

        Reduction of the aromatic A ring of the estra-
trienes and appropriate substitution at the 17--
position leads to compounds that show either androgenic or progestational activity. These 19-nor
steroids tend to have much better oral activity than
their 19-methylated counterparts.  Orally active
androgens have found some use both in replacement
therapy for androgen deficiency and as agents which
will reverse protein loss in various pathological
wasting diseases (as anabolic agents). Some contro-
versial use is also found in increasing the body mass
of professional athletes.  By far the largest clinical
application for the orally active progestins is as a
component part of oral contraceptives.

        Reduction of 19-nortestosterone *(23)*[7] with sodium
borohydride leads to a mixture of isomers consisting
largely of the 3β-alcohol *(24)*; the lack of stereospecificity can be traced back to the relative
remoteness of that 3-position from chiral centers
which could direct the incoming reagent.  Acylation
of diol *24* with acetic anhydride in the presence of

sodium acetate affords the anabolic agent *bolandiol diacetate (25).*[8]

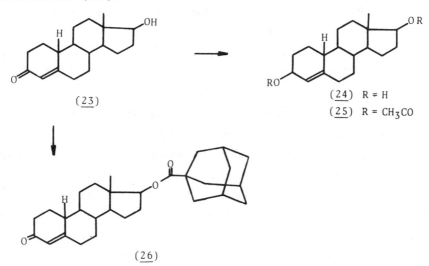

(23)

(24) R = H
(25) R = CH₃CO

(26)

A fairly common strategy for converting a drug to an agent which is excreted more slowly and may be longer acting pharmacologically consists of the preparation of a very lipophilic derivative. This is then administered by subcutaneous or intramuscular injection in an oil solution. The drug or its hydrolysis product then slowly leaches out of that oily depot to provide long-lasting levels in the blood. Reaction of 19-nortestosterone with adamantoyl chloride affords the longacting anabolic agent *bolmantalate (26).*[9] There is some evidence to suggest that this ester is not a prodrug, but has hormonal activity in its own right.

The presence of a 7α-methyl group has been found to potentiate anabolic activity. Acetylation of 19-nortestosterone affords the corresponding 17-acetate

(27). Treatment of this compound with chloranil
results in dehydrogenation at C-6,7 and thus formation
of the 4,6-diene-3-one moiety. Reaction of 28 with
methyl Grignard reagent in the presence of cuprous
bromide leads to conjugate (1,6) addition from the
bottom face of the molecule with concomitant loss of
the ester function from C-17 to give the 7α-methyl
derivative *(29)*. Oxidation of the alcohol at C-17
then affords diketone *30*. Condensation of that
product with pyrrolidine leads, because of the highly hindered
nature of the ketone at C-17, to selective formation
of the 3-enamine *(31)*. Addition of methylmagnesium
bromide followed by hydrolysis of the enamine function
gives *mibolerone (32)*.[10] This last has, interestingly,
recently been introduced as a canine oral contraceptive.

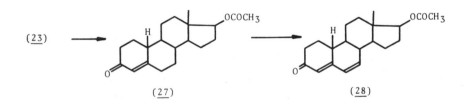

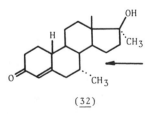

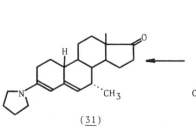

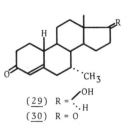

The formal replacement of the methyl group at C-
17 by ethynyl leads, in the 19-*nor* series, from compounds which show androgenic activity to agents active
as progestins.  The prototype for this series, and in
fact the compound used most widely in oral contraceptives, is *norethindrone (33)*. It is of note that
the analogue missing the ketone at C-3 retains this
activity.  Condensation of ethane dithiol with 19-
*nor*-testosterone affords the corresponding thioketal
*(34)*. Desulfurization with sodium in liquid ammonia
affords *35*. Oxidation affords the 17-ketone; reaction
with lithium acetylide gives the progestin *cingestol
(37)*.[11]  A similar scheme on the isomeric deconjugated
ketone *38* (obtained by hydrolyzing the enol ether
product from the Birch reduction of estradiol methyl
ether under mild conditions) gives *tigestol (39)*.[12]

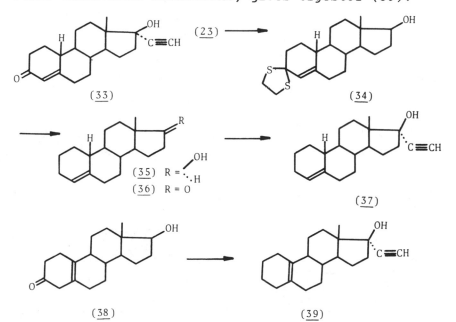

An unusual variation on this theme involves a
compound containing both extended conjugation involving the bond connecting rings AC and a haloacetylene
moiety.  Reaction of ketone _40_[13] with the anion
obtained by treatment of *cis* 1,2-dichloroethylene
with methyl lithium affords chloroacetylene *41*.  This
reagent can be generated either by formation of the
organometallic agent by abstraction of a proton
followed by loss of hydrogen chloride from the adduct
or, more likely, by elimination of HCl from the
ethylene followed by formation of the lithium reagent
from the resulting acetylene.  Hydrolysis of the enol
ether under mild conditions (acetic acid) affords the
unconjugated ketone *42*.  Treatment of that compound
in pyridine with bromine leads to the potent oral
progestin *ethynerone (44)*.[14]  This last reaction can
be rationalized by assuming that the first step
consists of addition of bromine to the double bond at
C-5,10 (*43*); double dehydrohalogenation will give the
observed product.  It is interesting to observe that
*44* does not enolize to give an aromatic A ring.

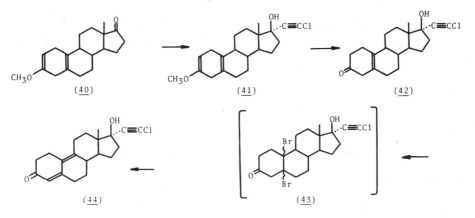

The potentiation observed in the 19-*nor* androgens
by inclusion of a C-7 methyl group is observed even
in the presence of the 17-ethynyl function.  Dehydrogenation of testosterone propionate (*45*) by means of
chloranil gives the corresponding 4,6-diene (*46*).
Conjugate addition of methyl magnesium bromide leads
to the 7α-methyl derivative *47* along with the 7β-
epimer.  Treatment of the major product with DDQ leads
in this case to the cross-conjugated 1,4-diene.  It
is likely that the direction of this second dehydrogenation is mandated by the presence of the methyl
group at C-7; this group may hinder the approach of
reagent to the center which would lead to the alternate diene.  The intermediate is then saponified and
alcohol at C-17 oxidized (*48*).  Elimination of the
angular methyl group at C-19 with consequent aromatization is achieved by treatment of the diene with
lithium in the presence of diphenyl;[15] there is thus
obtained 7α-methyl estrone (*49*).[16]  Methylation of
the phenolic hydroxyl group followed by reduction of
the 17-ketone gives *50*.  Birch reduction affords the
corresponding 2,5(10)-diene (*51*).  The hydroxyl at 17
is then oxidized by means of cyclohexanone and aluminum isopropoxide (Oppenauer oxidation) to give back
the 17-ketone (*52*).  Addition of lithium acetylide
proceeds to give the 17α-ethynyl derivative (*53*).
Hydrolysis of the enol ether under mild conditions
leads to the unconjugated ketone.  There is thus
obtained the anabolic agent *tibolone* (*54*).[17]

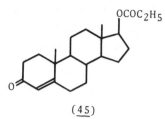

(45)

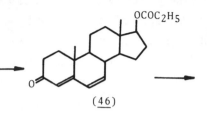

(46)

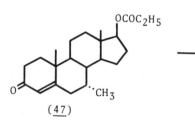

(47)

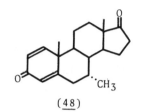

(48)

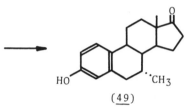

(49)

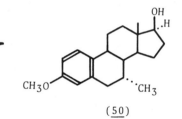

(50)

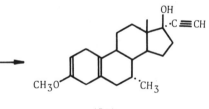

(51) R = $\overset{OH}{\underset{H}{\cdot}}$
(52) R = O

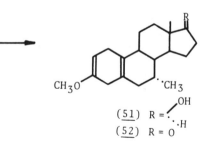

(53)

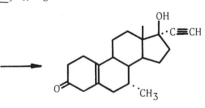

(54)

148

    Inclusion of a methyl group at the difficultly
accessible 11-position also proves compatible with
oral progestational activity in the 19-nor series.
Preparation of an agent incorporating this feature
starts with the 1,4-diene (55), corresponding to
adrenosterone.[18]  Due to the sterically hindered
nature of the carbonyl at C-11 and the low reactivity
of that at C-3, ketalization proceeds selectively at
C-17 (56); reduction of the 11-keto group by means of
lithium tri-t-butoxyaluminum hydride gives intermediate
57.  Aromatization by means of the lithium radical
anion from diphenyl gives intermediate 58.[19]
Methylation of the phenol (59) followed by oxidation
of the alcoholic hydroxyl at C-11 affords 60. Addition
of methyl Grignard reagent to that carbonyl group
serves to introduce the 11-methyl group (61).  It is
of note that the corresponding reaction in the 19-
methylated (androstrane) series proceeds with extreme
reluctance.  Deketalization gives the corresponding
17-ketone and acid catalyzed dehydration, followed by
catalytic reduction of the olefin (62), gives the
intermediate containing the 11β-methyl group (63).
That molecule is then subjected to the standard
carbonyl reduction, Birch reaction, oxidation,
ethynylation and, finally, hydrolysis sequence (see
50 to 53).  Hydrolysis of the enol ether under more
strenuous conditions than was employed with 53 gives
the conjugated ketone 65.  The carbonyl group is then
reduced to afford the corresponding 3β-alcohol (66).
Exhaustive acetylation affords the potent oral
progestin methynodiol diacetate (67).

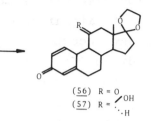

(55)

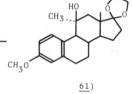

(56) R = O
(57) R = ⟨OH, H⟩

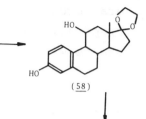

(58)

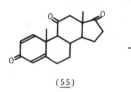

(62)

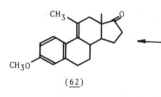

61)

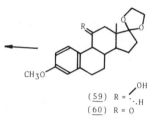

(59) R = ⟨OH, H⟩
(60) R = O

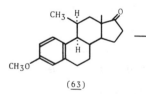

(63)

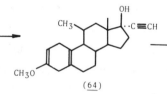

(64)

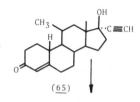

(65)

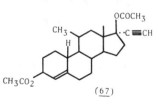

(67)

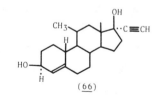

(66)

Elaboration of a commercially viable route for
total synthesis of 19-*nor* steroids led to the introduction of the totally synthetic product *norgestrel*
*(71)* as the progestational component of an oral
contraceptive.  As was observed in the "natural" 19-
*nor*-compounds, reduction of the 17-ethynyl group to 17-
ethyl affords compounds with androgenic/anabolic
activity. Oppenauer oxidation of the total synthesis
intermediate *68*[22] leads to the corresponding ketone.
Reaction with ethylmagnesium bromide gives the
expected condensation product.  It is of note that
reaction is much slower than in the 13-methyl series.
Hydrolysis with strong acid affords *norbolethone*
*(70)*.[21] The same compound can be obtained by selective
reduction of the ethynyl moiety of *norgestrel (71)*.

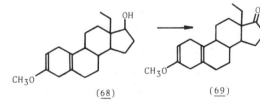

(68)

(69)

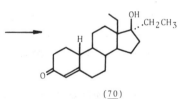

(70)

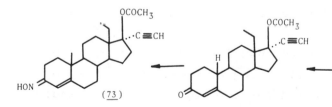

(73)

(72)

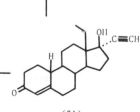

(71)

In much the same vein, acetylation of optically
active *d-norgestrel* by means of acetic anhydride and
tosic acid gives the 17-acetate *(72)*.   Reaction with
hydroxylamine hydrochloride in pyridine affords the
orally active progestin *dexnorgestrel acetime (73)*.[23]

The prevalence of 17-ethynyl carbinols among the
orally active 19-nor progestins can lead to the
impression that this is a necessary group for activity.
The good potency shown by a compound that possesses
the 17-hydroxy 17-acetyl moiety more characteristic of
the 19-methyl progestins indicates that the structure-
activity relationship is not quite that narrow. One
such compound, *gestonorone caproate (85)* is prepared
by oxidation of 16-hydropregnenolone *(74)*[24] to afford
the conjugated ketone *75*.   This is then converted to
the aromatic A-ring phenol *77* by the standard dehydro-
genation-aromatization scheme (see *47 to 49*).
Epoxidation of the double bond at C-16 by alkaline
peroxide gives the 16α,17α-oxide *78*.   Methylation of
the phenol affords the corresponding ether *(79)*.
*Trans-diaxial opening of the oxide by means of hydro-*
*gen bromide gives the bromohydrin 80;* halogen is then
removed reductively by means of zinc in acetic acid
*(81)*.   The carbonyl group at C-20 is next protected
against the reductive conditions of the subsequent
step by conversion to its ethylene ketal *(82)*. Birch
reduction leads in the usual way to the enol ether
*(83)*. Treatment with strong acid serves to remove
both the 20-ketal and the enol ether at C-3, leading
to conjugated ketone *84*. Treatment of this last intermediate with caproic anhydride and tosic acid affords

*gestonorone caproate (85).*[25]   The caproate function
not only contributes lipophilicity but, presumably,
Newman-type hinderence to saponification.

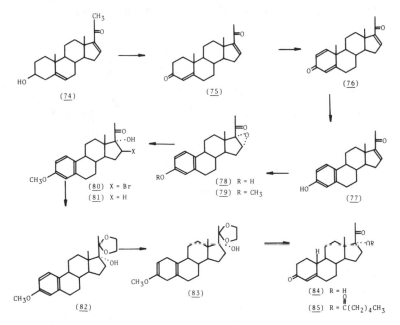

## 2.   ANDROSTANES

Additional unsaturation at C-1,2 is well known to
potentiate the action of both androgens and corticoids.
The former tend, however, to show poor oral activity
in the absence of an alkyl group at the 17-position.
Thus, they tend to be used mainly as injectable
agents.  As mentioned above, esterification with a
fatty chain leads to agents with long duration of
action. Thus, esterification of *86*[26] with the acid
chloride from undec-10-enoic acid gives the injectable
anabolic agent *boldenone 10-undecylenate (87).*[27]  An

enol ether, interestingly, can serve a similar
pharmacological purpose.  Thus, acetal interchange of
*86* with the diethyl acetal from cyclopentanone gives
*88;* pyrolysis leads to elimination of ethanol and
·formation of *quinbolone (89).*[28]

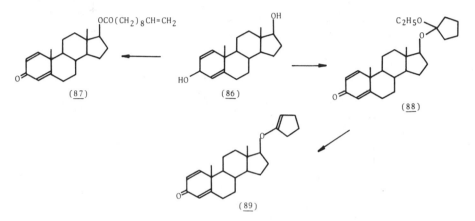

(87)          (86)          (88)

(89)

Neoplasms involving gonadal tissues are often
dependent on sex hormones for growth.  Depriving the
cancerous growth of hormonal stimulation frequently
slows its development. The past few years have seen
considerable application of hormone antagonists as
antineoplastic agents for treatment of such hormone-
dependent cancers.  *Bolasterone (91)* is known to be a
potent anabolic/androgenic agent; its 7β-isomer,
*calusterone,* has found some use in the treatment of
cancer. As originally prepared, conjugate addition of
methylmagnesium bromide to diene *90* affords a mixture
of *91 and 92* with the former predominating.
*Calusterone (92)* was separated by chromatography and
fractional crystallization.[29]

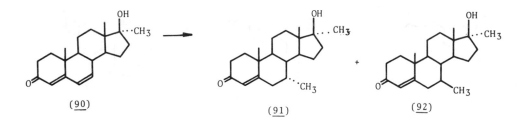

(90)                    (91)                    (92)

Formal isomerization of the double bond of
testosterone to the 1-position and methylation at the
2-position provides yet another anabolic/androgenic
agent.  Mannich condensation of the fully saturated
androstane derivative *93* with formaldehyde and dimethylamine gives aminoketone *94*.  A/B-trans steroids
normally enolize preferentially toward the 2-position,
explaining the regiospecificity of this reaction.
Catalytic reduction at elevated temperature affords
the 2α-methyl isomer *95*.  It is not at all unlikely
that the reaction proceeds via the 2-methylene intermediate.  The observed stereochemistry is no doubt
attributable to the fact that the product represents
the more stable equatorial isomer.  The initial
product would be expected to be the β-isomer but this
would experience a severe 1,3-diaxial non-bonded
interaction and epimerize via the enol. Bromination
of the ketone procéeds largely at the tertiary carbon
adjacent to the carbonyl *(96)*.  Dehydrohalogenation
by means of lithium carbonate in DMF affords *stenbolone
acetate (97)*.[30]  This product is readily separable
from a number of by-products by the fact that it
forms a water-soluble bisulfite adduct.

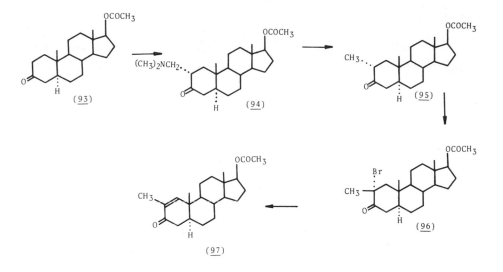

Contraction of the B-ring of the orally active
androgen 17-methyltestosterone, interestingly, leads
to a compound with antiandrogenic activity.  The
general method for preparation of such ring contracted
analogues was first developed using cholesterol
acetate *(98)* as a model.  Oxidation by means of
chromium trioxide affords keto acid *99* as the principal
product; this is then converted to the enol lactone
*100* by means of acetic anhydride.  Pyrolysis of that
enol lactone at 200°C gives the ring contracted
condensation product *101*.[31] The analogous 17-ketone
*102* is used as starting material for the antiandrogen.
Reaction with an excess of methylmagnesium bromide
affords the 17-methylcarbinol *103*; Oppenauer oxidation
affords *benorterone (104)*.[32]

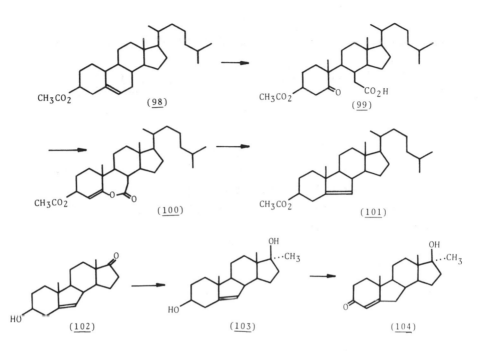

Fusion of a heterocyclic ring onto the A-ring of ethynyltestosterone leads to a compound with hormone antagonistic activity. Such agents find some use in those cases where either the given hormone is present in excessive amounts by malfunction of the particular endocrine gland or where it is desirable to suppress hormonal stimulation of some end organ. Condensation of 17-ethynyl testosterone *(105)* with ethyl formate in the presence of sodium methoxide gives the corresponding 2-hydroxymethylene derivative *(106)*. Reaction of that intermediate with hydroxylamine leads to the pituitary suppressant agent *danazol (107)*.[33]

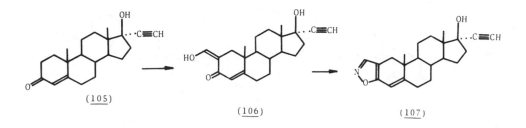

(105)          (106)          (107)

A somewhat related sequence leads to *trilostane*
(*111*), a compound that inhibits the adrenal gland;
more specifically the agent blocks some of the metabolic responses elicited by the adrenal hormone ACTH
in experimental animals.  Reaction of the hydroxymethylene derivative *108*, obtained from testosterone,
with hydroxylamine gives the corresponding isoxazole
(*109*).  Oxidation of the C-4,5 double bond by means

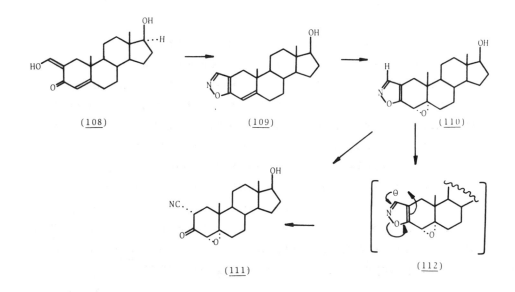

(108)          (109)          (110)

(111)                        (112)

of mCPBA proceeds from the less hindered side to give
the α-epoxide. Treatment of the intermediate *110* with
sodium methoxide leads to scission of the heterocycle
and formation of the corresponding cyanoketone *111*.
It is of interest that the epoxide is apparently
inert to these conditions; the nitrile is of course
readily epimerized, and thus assumes the more stable
α (equatorial) conformation.   There is thus obtained
*trilostane*.[34]   The ring opening can be rationalized
by assuming first formation of the anion *112*; electro-
cyclic rearrangement as shown gives the enolate anion
of *111*.

Fusion of a heterocyclic ring onto the A-ring of
a molecule which shows mainly progestational activity
leads to an antiinflammatory agent; this finding does
not seem to have been followed up to any extent.
Condensation of 17-ethynyl testosterone *(113)* with
ethyl formate in the presence of base gives the
corresponding 2-hydroxymethyl derivative *(114)*.
Reaction of that with p-fluorophenylhydrazine affords
the antiinflammatory pyrazolone *nivazol (115)*.[35]

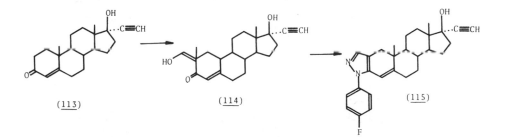

(113)                         (114)                         (115)

The antineoplastic agent *testolactone (121)*
appears to be obtained commercially by microbiological
transformation of either testosterone or progesterone.
The compound can be obtained synthetically, albeit in
low yield, starting from dehydroepiandrosterone
*(116a).*  Addition of bromine serves to protect the
double bond as the dibromide *(117).* Oxidation with
peracetic acid gives the Baeyer-Villiger product *118.*
The unsaturation at 5,6 is then restored by treatment
of the dibromide with sodium iodide *(119).*  This is
oxidized to the conjugated ketone *120* under Oppenauer
conditions.  (A real source of confusion exists in
the fact that *120* bears the trivial chemical name
testolactone while the same generic name is used to
denote *121.*)  Previous work, particularly on cortical
steroids, had shown that inclusion of additional
unsaturation in the A ring at 1,2 leads to a significant increase in potency.  Selenium dioxide is a
fairly specific reagent for achieving this transformation, and such treatment of *120* affords *testolactone (121).*[36]

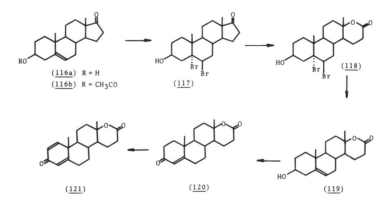

(116a) R = H
(116b) R = CH₃CO            (117)            (118)

(121)            (120)            (119)

It has been known for many years that elevated
levels of serum cholesterol are associated with
atherosclerosis, although the cause-effect relationship
remains unproven.  A rather straightforward therapeutic regimen intended for prevention or arrest of
the progress of this disease involves lowering levels
of serum cholesterol in the high-risk population.
Since a good part of the physiological cholesterol
load is provided by endogenous synthesis, agents that
inhibit this process should lower cholesterol levels
in the serum as an adjunct to dietary precautions,
although a compensatory increase in endogenous synthesis can combat this artifice.  One approach to
this therapeutic goal consists in providing false
substrates for enzyme systems involved in cholesterol
biosynthesis. Substitution of heteroatoms for carbon
has served to provide such enzyme antagonists in
other fields.  The strategy in the case at hand calls
for a cholesterol analogue containing nitrogen in the
side chain.  Shiff base formation between dehydroepiandrosterone acetate (*116b*) and 3-dimethylaminopropyl-
amine affords imine *122*.  Reduction (lithium aluminum
hydride) proceeds to give predominantly the β-amine
(*123*).  Further methylation by means of formic acid
and formaldehyde (Eschweiler-Clark reaction) leads to
*azacosterol* (*124*).[37]  Though the compound does lower
serum cholesterol in experimental animals it is not
used clinically in man.  The drug, not unexpectedly,
severely limits cholesterol availability in avian
species. Since egg formation in birds is dependent on
an abundant supply of cholesterol, *azacosterol* is, in

fact, an effective avian chemosterilant.  A glance at
the formula of cholesterol *(124a)* clearly shows the
bioisosterism used in the design of *124*.

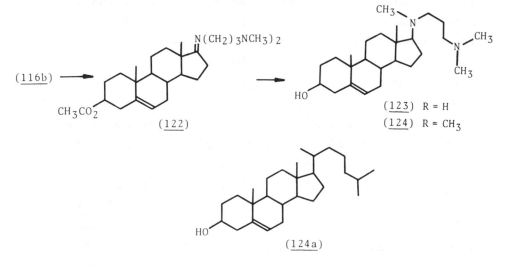

(116b) —→

(122)

(123)  R = H
(124)  R = CH₃

(124a)

     The crude toxin *curare*, used by South American
Indians to lend authority to their blow gun darts,
proved, because of its neuromuscular blocking activity,
to be of interest to surgeons. Structural analysis of
the mixture led to the erroneous conclusion that the
active agents possessed a pair of quaternary nitrogen
atoms with definite spacing because of the rigid
molecular framework.  Following the rationale based
on this belief led to a number of curarelike synthetic
agents in which the spacing is provided by aliphatic
chains; it is readily apparent that the rigid network
provided by a steroid would provide more accurate
location of the charged centers.  The synthesis of
one of these starts with conversion of *125* (probably

obtained by dehydration of the corresponding 3-
hydroxy compound) to the enol acetate *(126)*.  Epoxidation proceeds as expected from the α side to give
the bis epoxide *(127)*.  Both regio- and stereochemistry
of the subsequent reaction with piperidine are dictated
by the diaxial opening propensity of oxiranes; the
hemiacetal-like function left at C-17 spontaneously
reverts to the ketone to give *128*.  Reduction of that
ketone proceeds in the usual manner to afford *129*.
Acetylation of the hydroxyl groups *(130)*, followed by
quaterization with methyl bromide gives *pancuronium
bromide (131)*.[38]

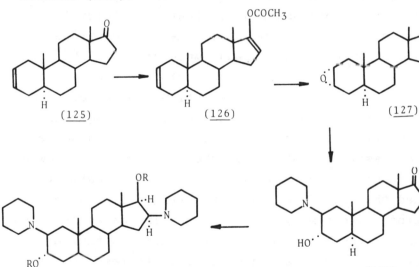

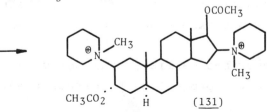

3.  PREGNANES

a.  11-Desoxy Derivatives

Progesterone, *132*, is, of course, the prototype
pregnane. This natural steroid plays an important
role in females in the intricate endocrine chain of
events involved in reproduction.  In essence, progesterone is one of the steroid hormones directly
involved in the timing of ovulation.  Very high
levels of progesterone are present in early pregnancy,
elaborated biosynthetically by a structure on the
ovary (the <u>corpus</u> <u>luteum</u>), and this inhibits ovulation
in the gravid female to prevent a superimposed pregnancy.  It is this observation that gave initial
direction to the development of the oral contraceptives.  As with the estrogens, much of the work
described below was carried out before a shadow fell
on this class of drugs.  In addition, there was some
evidence from human trials that a potent progestin
could provide contraceptive activity in the absence
of added estrogen.  Although the efficacy was somewhat
lower than for the combination Pill, the treatment
avoided the use of the suspect estrogenic component.
The finding that many potent progestins cause tumerous
lesions in the beagle on long-term administration
effectively laid this class of drugs to rest as far
as large-scale usage is concerned.  It can be argued
quite reasonably that this effect is restricted to
the beagle, but expert opinion is divided and use has
subsided.

As described earlier, oral activity can be
achieved in the progestins by either removing the 19-

methyl group or inclusion of an acyloxy group at the
17-position.  It is of interest that removal of the
oxygen function at C-3 is compatible with biological
activity in both series (see *37, 39*, this Chapter).
Thus, the 3-desoxy analogue of *medroxyprogesterone
acetate* shows very similar activity to the parent
substance.  Reaction of medroxyprogesterone *(133)*[39]
with ethanedithiol gives the corresponding thioketal
*(134)*.  Desulfurization by means of Raney nickel
leads to the 3-desoxy steroid *(135)*.  Treatment with
acetic acid in the presence of trifluoroacetic anhydride completes the synthesis of *angesterone acetate
(136)*.[40]

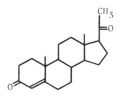

(132)

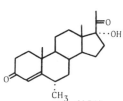

(133)

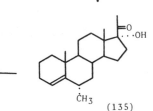

(134)

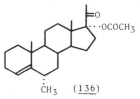

CH₃    (136)

(135)

*Chlormadinone acetate (137)*,[41] is an extremely
potent orally active progestin.  Treatment of this
compound with basic sodium borohydride serves to
reduce the ketone at C-3 to the corresponding 3-
carbinol (*138*; the regioselectivity is presumably due

to the more hindered environment about the 20-ketone).
Acetylation affords *clogestone (139).*[42] Further
dehydrogenation of the A ring of *chlormadinone* by
means of selenium dioxide affords *delmadinone acetate
(140).*[43]

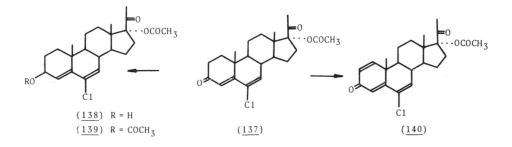

(138) R = H
(139) R = COCH₃                     (137)                      (140)

Fusion of a cyclopropyl ring onto the 1,2-
position of *chlormadinone* gives a compound which,
interestingly, shows mainly antiandrogenic activity.
Preparation of *cyproterone acetate (146)* starts by
reaction of triene *141* (obtainable from 17-acetoxy-
progesterone[44] by sequential dehydrogenations at C-
5,6 and C-1,2) with diazomethane affords the pyrazoline
*(142).* Pyrolysis leads to the cyclopropyl derivative
*(143)* by loss of nitrogen.[45] Oxidation by means of
perbenzoic acid gives the C-6,7 epoxide *(144).*
Regioselectivity in this reaction is probably due to
conjugate addition of peracid from the α side followed
by electron backflow and ejection of benzoate as
shown in *143a.* Reaction of that intermediate with
hydrogen chloride serves to open both the oxirane and
cyclopropyl rings. The intermediate chlorohydrin is
not observed as it undergoes spontaneous dehydration

to *145*.   Treatment of the chloromethyl derivative
with collidine serves to reform the cyclopropyl ring;
the reaction very probably goes by internal alkylation
of the anion generated by the base at the 2-position.
There is thus obtained *cyproterone acetate (146)*.[46]

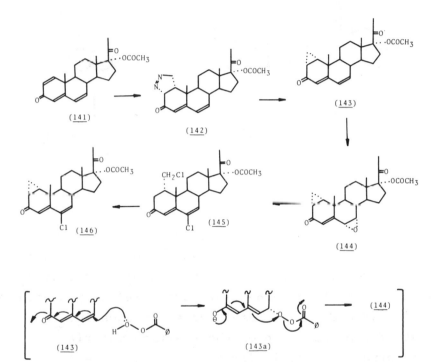

Inclusion of an additional fused cyclopropane
ring at C-16,17 gives a compound in which progestational activity is said to predominate.   Saponification of the acetate in *143* gives the corresponding 17-alcohol *(147)*.   Heating in refluxing quinoline
results in dehydration with formation of the
16,17-olefin *(148)*.   Reaction with diazomethane gives

the pyrazoline *(149)*, which on heating in acid affords
the biscyclopropyl derivative *(150)*.   This compound
is then taken on to the 6-chloro analogue by a sequence
identical to that used to prepare *146*.   There is thus
obtained the progestin *gestaclone (151)*.[47,48]

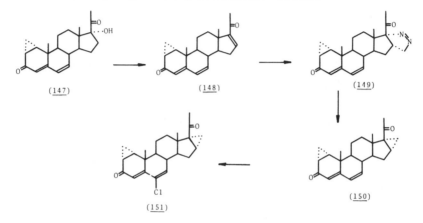

Substitution by a methyl group at the 16-position
is known to have a marked potentiating effect in the
corticosteroid series.   Combination of such a group
with the unsaturated 6-chloro group in the progesterone
series affords an extremely potent progestin.   One
route for preparation of the starting material for
this drug consists in first introducing the 17-
hydroxyl.   Thus, the ketone at C-17 in the progesterone
derivative *152* (obtainable from the corresponding
pregnenolone *165*) is converted to the enol acetate
*(153)*.   The next step in this so-called Gallagher
chemistry consists in conversion of the enol double
bond to the epoxide to give *154*.   Hydrolytic ring
opening gives initially the hydroxy hemiacetal acetate;
this quickly goes on to the hydroxy ketone *(155)*.

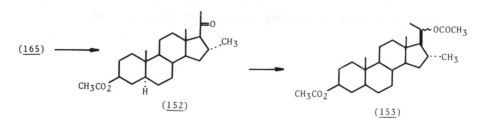

(165) ⟶ (152)

(153)

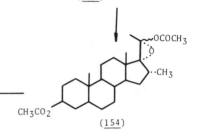

(154)

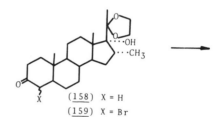

(155)

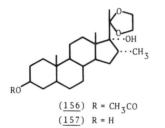

(156) R = CH₃CO
(157) R = H

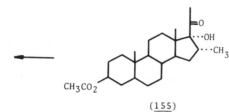

(158) X = H
(159) X = Br

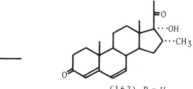

(162) R = H
(163) R = COCH₃

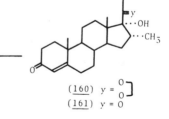

(160) y = $\begin{matrix} O \\ O \end{matrix}$ ⎤
(161) y = O

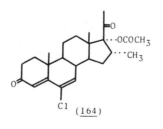

Cl (164)

169

After protection of the C-20 keto group as the dioxolane (156), the 3-acetyl group is saponified and the
resulting alcohol (157) is oxidized to the ketone
(158). Bromination (159) followed by dehydrobromination introduces the required 4-ene-3-one
functionality (160); removal of the ketal would then
afford the required starting material (161). Heating
of 161 in the presence of chloranil then introduces
the desired unsaturation at C-6,7. A sequence identical to that used to prepare 146 (epoxidation;
hydrogen chloride) is then used to introduce the 6-
chlorine atom[50] and the progestin clomegestone acetate
(164) results.

The analogue of 164 lacking unsaturation at C-6
and oxygen at C-17 unexpectedly shows antiestrogenic
rather than progestational activity. Pregnenolone
analogue 165[49] is starting material for this analogue
as well. Chlorination of the double bond by means of
chlorine in pyridine affords the dihalo derivative
166. The stereochemistry is best rationalized by
assuming chloronium ion formation on the less-hindered
α-side followed by diaxial opening of that ring by
chloride ion. Oxidation of the alcohol (167) affords
the 3-keto derivative (168), and reaction of that with
sodium acetate leads to dehydrochlorination, yielding
the enone (169). Exposure of that intermediate to
mild acid isomerizes the halogen substituent to the
more stable equatorial 6α-position and produces
clometherone (170).[51]

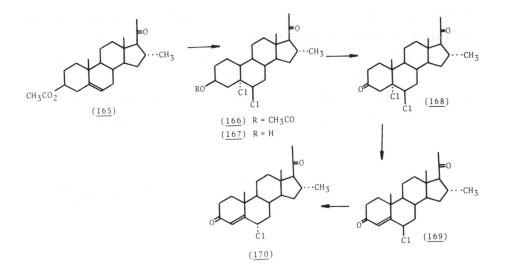

(165)

(166) R = CH₃CO
(167) R = H

(168)

(169)

(170)

Yet another observation that carries over from the corticoids to progestins is the potentiation observed by formation of acetonides from the 16,17-glycols. It is of note in this case that the parent glycol itself fails to show activity in the standard progestational assay. Treatment of the progesterone derivative *172* (available by oxidation of 16-dehydropregnenolone *(171)* with potassium permanganate) with acetone affords the 16,17-cyclic acetal *algestone acetonide (173)*;[52] in the same vein, reaction with acetophenone yields *algestone acetophenide (174)*.[53] Although formation of the latter involves the creation of a new chiral center, only one isomer is in fact isolated from the reaction. Since acetal formation is accomplished under thermodynamic conditions, the more stable isomer involving the least steric crowding

should prevail.  It has been proposed that the configuration of *174* is that which carries the aromatic
ring oriented away from the steroid molecule (*174a*).
Earlier work had shown that the presence of the 17-
hydroxyl substituent is crucial for oral activity in
the 21-carbon progestin series; progesterone itself

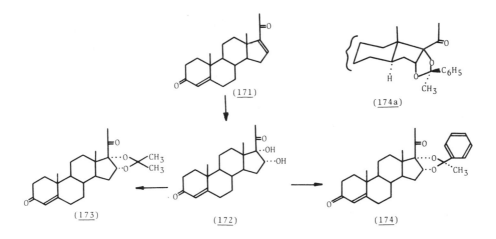

shows poor activity on oral administration.  This key
group can be replaced by halogen with retention of
oral activity.  Bromination of pregnenolone acetate
(*175a*) in acetic acid gives the tetrabromide *175b*.
Treatment with sodium iodide leads to both elimination
of the 5,6-dibromide grouping and displacement of the
α-keto halide at C-21 by iodine; there is obtained
dihalide *176*.  Reduction of the haloketone with
bisulfite gives the methylketone *177*;[54] the selectivity is probably due to both the greater reactivity
of iodine and the greater steric accessibility of

that group. Saponification to *178* followed by treatment
with peracid gives the 5,6-oxide *179*.  Diaxial ring
opening of the oxirane with HF leads to the *trans*-
fluorohydrin *180*.  Oxidation of the hydroxyl at C-3
by means of Jones reagent then affords hydroxyketone
*181*.  Treatment of this last with acid serves both to
generate the enone, by dehydration of the tertiary
carbinol, and to invert the fluoro group at C-6 to
the more stable equatorial, 6α-configuration.  There
is thus obtained *haloprogesterone (182)*.[55]

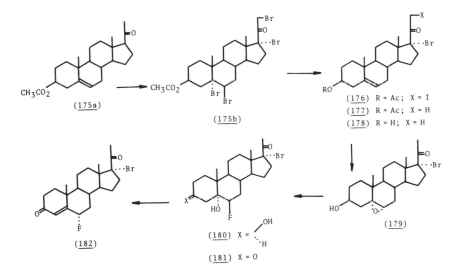

Aldosterone *(183)* is one of the key steroid
hormones involved in regulation of the body's mineral
and fluid balance. Excess levels of this steroid
quickly lead to marked retention of sodium chloride,
water and, often as a consequence, hypertension.  The
aldosterone antagonist *spironolactone (184)*[56] has
proven of great clinical value in blocking the effects

of hyperaldosteronism.  In addition, the drug has
proven an effective diuretic and antihypertensive
agent even in those cases where no gross excesses of
aldosterone can be demonstrated. It is of note that
the immediate chemical precursor of *spironolactone*
*(184)*, diene *185* was in fact found to be one of the
active metabolites of that drug in the body.  The
diene, *canrenone (185)* now constitutes a drug in its
own right.  Both this and the following aldosterone
antagonists are also available in the form of the
potassium salt of the ring-opened hydroxy acid; in
this case, *potassium canrenoate (186)*.

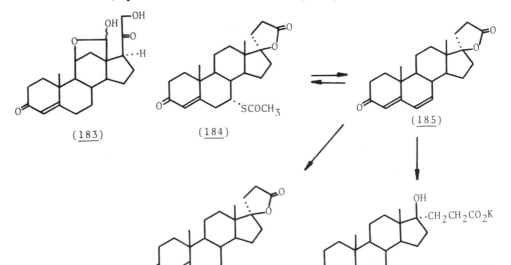

Cyclopropanation of the 4,6-diene function
proceeds selectively at the 5,6-double bond.  Thus,
reaction of *185* with the ylide from trimethyl sulfonium
iodide and sodium hydride, in DMSO, affords predominantly the α-cyclopropyl compound *(187)* accompanied

by traces of the β-isomer.  The lactone constitutes
the diuretic-antihypertensive *prorenone*;[57] the ring-
opened salt is known as *potassium prorenoate*.

Introduction of a carbomethoxy moiety at C-7
should afford a nonreversible counterpart of *184*.   To
effect this, addition of cyanide to the extended
conjugated system in *185* leads to addition of two
moles of the nucleophile; there is obtained the
unusual bicyclic intermediate *190*.  The reaction may
be rationalized by assuming that addition occurs
initially at the terminus of the system to give *188*
as expected.  This, however, under the reaction
conditions chosen, undergoes addition of the second
mole of cyanide which, of necessity, goes through
anion *189*; reaction of the negative charge at C-4
with the nitrile at C-7 would lead to the observed
product (*190*).  This can only happen following β-
addition of cyanide.  Hydrolysis of the imine function
proceeds to give diketone *191*.  A conformational
drawing (*191a*) shows that the molecule is by no means
as strained as the planar projection would suggest.
Reaction of *191* with methoxide reverses the formation
of the additional ring.  The reaction sequence probably
starts by addition of methoxide to the carbonyl group
(*192*); collapse of the alkoxide anion gives the
intermediate anion *193*, which neutralizes itself by
facile elimination of the excellent leaving group,
cyanide.  There is thus finally obtained *mexrenone*
(*194*);[58] the salt is known as *potassium mexrenoate*.

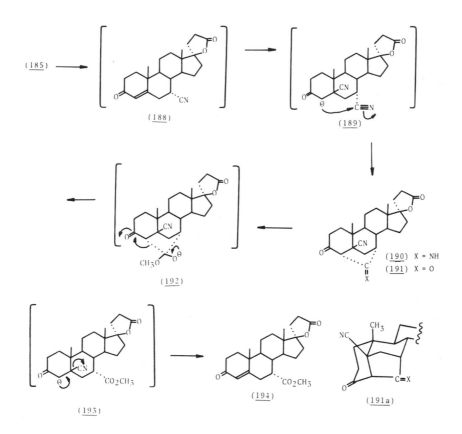

## b. 11-Oxygenated Pregnanes

The story of the discovery of the utility of cortisone
as an antiinflammatory agent has been told often enough
not to need full repetition here.[59] In brief, cortisone
is one of the more important hormonal steroids elaborated by the adrenal cortex; this steroid is intimately
involved in the regulation of a host of biological
processes such as, for example, regulation of glucose
utilization and mineral balance.  Administration of
doses far in excess of those required for hormonal

action were found to alleviate the symptoms of a
multitude of conditions marked by inflammation.  When
used for this purpose, the normal hormonal effects
are undesirable.  These side effects are, however,
seen to be natural extensions of the hormonal action.
Immediately following this discovery, an enormous
effort was mounted in the laboratories of the pharmaceutical industry aimed at separation of the antiinflammatory activity of these molecules from their
hormonal activities.  The most visible outcome of
this work was a tremendous increase in the milligram
potency achieved by various structural modifications.
Drugs were produced that, in addition, had changed
hormonal spectra; some such steroids had more pronounced effects on glucose metabolism ("glucocorticoids"), whereas others were more effective in
changing mineral balance ("mineralocorticoids").
Despite this, no steroid truly devoid of hormonal
activity rewarded these efforts.  The full realization
of the clinical deficiencies of the corticoids,
coupled with the increasing availability of nonsteroidal antiinflammatory agents, has led to a great
decrease in routine use of these drugs in medical
practice. It is for that primary reason that the
compounds discussed next failed to have greater
medical and economic impact.  It is of note that this
work represented an unparalleled effort on the part
of medicinal chemists, both as to the complexity of
the molecules involved and the length of the synthetic
schemes utilized.  In some ways this foreshadowed the
current prostaglandin programs, both in the goal

(splitting of activities) and in chemical sophisti-
cation (in fact, the same names often appear as
authors in the late steroid papers and early prostaglandin publications).

As has been mentioned, preparation of esters of
the C-17 hydroxyl group of selected progestins affords
compounds with prolonged action. Similar chemical
treatment of a corticoid would almost certainly lead
to an ester of the sterically more accessible primary
alcohol at C-21. In an interesting method for
achieving esterification of the more hindered and
less reactive tertiary 17-hydroxyl, *prednisolone*
*(195)*[59] is converted to a mixture of the diasteromeric
cyclic ortho esters *(196)* by ester interchange with
trimethyl ortho-pentanoate. Acid-catalyzed dioxolane
ring opening proceeds by protonation of the more

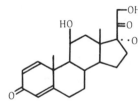

(195)

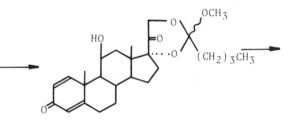

(196)

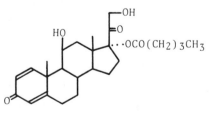

(197)

sterically accessible oxygen attached to the 21-
position. There is thus obtained *prednival (197)*.[60]
It is of interest that *197* rearranges to the 21-ester
on heating, representing an O-to-O acyl migration.

It was found quite early in the steroid effort
that inclusion of several groups, which singly poten-
tiated activity had an additive effect; for example,
a cortisone derivative that included both the unsaturation at C-1,2 and a methyl group at C-6 would be more
potent than the derivative that possessed either
group alone. Much of the chemical strategy thus
devolved on designing routes which would permit the
inclusion of combinations of potentiating groups.

Dehydration of cortisone *(198)* affords the diene
*199*. This is then converted to ketal *200*. The selectivity is due to hindrance about both the 11- and
20-carbonyl groups. The shift of the double bond to
the 5,6-position is characteristic of that particular
enone. Treatment of protected diene *200* with osmium
tetroxide results in selective oxidation of the
conjugated double bond at C-16,17 to afford the *cis*-
diol *(201)*. Reduction of the ketone at C-11 *(202)*
followed by hydrolysis of the ketal function gives
the intermediate *203*.[61a] Selenium dioxide has been
found empirically to dehydrogenate such 3-keto-4-ene
steroids to the corresponding 1,4-dienes. (See, for
example, *120-121* and *137-140*.) Thus in the case at
hand, reaction of *203* with selenium dioxide gives the
diene *204*.[61b] Reaction of the *cis*-diol function with
acetone forms the cyclic acetal and, thus, the corticoid *desonide (205)*.[62]

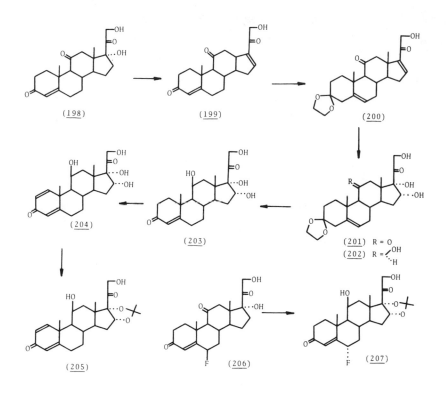

An analogous sequence starting with 6β-fluoro-
cortisone (206),[63] but omitting the selenium dioxide
dehydrogenation, affords *flurandrenolide (207)*.[64]

Microbiological oxidation has proven of enormous
value in steroid chemistry, often affording selective
means of functionalizing remote and chemically inacti-
vated positions. It will bear mentioning that the
11-oxygen for all commercially available corticoids
is in fact introduced by such a reaction carried out
on plant scale. Preparation of the 1-dehydro analogue
of 207 involves biooxidation to introduce the
16-hydroxyl. Incubation of 6α-fluoroprednisolone

(208)[63] with *Streptomyces roseochromogenes* effects
α-hydroxylation at the 16-position (209). Reaction
with acetone affords the corticoid *flunisolide* (210).[65]

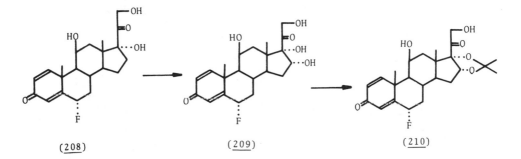

(208)                    (209)                    (210)

The 6-chloro-6-dehydro moiety apparently has a
similar potentiating effect on corticoids as it does
on progestins. One scheme for preparing the requisite
starting 6-chloro compound begins with the opening of
oxide *211* with hydrogen chloride to give halohydrin
*212*. Reduction of the 21-ester function by means of
lithium aluminum hydride, followed by acetylation,
gives *213*. Transformation of the 17,20-olefin to the
requisite hydroxyketone grouping is achieved by a
combination of osmium tetroxide and N-morpholine
oxideperoxide (NMOP) treatments. The reaction sequence
presumably starts by hydroxylation of the olefin via
the osmate ester; the secondary alcohol at C-20 is
then further oxidized to the ketone by the NMOP. The
latter also served to reoxidize the osmium reagent
from the dioxide to the tetroxide, allowing that
expensive and toxic reagent to be used in catalytic
quantities. Deketalization (215) followed by acid

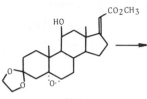

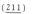

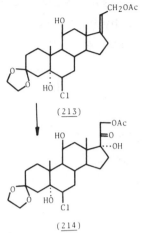

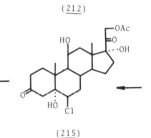

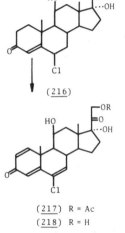

(217) R = Ac
(218) R = H

catalyzed dehydration affords the conjugated ketone
(216).[63] The remaining unsaturation at C-1 and C-6
is then introduced either by sequential treatment
with selenium dioxide and chloranil or under special
conditions with chloranil alone. Saponification of
the acetate affords the corticoid *cloprednol (218)*.[66]

Although oxygenation at C-11 seems to be required
for activity in the corticoid series, the presence of
that function is not incompatible with progestational
activity.[67] Thus, perhaps surprisingly in view of
some corticoids discussed below, mere lack of the
hydroxyl group at C-21 seems, in at least one case,

to give a compound which exhibits progestational
activity. Microbiological oxidation of diketone
epoxide *219* by means of *Rhizopus nigricans* affords
the corresponding 11α-hydroxy derivative *(220)*.
Dehydration of this via the mesylate *(221)* gives the
9,11-olefin *(222)*. Ring opening of the oxirane moiety
by means of hydrogen iodide gives the halohydrin *223*.
Treatment with zinc in acid serves to remove the
halogen reductively *(224)*; the 17-hydroxy group is
then acetylated by means of acetic anhydride in the
presence of tosic acid to give *225*.  The 11β-hydroxy-
9α-halo function is associated with most potent
corticoids; the manner of introduction used in this
case well illustrates the relatively standard sequence
used to incorporate this function.  Addition of the
elements of HOBr to the double bond is usually
accomplished by N-bromosuccinimide in aqueous base.
Both regio- and stereospecificity are no doubt guided
by the initial formation of the 9α,11α-bromonium ion,
followed by nucleophilic diaxial opening to give *226*.
Treatment of the bromohydrin with base leads to the
formation of the β-oxide *(227)* by intramolecular
displacement of halogen by the neighboring alkoxide
ion. Addition of hydrogen fluoride to the oxide proceeds with diaxial opening to afford the 9α-fluoro-
11β-hydroxy functional array. In the case at hand
there is formed the progestin *flurogestone acetate*
*(228)*.[69]  This drug has been in use for controlling
the estrus cycle in domestic animals under the name
Equamate®.

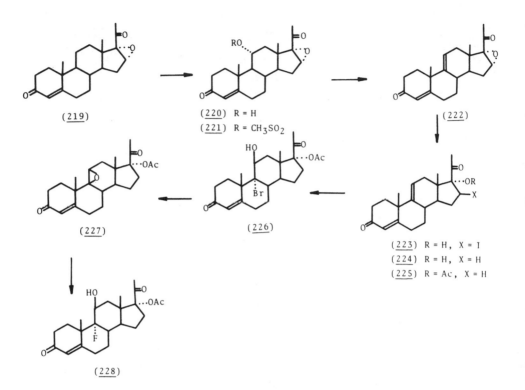

(219)

(220) R = H
(221) R = CH$_3$SO$_2$

(222)

(227)

(226)

(223) R = H, X = I
(224) R = H, X = H
(225) R = Ac, X = H

(228)

The presence of an additional carbon atom on the
dihydroxyacetone side chain is quite compatible with
antiinflammatory activity. Oxidation of 9α-fluopred-
nisolone (229)[70] by means of cupric acetate affords
the corresponding 21-aldehyde (230). Addition of
diazomethane to the aldehyde serves to lengthen the
side chain as the epoxide 231. Opening of the oxirane
ring with hydrogen bromide occurs regioselectively to
give the 22-bromo derivative (232). Heating of the
bromohydrin leads to loss of hydrogen bromide with
formation of the alpha diketone (233) (this reaction

can be rationalized as loss of HBr to give the enol
followed by ketonization).  Reduction of the side
chain diketo alcohol by means of yeast proceeds both
regio and stereospecifically to give the derivative
containing the 21α-hydroxyl group *(234)*.  Acetylation
under mild conditions then affords the antiinflammatory steroid *fluperolone acetate (235)*.[71]

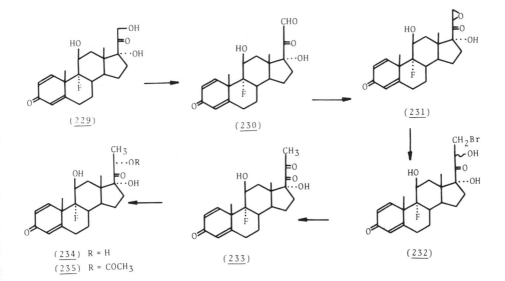

(229)          (230)          (231)

(234) R = H          (233)          (232)
(235) R = COCH₃

The potentiating effect of the 16-hydroxyl group
in the corticoid series has been mentioned previously.
The acetonide of such a steroid, *triamcinolone (237)*,
is in fact one of the more widely used corticosteroids.
The nature of the group used to form a ketal apparently
has only relatively minor influence on biological
activity.  Reaction of the 16,17-glycol *236*[72] with
3-butanone yields *amcinafal (238)*;[73] in the same vein
condensation with acetophenone leads to *amcinafide*

(239).[73]  The ketal stereochemistry is not specified.
Unsaturation in the A ring has been usually assumed
to be necessary for biological activity; the reader
will have noted the high prevalence of 1,4-dienes.
It is interesting therefore to note that the analogue
possessing a fully saturated A ring is apparently
quite active in its own right.   Thus, catalytic
reduction of *237* affords the corticoid *drocinonide*
(*240*).[74]

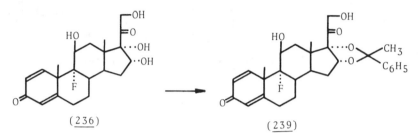

(*236*)                           (*239*)

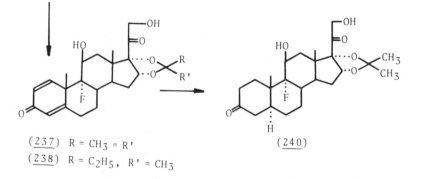

(*237*)  R = CH₃ = R'                (*240*)
(*238*)  R = C₂H₅,  R' = CH₃

     It is of interest that there exists a consi-
derable amount of flexibility as to the substituent
at C-21 in the acetonide series.  For example,
formation of the acetonide from *241*[72] affords intermediate *242*.  Reaction with methanesulfonyl chloride
gives the corresponding mesylate (*243*). Displacement

of the ester with lithium chloride in DMF gives the
corticoid *halcinonide (244)*.[75]

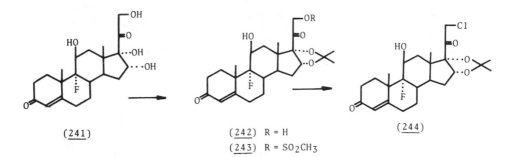

(241)                    (242) R = H                     (244)
                         (243) R = SO$_2$CH$_3$

The C-21 substituent can in fact be dispensed
with entirely. Perhaps because *descinolone acetonide
(254)* predates *244* by better than a decade, the
synthetic sequence reported for its preparation is
quite complex. Although *descinolone (253)* could in
principle be prepared in a few steps from some
currently available starting materials, such as *241*,
the original synthesis is presented for its heuristic
value.

Epoxyketone *245* is readily available from 16-
dehydropregnenolone via several steps, including a
crucial microbiological 11α-hydroxylation. Dehydration
of *245* gives the 9,11-olefin *246*. The alcohol at
C-21 is then converted to the mesylate *(247)*, and
this is reduced to give the methyl ketone *(248)*. The
olefin is then converted to the 9α-fluoro-11β-hydroxy
array *(250)* by the standard sequence [addition of
HOBr, closure to the oxirane *(249)*, opening with HF].
Note that the reactivity of the epoxides in *249* is

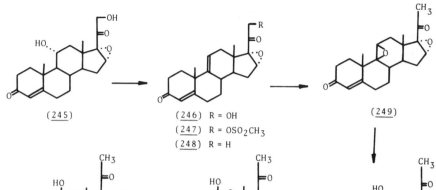

(245)

(246) R = OH
(247) R = OSO$_2$CH$_3$
(248) R = H

(249)

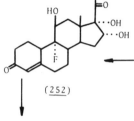

(252)

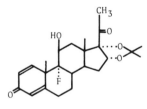

(251)

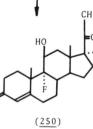

(250)

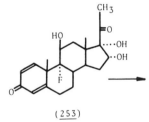

(253)

(254)

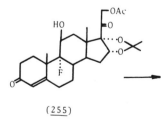

(255)

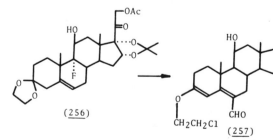

(256)

CH$_2$CH$_2$Cl
(257)

188

sufficiently different so that reaction occurs regioselectively at C-9,11. The remaining major transformation is the establishment of the 16α,17α-glycol
function; this cannot be readily achieved from *250*
since this would demand the *cis*-opening of an oxirane.
Deoxygenation of the epoxide with chromous chloride
gives back the 16,17-olefin *(251)*. In effect the
epoxide has been used in this sequence as a protecting
group for an olefin. Hydroxylation with osmium
tetroxide gives the desired glycol *(252)*; microbiological dehydrogenation (using *Nocardia corallina*)
serves to introduce the double bond at C-1 *(253)*.
Reaction with acetone finally affords *descinolone
acetonide (254)*,[76] an antiinflammatory agent.

Although the Vilsmeier reaction is known best in
aromatic systems, aliphatic olefins also undergo
formylation. Synthesis of *formocortal (257)* involves
such a step. Formation of the monoketal of *255*
involves the 3-ketone function with the familiar
concomitant shift of the double bond to C-5,6.
Reaction of *256* with phosphorous oxychloride and DMF
involves first formylation at the 6-position; opening
of the ketal to the enol ether by the HCl produced in
the Vilsmeier reaction would afford a hydroxyethyl
side chain at C-3. This is no doubt converted to a
chloroethyl group by excess oxychloride. There is
thus obtained the antiinflammatory agent *formocortal
(257)*.[77]

As is the case with other classes of steroids,
inclusion of nitrogen atoms into corticoids has met
with only limited pharmacological success. Compounds

containing a pyrazole ring fused onto the A ring
have, however, shown sufficient activity to merit
generic names.  Synthesis of the requisite intermediate for its incorporation starts with the protection of the dihydroxyacetone side chain.  Reaction of
258 with formaldehyde gives the internal double
acetal 259.  (This bismethylenedioxyether-protected
(259a) function is known as BMD for short.)  Dehydrogenation by means of chloroanil proceeds in the usual
way to give the 4,6-diene (260).  Formylation with
ethyl formate and sodium hydride leads to 261.

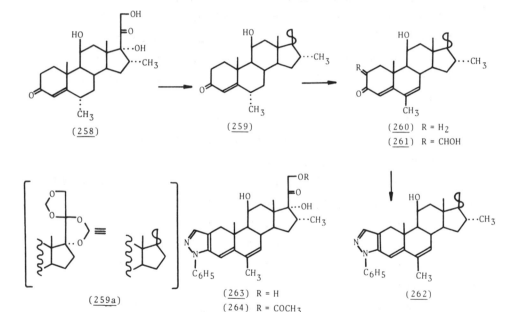

Condensation with phenylhydrazine results in phenyl-
pyrazole 262.  The regiospecificity results from
intermediate phenylhydrazone formation of the more

reactive aldehyde function. The sequence is completed
by deprotection of the cortical side chain by acid
hydrolysis (263), followed by acetylation of the
21-hydroxy group. There is thus obtained the corticoid
*cortivazol (264).*[78]

Inclusion of halogen, particularly fluorine, at
either the C-6 or C-9 positions in the cortisone
molecule is well known to increase potency. Combination of these potentiating groups in the same molecule
in general leads to an additive influence on potency.
The synthesis of one such compound, *difluprednate*
*(271),* starts with a scheme analogous to that used to
prepare *197.* The C-17,21 diol *265* is first converted
to the cyclic ortho-ester (266) by means of methyl
ortho-butyrate. Cautious hydrolysis affords the
17-butyrate ester (267). Exhaustive acetylation
leads to reaction not only at C-21, but formation of
the enol acetate at C-3 as well (268). Reaction of
that intermediate with perchloryl fluoride (FClO$_3$)
leads to halogenation at the terminus of the electron-
rich diene system. Work-up gives a mixture of the
epimeric 6-fluoro compounds; equilibration in acid
provides the more stable equatorial 6α-isomer (269).
The 9,11-diene is then taken on to the 9α-fluoro-11β-
hydroxy function by the standard reaction sequence
(270). Dehydrogenation by means of DDQ completes the
synthesis of *difluprednate (271).*[79]

Omission of the 17-hydroxyl group in the 6,9-
dihalo compounds apparently does not lead to loss of
biological activity. Dehydration of the 6α-fluoro-17-
desoxy intermediate *272*[80] by means of NBS in pyridine

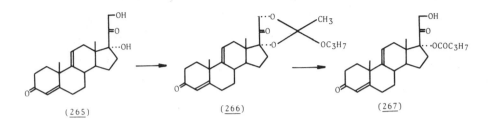

(265)                    (266)                    (267)

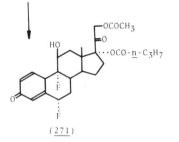

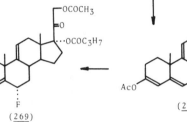

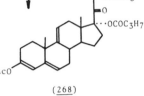

(270)                    (269)                    (268)

(271)

leads to the 9,11-olefin *(273)*. This is then converted
to the halohydrin by the standard sequence.  Microbiological dehydrogenation of the A ring leads to the
1,4-diene.   There is thus obtained the antiinflammatory
steroid *diflucortolone (275)*.[81]

Although the most common substituent found at
the C-9 position in the commercially available corticoids is fluorine, the initial observation of the

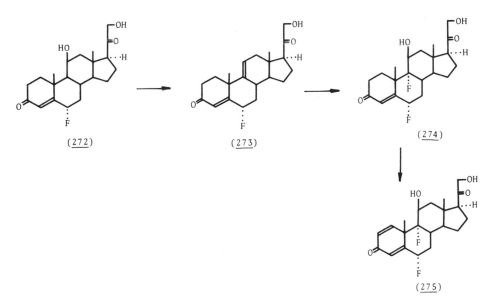

potentiating effect of halogen was in fact made with
chlorine at that spot.  It is thus of interest to
note that one of the more recent 17-desoxy-6,9-dihalo
cortocoids contains chlorine at C-9.  Starting material
for that compound is 16-methyl steroid *276*.[82]  In
distinct contrast to previous work, the desired
halohydrin is introduced in a convenient single step
rather than by the usual three-step sequence.  Thus,
reaction of the olefin with tertiary butyl hypo-
chlorite in the presence of perchloric acid affords
directly the 9α-chloro-11β-hydroxy function and,
thus, *clocortolone (277)*, an antiinflammatory agent.
It is not unlikely that the actual reagent is HOCl;
attack on the 9,11-olefin by Cl$^+$ would occur from the
less hindered side to give the 9α,11α-chloronium
intermediate.  Attack of OH to give diaxial ring
opening would lead to the observed halohydrin.

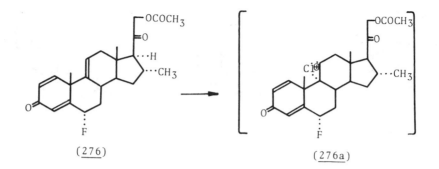

(276)                          (276a)

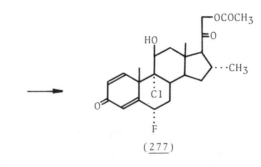

(277)

The scheme required to prepare the potent tri-
fluoro corticoid *cormethasone acetate (292)* illustrates the synthetic complexities involved in some of
this work.  Sequential acetylation of the pregnenolone
derivative *278* with first acetic anhydride in pyridine
and then acetic anhydride in the presence of tosic
acid affords diacetate *279*.  Reaction of that intermediate with nitrosyl fluoride results initially in
addition of the reagent to the 5,6-olefin moiety to
afford the fluoro oxime; reaction with a second mole
of reagent at nitrogen gives the nitroimine derivative
*280;* passage over alumina serves to hydrolyze the
imine function to the corresponding 6-ketone *(281).*

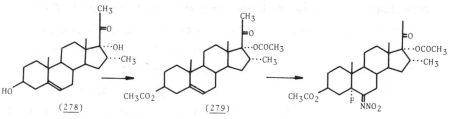

(278)     CH₃CO₂     (279)

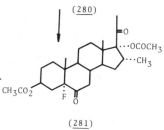

(280)

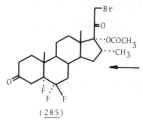

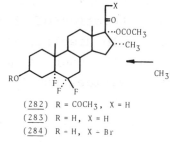

CH₃CO₂    (281)

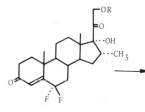

(285)

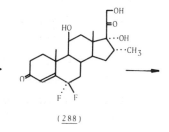

(282) R = COCH₃, X = H
(283) R = H, X = H
(284) R = H, X - Br

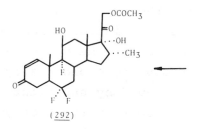

(286) R = COCH₃
(287) R = H

(288)

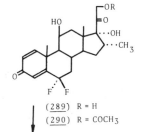

(289) R = H
(290) R = COCH₃

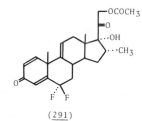

(292)

(291)

195

Sulfur tetrafluoride in hydrogen fluoride has been
developed as a selective and general reagent for
converting ketones to the corresponding difluoromethylene groups. Application of that reaction to *281*
gives the desired 6,6-difluoro derivative *282*. The
less-hindered acetate at C-3 is then hydrolyzed
selectively (to *283*); bromination in dioxane leads to
the 21-bromo derivative *284*. Jones oxidation gives
the 3-ketone *(285)*. Reaction of that compound with
silver acetate serves to displace the bromine by
acetate, to introduce the enone function by elimination of hydrogen fluoride, and to hydrolyze the
17-acetate. There is thus obtained *286*. Saponification of the remaining 21-acetate gives the
desired intermediate *287*. Successive microbiological
oxidation with *Curvularia lunata* and *Arthrobacter
simplex* serves to introduce respectively the 11β-
hydroxyl *(288)* and 1-olefin functions *(289)*.
Reacetylation *(290)* followed by dehydration gives the
required 9,11-olefin *(291)*. This is converted to the
9,11-fluorohydrin by the standard sequence to afford
finally *cormethasone acetate (292)*.[83]

The recurring theme in work on corticoids discussed thus far  with the exception of the 17-desoxy
compounds consisted in the introduction of additional
functions to the basic cortisone molecule. Some
further success in producing biologically active
molecules has been achieved by substituting unnatural
functions for those present in the protoype molecule.
Thus the hydroxyl groups at both C-11 and C-21 can be
replaced by halogen with retention of activity.

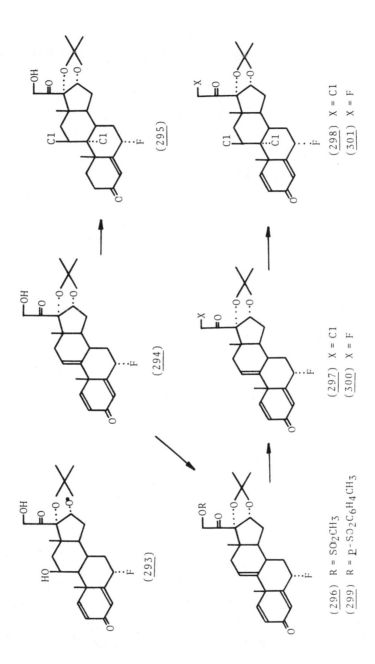

(293)

(294)

(295)

(296)  R = SO₂CH₃
(299)  R = p-SO₂C₆H₄CH₃

(297)  X = Cl
(300)  X = F

(298)  X = Cl
(301)  X = F

Reaction of the olefin (294), corresponding to *fludro-cortide (293)*,[84] with chlorine affords directly *flu-cloronide (295)*.[85] The stereochemistry can, as in the case of 277, be rationalized by invoking the inter-mediacy of the 9α,11α-chloronium ion. Reaction of 294 with methanesulfonyl chloride affords the corres-ponding mesylate (296); displacement of the ester by means of lithium chloride affords the 21-chloro intermediate (297). Addition of chlorine to the 9,11-double bond gives *triclonide (298)*.[86] A similar sequence on the tosylate (299), leading through the intermediate fluoride (300), gives the antiinflam-matory agent *tralonide (301)*.[87]

Antiinflammatory activity also persists in the absence of oxygen at either C-17 or C-21. In this case, unlike those in which those positions are occupied by halogen, the possibility exists that these are in fact prodrugs. That is, the compounds may have no intrinsic biological activity but need to be hydroxylated to the active entities in vivo. The synthetic sequence starts by formation of the bisketal 303 from 11α-acetoxy progesterone (302). Epoxidation affords predominantly the 5α,6α-oxide (304). Reaction with methylmagnesium bromide both opens the oxiran and cleaves the ester (305). Successive treatment with aqueous acid and base serves to hydrolyze the ketal groups and dehydrate the resulting β-hydroxy-ketone (306). The α,β-unsaturated function provides a means for epimerization of the 6β-methyl group to 6α. There now remains the task of inverting the configuration at C-11 as well. Oxidation proceeds in

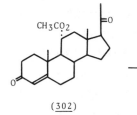

(302)

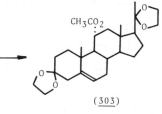

(303)

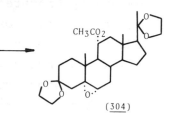

(304)

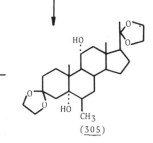

(305)

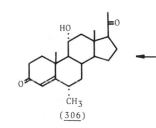

(306)

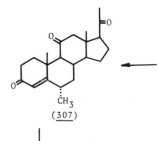

(307)

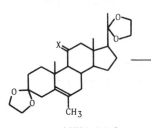

(308) X = O

(309) X =  OH ···H

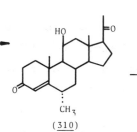

(310)

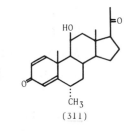

(311)

199

straightforward manner to give the 11-ketone *(307)*;
the highly hindered nature of the 11ketone permits
selective ketal formation at C-3 and C-20 *(308)*.
Reduction by means of lithium aluminum hydride *(309)*,
followed by hydrolysis of the ketal groups affords
antiinflammatory steroid *medrysone (310)*.[88] The
analogue containing additional unsaturation at C-1,
*endrysone (311)*, can presumably be obtained from *310*
by any one of the standard dehydrogenation schemes.


REFERENCES

1.  Y. Lefebvre, U. S. Patent 3,428,627 (1969).

2.  V. Prelog, L. Ruzicka and P. Wieland, *Helv.
    Chim. Acta*, *27*, 250 (1944).

3.  J. De Visser, Dutch Patent 95,275 (1960).

4.  R. E. Brown, D. M. Lustgarten, R. J. Stanaback,
    M. W. Osborne and R. I. Meltzer, *J. Med. Chem.*,
    *7*, 232 (1964).

5.  R. Clarkson, *J. Chem. Soc.*, 4900 (1965).

6.  Anon., Belgian Patent 647,699 (1964).

7.  See D. Lednicer and L. A. Mitscher, Organic
    Chemistry of Drug Synthesis, Vol. I, p. 164
    (1975).

8.  F. B. Colton, U. S. Patent 2,843,608 (1958).

9.  R. T. Rapala, Belgian Patent 666,469 (1966);
    *Chem. Abstr.*, *65:* 5506h (1966).

10. J. C. Babcock and J. A. Campbell, Belgian Patent
    610,385 (1962); *Chem. Abstr.*, *57:* 13834 (1962).

11. M. S. de Winter, C. M. Siegmann and S. A.

Szpilfogel, *Chem. Ind.*, 905 (1959).

12.  Anon., British Patent 841,411 (1960).

13.  See D. Lednicer and L. A. Mitscher, Organic Chemistry of Drug Synthesis, Vol. I, p. 165 (1975).

14.  J. Fried and T. S. Bry, U. S. Patent 3,096,353 (1963).

15.  H. L. Dryden, Jr., G. N. Webber and J. Wieczorek, *J. Am. Chem. Soc.*, *86*, 742 (1964).

16.  P. Wieland and G. Anner, *Helv. Chim. Acta.*, *50*, 289 (1967).

17.  Anon., Dutch Patent 6,406,797 (1965); *Chem. Abstr.*, *64:* 12759b (1966).

18.  D. Lednicer and L. A. Mitscher, Organic Chemistry of Drug Synthesis, Vol. I, p. 177 (1975).

19.  J. S. Baran, *J. Med. Chem.*, *10*, 1188 (1967).

20.  J. S. Baran, H. D. Lennon, S. E. Mares and E. F. Nutting, *Experientia*, *26*, 762 (1970).

21.  H. Smith, G. A. Hughes, G. H. Douglas, G. R. Wendt, G. C. Buzby, Jr., R. A. Edren, J. Fisher, T. Foell, G. Gadstry, D. Hartley, D. Herst, A. B. A. Jansen, K. Ledig, B. J. McLoughlin, J. McMenamin, T. W. Pattison, P. C. Phillips, R. Rees, J. Siddall, J. Sinda, L. L. Smith, J. Tokolics and D. H. P. Watson, *J. Chem. Soc.*, 4472 (1964).

22.  D. Lednicer and L. A. Mitscher, Organic Chemistry of Drug Synthesis, Vol. I, p. 168 (1975).

23.  Anon., British Patent 1,123,104 (1968); *Chem. Abstr.*, *70:* 4410b (1969).

24.  D. Lednicer and L. A. Mitscher, Organic

Chemistry of Drug Synthesis, Vol. I, p. 157 (1975).

25. A. Popper, K. Prezewowsky, R. Wiechert, H. Gibian and G. Raspe, *Arzneimittelforsh.*, *19*, 352 (1969).

26. C. Meystre, H. Frey, W. Voserand and A. Wettstein, *Helv. Chim. Acta*, *39*, 734 (1956).

27. Anon., Belgian Patent 623,277 (1963).

28. A. Ercoli, R. Gardi and R. Vitali, *Chem. Ind.*, 1284 (1962).

29. J. C. Babcock and J. A. Campbell, U. S. Patent 3,341,557 (1967).

30. R. E. Counsell, P. D. Klimstra and F. B. Colton, *J. Org. Chem.*, *27*, 248 (1962); R. Mauli, J. H. Ringold and C. Djerassi, *J. Am. Chem. Soc.*, *82*, 5494 (1960).

31. F. Sorm and H. Dykova, *Coll. Czech. Chem. Commun.*, *13*, 407 (1946).

32. J. Joska, J. Fakjos and F. Sorm, *Chem. Ind.*, 1665 (1958).

33. A. J. Manson, F.W. Stonner, H. C. Neumann, R. G. Christiansen, R. L. Clarke, J. H. Ackerman, D. F. Page, J. W. Dean, D. K. Phillips, G. O. Potts, A. Arnold, A. L. Beyler and R. O. Clinton, *J. Med. Chem.*, *6*, 1 (1963).

34. H. C. Neumann, G. O. Potts, W. T. Ryan and F. W. Stonner, *J. Med. Chem.*, *13*, 948 (1970).

35. F. W. Stoner, S. African Patent 68 04,986 (1969); Chem.

36. J. M. Nascimento and M. H. Venda, *Rev. Port. Farm.*, *13*, 472 (1963); *Chem. Abstr.*, *61*: 3163a (1964).

37.  R. E. Counsell, P. D. Klimstra and R. E. Ranney,
     *J. Med. Chem.*, *5*, 1224 (1962).

38.  W. R. Buckett, C. L. Hewett and D. S. Savage,
     *Chim. Ther.*, *2*, 186 (1967).

39.  See D. Lednicer and L. A. Mitscher, Organic
     Chemistry of Drug Synthesis, Vol. I, p. 181
     (1975).

40.  Anon., Belgian Patent 624,370 (1963); *Chem.*
     *Abstr.*, *60:* 10764g (1964).

41.  See D. Lednicer and L. A. Mitscher, Organic
     Chemistry of Drug Synthesis, Vol. I, p. 181
     (1975).

42.  Anon., Belgian Patent 646,957 (1964).

43.  H. J. Ringold, E. Batres, A. Bowers, J. Edwards
     and J. Zderic, *J. Am. Chem. Soc.*, *81*, 3485 (1959).

44.  See D. Lednicer and L. A. Mitscher, Organic
     Chemistry of Drug Synthesis, Vol. I, p. 179
     (1975).

45.  R. Wiechert, E. Kaspar and M. Schenck, German
     Patent 1,072,991 (1960).

46.  R. Wiechert, U. S. Patent 3,234,093 (1966).

47.  Anon., British Patent 1,095,958 (1967); *Chem.*
     *Abstr.*, *69:* 27645a (1968).

48.  H. Gries' and J. Hader, German Patent 1,286,039
     (1969); *Chem. Abstr.*, *70:* 88115v (1969).

49.  See D. Lednicer and L. A. Mitscher, Organic
     Chemistry of Drug Synthesis, Vol. I, p. 200
     (1975).

50.  Anon., Belgian Patent 621,981 (1963).

51.  R. T. Rapala and M. J. Murray, Jr., *J. Med. Chem.*,
     *5*, 1049 (1962).

52.  G. Cooley, B. Ellis, F. Hartly and V. Petrow, *J.
     Chem. Soc.*, 4373 (1955).

53.  J. Fried, E. F. Sabo, P. Grabowich, L. J. Lerner,
     W. W. Kessler, D. M. Brennan and A. Borman, *Chem.
     Ind.*, 465 (1961).

54.  P. L. Julian and W. J. Karpel, *J. Am. Chem. Soc.*,
     *72*, 362 (1950).

55.  J. S. Mills, O. Candiani and C. Djerassi, *J. Org.
     Chem.*, *25*, 1056 (1960).

56.  See D. Lednicer and L. A. Mitscher, Organic
     Chemistry of Drug Synthesis, Vol. I, p. 207
     (1975).

57.  Anon., Belgian Patent 730,163 (1969).

58.  R. M. Weier and L. M. Hoffman, *J. Med. Chem.*, *18*,
     817 (1975).

59.  See D. Lednicer and L. A. Mitscher, Organic
     Chemistry of Drug Synthesis, Vol. I, p. 192
     (1975).

60.  R. Gardi, R. Vitali and A. Ercoli, *Tet. Lett.*
     448 (1961).

61a. W. S. Allen and S. Bernstein, *J. Am. Chem. Soc.*,
     *78*, 1909 (1956).

61b. S. Bernstein, R. H. Lenhard, W. S. Allen, M.
     Heller, R. Littell, S. M. Stolar, K. I. Feldman
     and R. H. Blank, *J. Am. Chem. Soc.*, *81*, 1689
     (1959).

62.  S. Bernstein, R. Littell, J. J. Brown and I.
     Ringler, *J. Am. Chem. Soc.*, *81*, 4573 (1959).

63. J. A. Hogg and G. B. Spero, U. S. Patent 2,841,600 (1958); Organic Chemistry of Drug Synthesis, Vol. I, p. 195 (1975).

64. H. J. Ringold, J. A. Zderic, C. Djerassi and A. Bowers, German Patent 1,131,213 (1962); *Chem. Abstr.*, *58:* 10281c (1963).

65. Anon., British Patent 933,867 (1963).

66. Anon., French Patent 1,271,981 (1962); *Chem. Abstr.*, *58:* 11448a (1963).

67. See D. Lednicer and L. A. Mitscher, Organic Chemistry of Drug Synthesis, Vol. I, p. 180 (1975).

68. R. M. Dodson and C. Bergstrom, U. S. Patent 2,705,711 (1955); *Chem. Abstr.*, *50:* 5045f (1956).

69. C. Bergstrom, R. T. Nicholson, R. L. Elton and R. M. Dodson, *J. Am. Chem. Soc.*, *81*, 4432 (1959).

70. See D. Lednicer and L. A. Mitscher, Organic Chemistry of Drug Synthesis, Vol. I, p. 193 (1975).

71. E. J. Agnello, S. K. Figdor, G. M. K. Hughes, H. W. Ordway, R. Pinson, Jr., B. M. Bloom and G. D. Laubach, *J. Org. Chem.*, *28*, 1531 (1963).

72. See D. Lednicer and L. A. Mitscher, Organic Chemistry of Drug Synthesis, Vol. I, p. 201 (1975).

73. J. Fried, A. Borman, W. B. Kessler, P. Grabowich and E. F. Sabo, *J. Am. Chem. Soc.*, *80*, 2339 (1958).

74. J. Fried, U. S. Patent 3,053,836 (1962).

75. L. T. Difazio and M. A. Augustine, German Patent 2,355,710 (1974); *Chem. Abstr.*, *81:* 91807e (1974).

76.  S. Bernstein, J. J. Brown, L. I. Friedman and N.
     E. Rigler, *J. Am. Chem. Soc.*, *81*, 4956 (1959).

77.  G. Baldratti, B. Camerino, A. Consonni, F.
     Facciano, F. Mancini, U. Pallini, B. Pateli, R.
     Sciaky, G. K. Suchowsky and F. Tani, *Experientia*,
     *22*, 468 (1966).

78.  H. J. Fried, H. Mrozik, G. E. Arth, T. S. Bry,
     N. G. Steinberg, M. Tishler, R. Hirschmann and S.
     L. Steelman, *J. Am. Chem. Soc.*, *85*, 236 (1963).

79.  A. Ercoli and R. Gardi, S. African Patent
     68 03,686 (1968).

80.  For preparation of the corresponding 16-methyl
     analogue, see D. Lednicer and L. A. Mitscher,
     Organic Chemistry of Drug Synthesis, Vol. I, p.
     205 (1975).

81.  J. A. Campbell, J. C. Babcock and J. A. Hogg,
     U. S. Patent 2,876,219 (1959).

82.  E. Kaspar and R. Phillippson, U. S. Patent
     3,729,495 (1973).

83.  R. M. Scribner, U. S. Patent 3,767,684 (1973).

84.  See D. Lednicer and L. A. Mitscher, Organic
     Chemistry of Drug Synthesis, Vol. I, p. 202
     (1975).

85.  A.Bowers, U. S. Patent 3,201,391 (1965). 86.
     J. H. Fried, German Patent 1,917,082 (1969);
     *Chem. Abstr.*, *72*: 67206b (1970).

87.  J. H. Fried, S. African Patent 68 00,282 (1968);
     *Chem. Abstr.*, *70*: 58146p (1969).

88.  G. B. Spero and J. L. Thompson, U. S. Patent
     2,968,655 (1961).

# 7

# Polycyclic Aromatic and Hydroaromatic Compounds

The ring systems covered in this chapter provide the molecular framework upon which the necessary functionality for a diverse range of pharmacologically active agents are assembled.  Intrinsic agonist activity is rarely, if ever, attributable to the ring system itself among this class, but often replacement or "simplification" by omission of rings leads to a serious decrease in activity.  This is generally considered to be due to a considerable alteration in lipid/water solubility ratio, a deleterious alteration in the spatial arrangement of the functions necessary to fire the receptor, a change in the pK such that altered intracellular concentrations are achieved, or some such factor.  This lack of intrinsic pharmacophoric action is demonstrated clearly by the indanes in the first section.  Of the six substances covered, each has a different main pharmacological action!

207

## 1.   INDANES AND INDENES

Of a series of indanylthiocarbamates, *tolindate* (2)
had significant antifungal properties.  It is prepared simply from 5-indanyl thionochloroformate (1) by
reaction with N-methyl-m-toluidine.[1] It presumably
joins the fairly large family of organic compounds
having sulfur divalently bound to carbon which are
useful topical agents for dermatophytes.

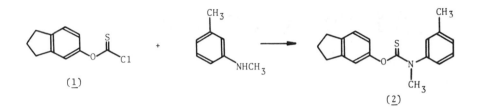

When indan-2-one (3) forms a Schiff's base with
aniline and this is reduced with sodium borohydride,
the aminoindane 4 is found.  The acidic hydrogen is
removed with sodium hydride and this is in turn
reacted with 3-diethylaminopropyl chloride to complete
the synthesis of *aprindine* (5), an antiarrythmic
agent.[2]

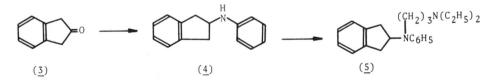

When l-phenylindene (6) is treated successively
with n-butyl lithium and dimethyl β-chloroethylamine,
*indriline* (7), a central stimulant, is formed along
with inactive isomer 8, both presumably arising via
reaction with the intermediate aziridinium ion.[3]

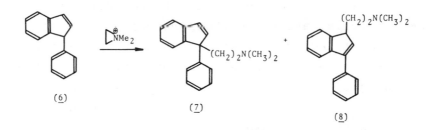

(6)          (7)          (8)

Reaction of p-fluorobenzyl chloride with the
anion of diethylmethylmalonate ester followed by
saponification and decarboxylation leads to acid 9.
Polyphosphoric acid cyclization leads to indanone 10.
A Reformatsky reaction with zinc amalgam and bromoacetic ester leads to carbinol 11 which is then

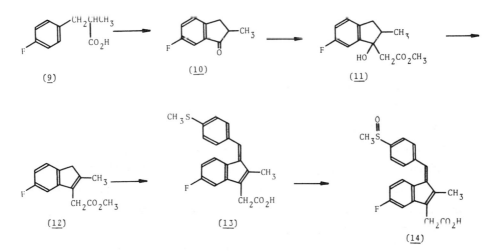

(9)          (10)          (11)

(12)          (13)          (14)

dehydrated with tosic acid to indene 12.  The active
methylene group of 12 is condensed with p-thiomethyl-
benzaldehyde, using sodium methoxide as catalyst, and
then saponified to give Z-isomer 13 which is in turn

oxidized with sodium metaperiodate to sulfoxide *14*, the antiinflammatory agent *sulindac*.[4]

Phenyl indandiones with an acidic hydrogen often interfere with clot formation. When electron with-drawing groups are present in the p-position, acidity is increased and activity goes up. The opposite effect is seen with electron-donating substituents. Synthe-sized in the usual way, the anticoagulant *bromindione* *(15)* results from sodium acetate-catalyzed conden-sation of phthalic anhydride and p-α-bromophenyl-acetic acid.[5]

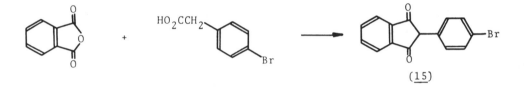

(15)

An analgesic compound that does not completely embody the essential structural features of the classical morphine rule is *dimefadane (19)*. Friedel-Crafts alkylation of benzene with cinnamic acid using a Lewis acid catalyst gives β,β-diphenylacetic acid *(16)*, which is cyclized to indanone *17*. Heating with ammonium formate (Leuckart reaction) produces indanylamine 18 in a more efficient manner than does hydrogenation of the oxime. Heating with formalde-hydeformic acid (Eschweiler-Clark reaction) then produces *dimefadane (19)*,[6] an analgesic with about the same potency as codeine but without much of the

untoward gastrointestinal side effects of the natural
product.

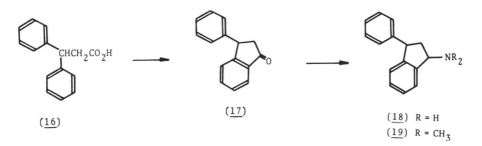

(16)

(17)

(18) R = H
(19) R = CH₃

## 2.    NAPHTHALENES

An analogue of *tolindate (2)* which has had greater
success as an antifungal drug is *tolnaftate (20)*.
The synthesis follows the usual path, condensing
β-naphthol with $Cl_2CS$ and then reacting the resulting
chlorothioformate with N-methyl-m-toluidine.[7]

It will be recalled that certain local anesthetic amides, such as *procainamide* and *lidocaine*,
are active antiarrythmic agents.  Annelation of a
second aromatic ring is consistent with bioactivity.
*Bunaftine (21)* is such an agent, prepared simply from
reaction of the acid chloride of 1-naphthoic acid and
β-dimethylaminoethylbutylamine.[7]

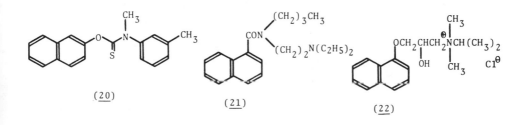

(20)

(21)

(22)

Interestingly, when *propranolol* is quaternized
with methyl chloride, it loses its β-blocker activity
and becomes the antiarrythmic agent *pranolium chloride*
*(22)*.[8]

A number of amidines have anthelmintic activity.
*Bunamidine (25)*, indicated for treatment of human
pinworm infestations, is prepared from α-naphthylhexyl-
ether *(23)* by Friedel-Crafts type reaction with
cyanogen bromide and aluminum chloride to give nitrile
*(24)*.  This, then, is reacted with the magnesium
bromide salt of di-n̲-propylamine leading to the naph-
thamidine structure *(25)*.[9]-

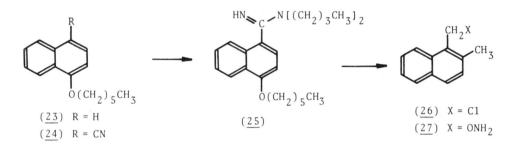

(23) R = H
(24) R = CN

(25)

(26) X = Cl
(27) X = ONH₂

Muscle relaxant activity is found in the aminoxy-
methylnaphthalene structure of *nafomine (27)*.  The
synthesis proceeds from 1-chloromethyl-2-methylnaph-
thalene *(26)*, which is reacted with N̲-carbethoxy-
hydroxylamine and base.  In this way, the basic
nitrogen is protected as the carbamate.  Loss of the
carbethoxy group either during reaction or on workup
affords *nafomine (27)*.[10]

Certain ethanolamine analogues are active as CNS stimulants if they can be transported across the blood-brain barrier.  One technique for bringing this about is to esterify them.  One agent designed for this purpose, but which is more interesting as a vasodilator, is *nafronyl (29)*.[11]  The acid component is synthesized by condensing furfuryl chloride and methyl malonate followed by catalytic reduction, alkylation with 1-chloromethylnaphthalene and saponi-fication/decarboxylation to give *28*.[12]  Esterification with N,N-diethylethanolamine produces *nafronyl (29)*.

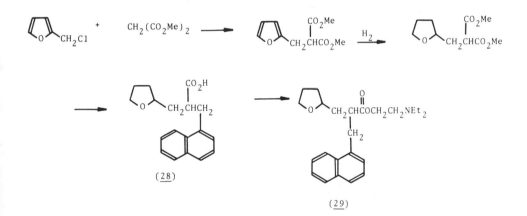

A number of products in which one of the naph-thalene rings has been reduced have interesting pharmacological properties.  Reaction of tetralone *30* with dimethylamine under $TiCl_4$ catalysis produces the corresponding enamine *(31)*.  Reaction with formic acid at room temperature effects reduction of the

eneamine double bond to product the tranquilizer and
anti-Parkinsonian agent, *lometraline (32).*[13].

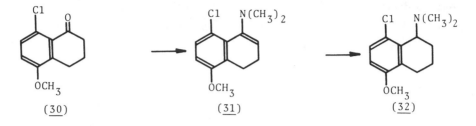

(30)                    (31)                    (32)

Branched aryloxyacetic acids often have hypo-
chloesterolemic activity.  When tetralol *33* is reacted
with phenol in a Friedel-Crafts reaction, α-tetralin
derivative *34* is formed.  This is reacted with ethyl
α-bromoisobutyrate and saponified to produce the
hypolipidemic agent, *nafenopin (35).*[14]

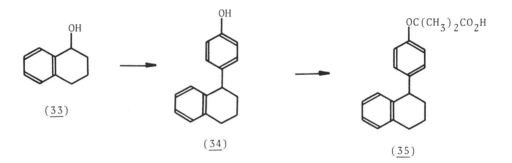

(33)                    (34)                    (35)

As noted above, phenylethanolamines are usually
β-adrenergic agonists, whereas phenylpropanolamines
show antagonist activity.  A small series of phenylethanolamine blockers is, however, known.  When the
haloatom of ω-bromo-5,6,7,8-tetrahydro-2-acetonaphth-
one *(36)* is displaced with isopropylamine and the

carbonyl group is reduced catalytically, the adrenergic blocking agent *bunitridine* (37) is produced.[15]

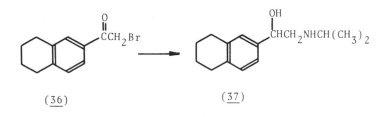

(36)                                      (37)

A number of tetralins with the appropriate side
chains have β-adrenergic blocking activity.  Presumably, the tetralin ring provides greater lipid solubility than the corresponding benzenes.  *Bunolol (41)*
is synthesized from phenolic tetralone (38) by sequential reaction with 2,3-dihydroxypropyl chloride (to
39), tosyl chloride (to 40), and t-butylamine to give
*bunolol.*[16]  Restoration of a considerable amount of
the water solubility of this small group of drugs is
accomplised by incorporating a glycol moiety in the
reduced ring.  When 5,8-dihydronaphthol (42) is
acetylated and then hydroxylated via the Woodward

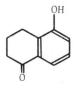                    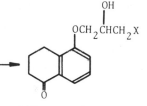

(38)                      (39)  X = OH
                          (40)  X = $OSO_2C_6H_4CH_3$
                          (41)  X = $NHC(CH_3)_3$

modification of the Prevost process (silver acetate
and iodine), glycol _43_ is formed.  The rest of the
molecule is constructed in the usual way involving
the sequence: saponification to the phenol, alkylation
with epichlorohydrin, and displacement with _t_-butyl-
amine to produce _nadolol (44)_, a β-adrenergic blocking agent.[17]

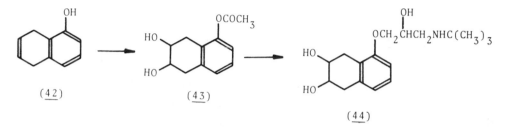

Despite the best efforts of the World Health
Organization, malaria remains a widespread tropical
disease with substantial mortality.  Of the many
structural types explored in attempts to find prophy-
lactic and chemotherapeutic agents, some have been
naphthoquinones.  During World War II, a large number
of such quinones with aliphatic side chains were
investigated. Several were active in ducks but not in
man, and the reason for this difference was traced to
man's ability to inactivate these materials by
hydroxylation.  To counter this, some agents with
relatively very large hydrocarbon sidechains were
made.  For example, acylation of cyclohexanone enamine
45 with dihydrocinnamoyl chloride produced 46, which
underwent ring-opening diketone cleavage with base to
give acid 47. Wolff-Kishner reduction and hydrogenation

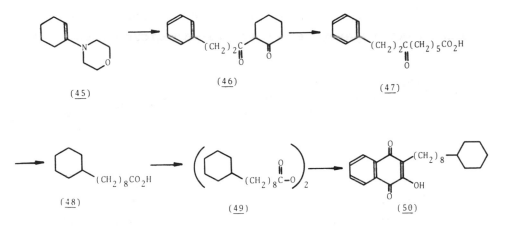

(45)    (46)    (47)

(48)    (49)    (50)

over a platinum catalyst produced saturated acid *48*
that was converted to the acid chloride with $SOCl_2$
and then to the acyl peroxide *(49)* with $H_2O_2$ and
pyridine.  Heating *49* in acetic acid along with 2-
hydroxynaphthoquinone resulted in radical formation
and alkylation to produce the antimalarial agent,
*menoctone (50).*[18]

### 3.   FLUORENES

Many nonsteroidal antiinflammatory agents are acids
and are believed to act by inhibiting prostaglandin
synthesis.  The synthesis of one such agent, *cicloprofen*
*(53)*, is illustrative. When fluorene *51* is acylated
by ethyl oxalylchloride and $AlCl_3$, ketoester *52*
results.  Reaction with methyl Grignard reagent, acid
dehydration of the tertiary carbinol, and catalytic
reduction of the resulting terminal olefinic linkage
produces the antiinflammatory agent, *cicloprofen*

(53).[19]  Elements of the structure of *ibuprofen* and
its congeners are clearly visible in *cicloprofen*.

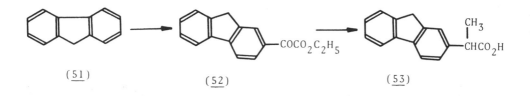

(51)                    (52)                    (53)

A number of amines are also nonsteroidal antiinflammatory agents.  One such agent was uncovered
while searching for estrogenic substances.
9-Fluorenone *(54)* undergoes Grignard addition and
dehydration with p-bromobenzylmagnesium bromide to
give 55.  Displacement of halogen with CuCN gives
nitrile 56, which can be converted to the amidine in
the usual way. Reaction with ethanol under acid-
catalyzed anhydrous conditions leads to iminoether 57
which undergoes displacement with liquid ammonia to
give the antiinflammatory agent, *paranyline (58)*.[20]

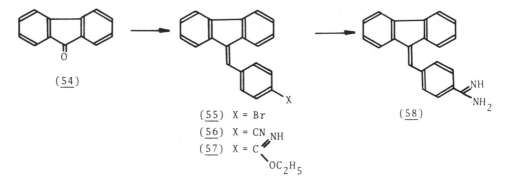

(54)

(55)  X = Br                    (58)
(56)  X = CN
(57)  X = C

One substance intended to be an antiinflammatory
agent has achieved much greater prominence because it

is an interferon inducer and is therefore protective
against viral infections. This drug is *tilorone*
*(63)*.[21] In its synthesis, fluorene *(51)* is sulfonated
and converted to its potassium salt *(59)*.  This is
oxidized with $KMnO_4$ to the fluorenone *(60)*.  Upon KOH
fusion, nucleophilic substitution to the *bis*-phenol
occurs, accompanied by ring cleavage, to give *61*.
Friedel-Crafts cyclization ($ZnCl_2$) restores the
fluorenone system *(62)*.  Ether formation with β-
bromotriethylamine (probably via the aziridinium)
produces *tilorone (63)*.

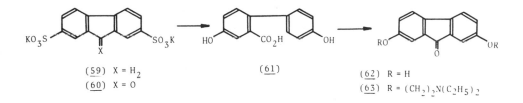

(<u>59</u>) X = $H_2$             (<u>61</u>)
(<u>60</u>) X = O                                    (<u>62</u>) R = H
                                                     (<u>63</u>) R = $(CH_2)_2N(C_2H_5)_2$

### 4.  ANTHRACENES

Anthracenes are planar by virtue of the necessity of
maintaining aromaticity.  When the central ring is
reduced, an overall "butterfly" conformation is
achieved.  For reasons that are not yet understood at
the molecular level, this conformation is often
associated with central antidepressant activity.

The methylene group of anthrone *64* is acidic by
virtue of doubly vinylic activation by the carbonyl
group.  Thus, treatment with methyl iodide and base
leads to the 9,9-dimethyl derivative *65*.  Grignard
reaction with δ-dimethylaminopropyl magnesium chloride

gives tertiary carbinol *66* and subsequent acid dehydration produces *melitracen (67)*, an antidepressant.[22]

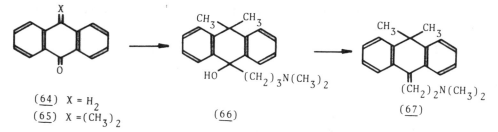

(64) X = H₂
(65) X =(CH₃)₂                    (66)                    (67)

The same nonpolar conformation can be achieved
by conversion to bicyclic structures. 1,4-Cyclo-
addition of ethylene to anthracene-9-carboxylic acid
gives acid *68*. Successive conversion to the N-
methylamide, via the acid chloride, followed by
reduction with lithium aluminum hydride produced
*benzoctamine (69)*, a sedative and muscle relaxant.[23]

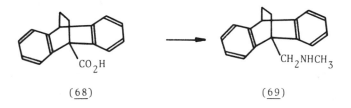

(68)                    (69)

Lengthening the side chain produces the antidepressant *maprotiline (73)*, which has a topological
relationship to the clinically useful tricyclic antidepressants. The requisite acid is constructed by
conjugate addition of the carbanion of anthrone *(64)*
to acrylonitrile, followed by hydrolysis to give *70*.
Reduction of the carbonyl group with zinc and ammonia
gives anthracene *71* by dehydration of the intermediate

alcohol function.   Diels-Alder reaction with ethylene
gives *72*, which is converted to *maprotiline* *(73)*[23] by
the same three-step sequence as used for *benzoctamine*.

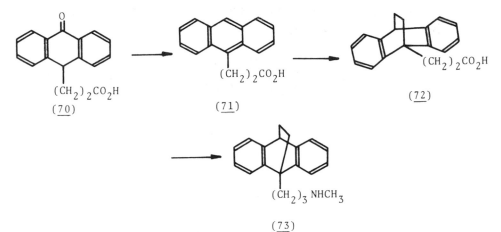

(CH$_2$)$_2$CO$_2$H
(70)

(CH$_2$)$_2$CO$_2$H
(71)

(CH$_2$)$_2$CO$_2$H
(72)

(CH$_2$)$_3$NHCH$_3$
(73)

5.   DIBENZOCYCLOHEPTANES AND DIBENZOCYCLOHEPTENES
Drugs in this structural class have effected a revolu-
tion in the treatment of severely depressed patients
such that deinstitutionalization is a feasible public
policy.   The compounds often show other CNS activities
which depend on the length of the side chain.   One-
carbon chains generally lead to anticonvulsant activity; amines separated from the nucleus by three
carbons usually convey antidepressant activity.
Selected examples possess significant anticholinergic
activity.

Reaction of chlorodibenzocycloheptatriene *74*
with butyl lithium, followed by carbonation produces
acid *75*, which is converted by ammonia, via the acid
chloride, to *citenamide* *(76)*, an anticonvulsant.[24]
The partially saturated analogue *77* is prepared

essentially the same way from chlorodibenzocyclo-
heptadiene and is *cyheptamide*, also an anticonvulsant.[25]  In the dihydro series the two benzene rings
are not only out of plane, but also helical with
respect to one another.

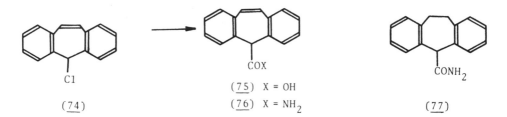

(74)

(75) X = OH
(76) X = NH$_2$

(77)

    Base-catalyzed condensation between phenylacetic
acid and phthalic acid produces enol lactone *78*,
which is reduced to benzoate *79* with HI and phosphorous.  Friedel-Crafts cyclization by polyphosphoric
acid followed by reduction produces alcohol *80*.  This
alcohol forms ethers exceedingly easily, probably *via*
the carbonium ion.  Treatment with N-methyl-4--
piperidinol in the presence of acid leads to the
antidepressant *hepzidine (81)*.[26]

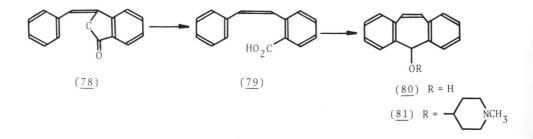

(78)                    (79)

(80)  R = H

(81)  R =

Inclusion of an acetylenic linkage as part of
the side chain is apparently consistent with antidepressant activity. Reaction of propargyl magnesium
bromide with dibenzocycloheptadieneone leads to
carbinol *82*.  A Mannich reaction with formaldehyde
and dimethylamine leads to *83* which, upon dehydration
with SOCl$_2$ and pyridine, was transformed into
*intriptyline (84)*, an antidepressant.[27]

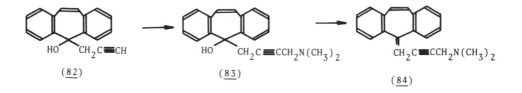

(82)                    (83)                    (84)

Rigidity can be achieved with retention of the
overall molecular conformation by use of a cyclopropyl ring in place of the olefinic bond bridging
the two benzenes.  Treatment of dibenzocyclohepta-
trieneone with dichlorocarbene generated from di-
chloroacetic ester and sodium ethoxide gives addition
product *85*.  Reaction with cyclopropyl Grignard
reagent gives carbinol *86* from which the *gem*-dihalo-
atoms are removed by lithium and t-butanol to give
*87*.  Reaction of the latter with HCl generates
chloride *88* via the intermediate cation *(87a)*.
Chloride displacement with methylamine completes the
synthesis of antidepressant *octriptyline (89)*.[28]

Incorporation of the side chain amino group into
a ring leads to tranquilizers.  This is of special
interest in that the amino group is now separated

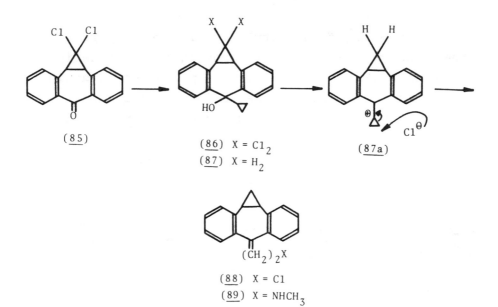

(85)

(86) X = Cl$_2$
(87) X = H$_2$

(87a)

(88) X = Cl
(89) X = NHCH$_3$

from the tricyclic ring system by a smaller distance than is common to the other agents discussed. Reaction of amine *90* with δ-lactone *91* gives hydroxyamide *92*. Cyclodehydration proceeds apparently through the expected Bischler-Napieralski intermediate *93* which cyclizes further to imine *94*. Reduction with sodium borohydride or hydrogenation with platinum catalyst produces the undesired *cis* isomer. On the other hand, zinc and acetic acid reduction leads to the thermodynamically stable *trans* product, the minor tranquilizer *taclamine (95)*.[29] The apparent conformation of *taclamine* is *96*.

An alternate means of forming *96* arises from reaction of imine *97* with methylvinylketone in a variant of the Robinson annulation reaction. This

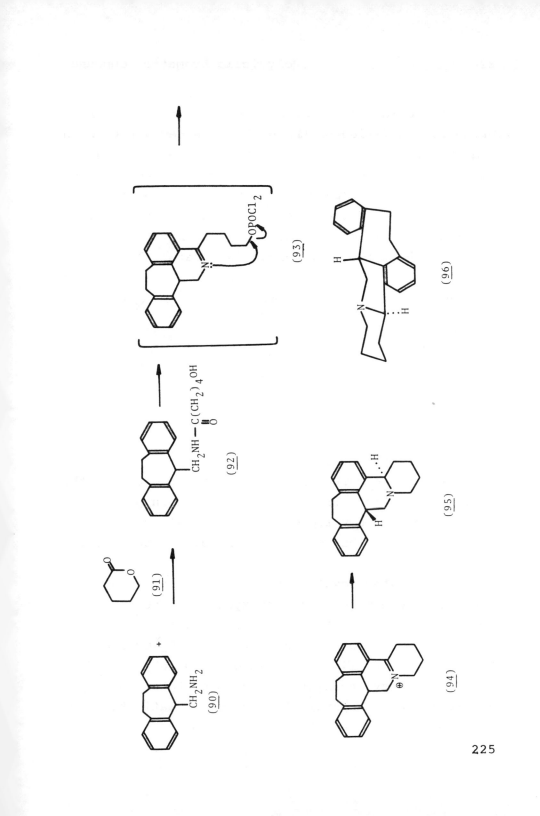

(90)

(91)

(92)

(93)

(94)

(95)

(96)

can proceed in two directions, but *98* is the major
product.  Formation of the dithiolane derivative with
$(CH_2SH)_2$ and $BF_3$ followed by Raney nickel desulfurization also leads to *taclamine*.  The availability of
ketone *98* makes it possible to prepare more highly
functionalized derivatives. Addition, for example, of
t-butyl lithium leads to tranquilizer *butaclamol*
*(99)*.[30]  The large alkyl group is equatorial.

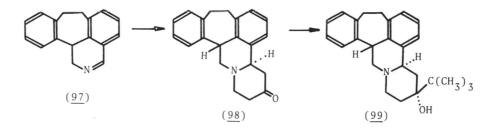

(97)                    (98)                    (99)

## 6.    TETRACYCLINES

Still among the most frequently prescribed drugs, the
antibiotic tetracyclines have decreased in popularity
recently due to development of bacterial resistance
in the clinic.  The search for improved agents goes
on.

     When oxytetracycline *(100)* is reacted with
<u>N</u>-chlorosuccinimide in dimethoxyethane, the active
methine group at $C_{11a}$ reacts and, apparently, there
is formed a hemiketal bond between the $C_6$-OH and the
$C_{12}$-ketogroup *(101)*.  Dehydration with anhydrous HF
of the tertiary, benzylic $C_6$-OH group takes an
exocyclic course, partially because aromatization to

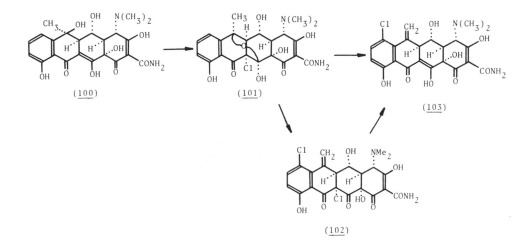

the naphthalene system is forbidden by the presence
of the blocking $C_{11a}$-chlorine atom.  The product is
sufficiently stable to allow electrophilic aromatic
substitution.  Reaction with N-chlorosuccinimide in
liquid HF results in formation of the 7,11a-dichloro-
6-methylene analogue (102).  When the latter is
subjected to chemical reduction (with sodium bisulfite,
for example), the labile $C_{11a}$-Cl atom is removed and
meclocycline (103) is formed.  This broad spectrum
antibiotic is about six times more potent in vitro
against Klebsiella pneumoniae than methacycline
itself.[31]

Nitro derivative *104* is an undesired side product
in the synthesis of *minocycline*.[32]  Upon catalytic
reduction it is converted to the corresponding aniline,
*amicycline (104)*. This substance is slightly less
than half as active *in vitro* against *Staphylococcus
aureus* than chlortetracycline *(100)*, but is nearly
twice as active as its $C_7$ isomer.[33,34]

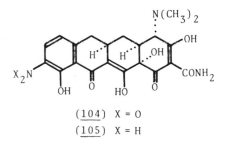

(104) X = O
(105) X = H

## REFERENCES

1.  B. Elpern and J. B. Youlus, U. S. Patent
    3,509,200 (1970); *Chem. Abstr.*, *73:* 14,546b
    (1970).
2.  P. Vanhoff and P. Clarebout, German Patent
    2,060,721 (1971); *Chem. Abstr.*, *75:* 76,463x
    (1971).
3.  A. Kandel and P. M. Lish, Belgian Patent 667,739
    (1966); *Chem. Abstr.*, *65:* 8,844c (1966).
4.  T. Y. Shen, B. E. Witzel, H. Jones, B. O. Linn
    and R. B. Greenwald, German Patent 2,039,426
    (1971); *Chem. Abstr.*, *74:* 141,379x (1971).
5.  G. Cavallini, E. Milla, E. Grumelli and F.
    Ravenna, *Il Farmaco, Ed. Sci.*, *10*, 710 (1955).

6. J. A. Barltrop, R. M. Achison, P. G. Philpott, K. E. MacPhee and J. S. Hunt, *J. Chem. Soc.*, 2928 (1956).

7. T. Noguchi, Y. Hashimoto, K. Miyazaki and A. Kaji, *Yakugaku Zasshi*, *88*, 335 (1968).

8. M. Giannini, P. Boni, M. Fedi and G. Bonacchi, *Il Farmaco, Ed. Sci.*, *28*, 429 (1973).

9. B. R. Luchesi, German Patent 2,333,965 (1974); *Chem. Abstr.*, *80:* 95,610n (1974).

10. M. Harfenist, R. B. Burrows, R. Baltzly, E. Pederson, G. R. Hunt, S. Gurbaxani, J. E. D. Keeling and O. O. Standen, *J. Med. Chem.*, *14*, 97 (1971).

11. W. R. McGrath and E. M. Roberts, Belgian Patent 654,632 (1965); *Chem. Abstr.*, *65:* 669c (1966).

12. E. Szarvasi, L. Neuvy and L. Fontaine, *Compt. Rend.*, *260*, 920 (1965).

13. E. Szarvasi and L. Neuvy, Bull. *Soc. Chim. Fr.*, 1343 (1962).

14. R. Sarges, German Patent 2,018,135 (1970); *Chem. Abstr.*, *74:* 22,601b (1971).

15. Anon., Dutch Patent 6,413,268 (1965); *Chem. Abstr.*, *63:* 13,178c (1965).

16. Anon., French Patent 1,390,056 (1965); *Chem. Abstr.*, *62:* 16,162d (1965).

17. E. J. Merrill, *J. Pharm. Sci.*, *60*, 1589 (1971).

18. F. P. Hauck, C. M. Cimarusti and V. L. Narayanan, German Patent 2,258,995 (1973); *Chem. Abstr.*, *79:* 53,096y (1973).

19. L. F. Fieser, J. P. Schirmer, S. Archer, R. R.

Lorenz and P. Pfaffenbach, *J. Med. Chem.*, *10*, 513 (1967).

20. E. Stiller, P. A. Diassi, D. Gerschutz, D. Meikle, J. Moetz, P. A. Principe and S. D. Levine, *J. Med. Chem.*, *15*, 1029 (1972).

21. R. E. Allen, E. L. Schumann, W. C. Day and M. G. Van Campen Jr., *J. Am. Chem. Soc.*, *80*, 591 (1958).

22. E. R. Andrews, R. W. Fleming, J. M. Grisar, J. C. Kihm, D. L. Wenstrup and G. D. Mayer, *J. Med. Chem.*, *17*, 882 (1974).

23. T. Holm, *Acta Chem. Scand.*, *17*, 2437 (1963).

24. M. Wilhelm and P. Schmidt, *Helv. Chim. Acta*, *52*, 1385 (1969).

25. M. A. Davis, S. O. Winthrop, R. A. Thomas, F. Herr, M.P. Charest and R. Gaudry, *J. Med. Chem.*, *7*, 88 (1964).

26. M. A. Davis, S. O. Winthrop, J. Stewart, F. A. Sunahara and F. Herr, *J. Med. Chem.*, *6*, 251 (1963).

27. C. Van der Stelt, A. F. Harms and W. T. Nauta, *J. Med. Chem.*, *4*, 335 (1961).

28. J. F. Cavalla and A. C. White, British Patent 1,406,481 (1975); *Chem. Abstr.*, *84:* 4,744c (1976).

29. W. E. Coyne and J. W. Cusic, *J. Med. Chem.*, *17*, 72 (1974).

30. F. T. Bruderlein, L. G. Humber and K. Pelz, *Can J. Chem.*, *52*, 2119 (1974).

31. F. T. Bruderlein, L. G. Humber and K. Voith, *J. Med. Chem.*, *18*, 185 (1975).

32.  R. K. Blackwood, J. J. Beereboom, H. H. Rennhard,
     M. Schach von Wittenau and C. R. Stephens, J.
     *Am. Chem. Soc.*, *83*, 2773 (1961).
33.  D. Lednicer and L. A. Mitscher, Organic Chemistry
     of Drug Synthesis, Vol. I, p. 215 (1977).
34.  J. H. Boothe, J. J. Hlavka, J. P. Petisi and J.
     L. Spencer, *J. Am. Chem. Soc.*, *82*, 1253 (1960).
35.  J. Petisi, J. L. Spencer, J. J. Hlavka and J. H.
     Boothe, *J. Med. Chem.*, *5*, 538 (1962).

# 8

# Five-Membered Heterocycles

Heterocyclic compounds occupy a central position
among those molecules that make life possible.  In
support, one need only mention the molecular basis of
continuation of a given species, *i.e.*, the heterocyclic purines and pyrimidines that form the building
blocks of DNA and RNA.  This realization, along with
some early adventitious successes with heterocyclic
drugs and the frequency with which the active principles of the important vegetable drugs of antiquity
turned out to be heterocycles have led the medicinal
chemist to devote a good deal of attention to this
class of compounds as a source of potential therapeutic agents.  Perhaps as a result of this, somewhat
over half the organic drugs to have been assigned
generic names are heterocyclic molecules.  It does
not, however, follow that all biologically active
molecules that contain a heterocyclic moiety owe

232

their activity to that fragment.  As will be seen
below, some classes of heterocycles do share a common
biological response; in those cases it is of course a
fair assumption that the heterocycle is a significant
part of the pharmacophore.  Cases are equally frequent,
however, where it is apparent that the ring contributes little of a specific nature to the activity.  A
relatively neutral heterocyclic ring can often be
substituted for a benzene ring with little qualitative
effect on biological activity.  For example, medicinal
chemists often substitute a thiophene ring for a
benzene ring in a drug.  This practice is the venerable
device of biological isosterism.

### 1.   DERIVATIVES OF PYRROLE
Molecules whose sole heterocyclic moiety consists of
a pyrrolidine ring are dealt with elsewhere in this
book.  There is a wealth of evidence to indicate that
N-alkylpyrrolidine is usually a surrogate for a
tertiary amine.

    The large class of antiinflammatory phenylacetic
acids are treated at some length in Chapter 4.  A
number of these agents consist of acetic or propionic
acids substituted by an aroyl group.  It is of interest
that the central benzene ring of these molecules can
be replaced by pyrrole with retention of activity.
For example, Mannich reaction of N-methylpyrrole
affords the corresponding dimethylaminomethyl derivative (2) and treatment with methyl iodide affords the
quaternary salt (3).  Displacement of the quaternary
amine by means of cyanide leads to the substituted

acetonitrile 4.[1]  Friedel-Crafts acylation of that
intermediate with the acid chloride from p-toluic
acid gives a mixture of the 4-aryl ketone and the
desired ketone 5.   Hydrolysis with sodium hydroxide
completes the synthesis of the antiinflammatory agent
tolmetin (6).[2]

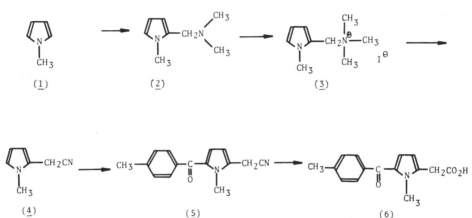

The wide latitude of structural variation
consistent with bioactivity in this series is illustrated by the observation that antiinflammatory
activity is maintained even when the second aromatic
group is attached directly to the pyrrole nitrogen
rather than to the heterocyclic ring via a carbonyl
group as in the previous case.  Condensation of p-
chloroaniline with hexane-2,5-dione (or its dimethoxy-
tetrahydrofuran equivalent) affords pyrrole 7.   The
acetic acid side chain is then elaborated as above.
Thus, Mannich reaction leads to the dimethylaminomethyl
derivative 8, which is in turn methylated (9); the
quaternary nitrogen replaced by cyanide to afford 10.
Hydrolysis of the nitrile then gives clopirac (11).[3]

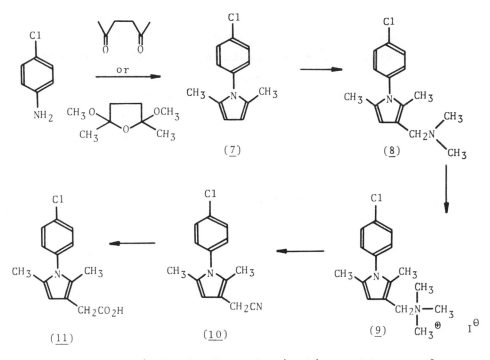

(7)        (8)

(11)        (10)        (9)

A change in both the substitution pattern and the oxidation state of the heterocyclic ring leads to a compound that exhibits antidepressant activity. This agent, *cotinine (13)*, is found in nature as a product from the autoxidation of nicotine *(12)* (note the anagram). The compound can also be obtained in decidedly modest yield by oxidation of nicotine with hydrogen peroxide.[4]

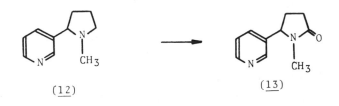

(12)        (13)

A more highly substituted pyrrolidone, *doxapram*,
shows activity as a respiratory stimulant.  Preparation of this agent involves an interesting rearrangement, which in effect results in a ring exchange
reaction.  Alkylation of the anion from diphenylaceto-
nitrile with the chloropyrrolidine *14* affords *15*.
Hydrolysis of the nitrile function leads to the

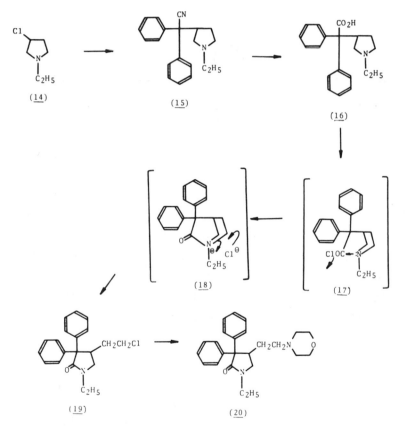

expected acid *16*.  Treatment of *16* with thionyl chloride presumably gives first the acid chloride *17*;
internal acylation would then lead to the bicyclic

quaternary ammonium salt *18*.   Attack on the two-carbon
bridge by the gegenion would afford the observed
chloroethyl pyrrolidone *19*.   (Regioselectivity may be
due to the hindered environment about the one carbon
bridge.)   Displacement of chlorine by morpholine
completes the synthesis of *doxapram* (*20*).[5]

The discovery of the sedative/hynoptic activity
of derivatives of barbituric acid has led to very
extensive dissections of that molecule.   One outcome
of this work is the realization that acylurea and
acylamide derivatives often exhibit CNS depressant
activity.   A fair number of such molecules have been
prepared that contain a succinimide or glutarimide
pharmacophore.   For example, Michael addition of
cyanide to the stereochemically undefined cinnamate
*21* affords intermediate *22*.   Acid hydrolysis leads
directly to the tranquilizer *fenimide* (*23*).[6]   Although
the stereochemistry of this compound is not specified,
the fact that the ethyl group resides on an enolizable
center makes it probable that this is in fact the
thermodynamically more stable isomer.

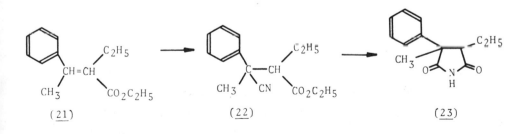

(21)                          (22)                          (23)

## 2. DERIVATIVES OF FURAN

Many carbonyl derivatives of 5-nitrofurfural exhibit
bacteriostatic activity. For example, the oxime,
*nifuroxime*, has found some clinical use in the treatment of infections of the gastrointestinal and urinary
tract. An impressive amount of work has been devoted
to such derivatives in attempts to alter both their
distribution and pharmacodynamics by modification of
the substituents on the imine nitrogen. Much of this
was detailed in the earlier volume. By way of additional examples, reaction of 5-nitrofurfural *(24)*
with N-(2-hydroxyethyl)hydroxylamine gives the antimicrobial agent *nitrofuratrone (25)*,[7] probably the
only nitrone to have been assigned a generic name.
In a similar vein condensation with 2-ethylsemi-
carbazide leads to the semicarbazone *nitfursemizone*
*(26)*,[8] an antiprotozoal agent for use in poultry.

$$O_2N \overset{\text{O}}{\underset{\uparrow}{\text{CH=N}}}CH_2CH_2OH \quad \longleftarrow \quad O_2N \overset{}{\text{CHO}} \quad \longrightarrow \quad O_2N \overset{\text{O}^-}{\underset{C_2H_5}{\text{CH=NN}\overset{\text{O}}{\overset{\|}{\text{C}}}NH_2}}$$

(25)                         (24)                         (26)

N-Aminoimidazolinones have found extensive use
as synthons for such nitrofurans. Reaction of an
appropriate 1,2-diamine *(27, 31)* with urea gives the
desired heterocycle *(28, 32)*. Nitrosation with

nitrous acid, followed by reduction of the intermediate
(*29, 33*) with zinc, gives the desired hydrazine (*30,
34*).   Condensation of *30* with *24* affords *nifurdazil*
(*35*).[9]  In a modification of the usual scheme, condensation of *34* with furfuraldehyde gives the hydrazone
*36*.   Nitration of that intermediate affords *nifurimide*
(*37*).[10]

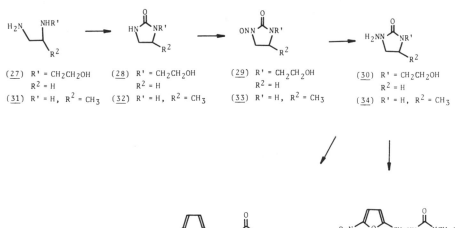

(27)  R' = CH₂CH₂OH       (28)  R' = CH₂CH₂OH        (29)  R' = CH₂CH₂OH          (30)  R' = CH₂CH₂OH
      R² = H                     R² = H                     R² = H                        R² = H
(31)  R' = H, R² = CH₃    (32)  R' = H, R² = CH₃     (33)  R' = H, R² = CH₃        (34)  R' = H, R² = CH₃

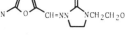

(36)  X = H                              (35)
(37)  X = NO₂

It is of interest that antibacterial activity
can be retained even when the imine carbon-nitrogen
bond is replaced by a carbon to carbon double bond.
Base-catalyzed condensation of 5-nitrofurfuraldehyde
(*24*) with 2,6-dimethylpyridine (*38*) affords olefin
*39*.   Treatment of this compound with hydrogen peroxide
gives the corresponding N-oxide (*40*).   Heating of

that intermediate in acetic anhydride leads to acetoxy-
lation of the 2-methyl group by the Polonovski reaction.
Hydrolysis of the ester group affords *nifurpirinol*
(*42*).[11]

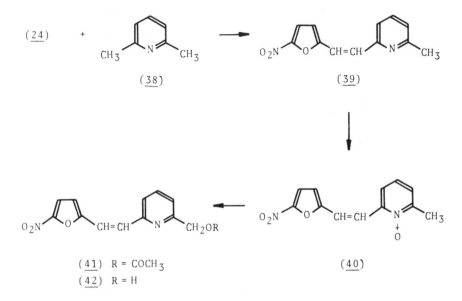

(*24*)     +                    (*38*)                                    (*39*)

(*41*)  R = COCH₃                              (*40*)
(*42*)  R = H

Taking the spacer ethylene moiety out and attach-
ing a heterocyclic ring directly to the nitrofuran
ring also results in an active antimicrobial agent.
Condensation of bromoketone *43* (obtainable by halogenation of the corresponding acetylnitrofuran) with
thiourea gives the aminothiazole *44*.  Although the
detailed mechanism of this well known method for
forming thiazoles is still under discussion, the
reaction at least formally represents conversion of
the ketone to an imine and displacement of the halogen
by sulfur.  Next, the primary amine is nitrosated

*(45)*, and this intermediate is reduced to the hydrazine *(46)*. Acylation of the more basic terminal
nitrogen with formic acid completes the synthesis of
the antimicrobial agent *nifurthiazole (47)*.[12]

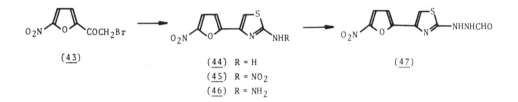

(43)

(44) R = H
(45) R = NO$_2$
(46) R = NH$_2$

(47)

Interposition of a phenyl ring between the furan
and the nitro group radically changes the biological
activity; product from this formal replacement is in
fact a centrally acting muscle relaxant. In order to
prepare the target lead, reaction of the diazonium
salt *(49)* from p-nitroaniline *(48)* with furfural
using cupric chloride as catalyst affords the coupling
product 50. In a convergent synthesis, glycine
derivative 51 is converted to the urea 52. Acid-
catalyzed cyclization leads to aminohydantoin 53.
Semicarbazone formation from aldehyde 50 with hydrazine
derivative 53 affords *dantrolene (54)*.[13]

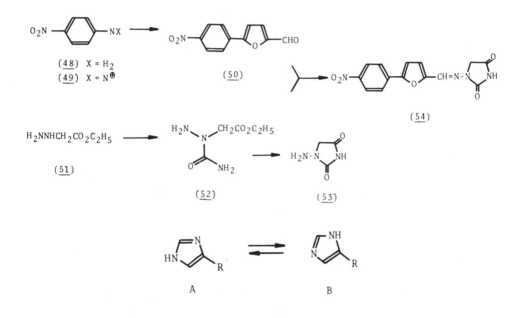

(48) X = H₂
(49) X = N⊕

(50)

(54)

(51)

(52)

(53)

A                    B

## 3. DERIVATIVES OF IMIDAZOLE

In its various oxidation states, the imidazole nucleus
has proven to be an unusually fertile source of
medicinal agents. Nitroimidazoles are very often
associated with antimicrobial activity, whereas
imidazolines are often present in drugs acting as
adrenergic agents. These considerations suggest, as
a working hypothesis, that these particular imidazole
derivatives are integral parts of the respective
pharmacophores.

While nitrofurans are often prepared as antibacterial agents, nitroimidazole forms the basis for
an extensive class of agents used in the treatment of
infections by the protozoans. Unlike bacterial infections, protozoal infections are seldom
life-threatening.  The physical discomfort occasioned
by such infections is, however, of sufficient
importance to provide a useful therapeutic place for
antiprotozoal agents.  A particularly common set of
such conditions are parasitic infections of the
genitalia caused by *Trichomonas vaginalis*.  These
disorders are called trichomoniasis.

One of the problems complicating the chemistry
of the imidazoles needed for preparing these agents
is their structural ambiguity.  Imidazoles undergo a
facile tautomeric equilibrium involving a shift of
the proton on nitrogen so that it is sometimes difficult to assign unambiguous structures to unsymmetri-
cally substituted derivatives.  Most drugs containing
this ring system are alkylated on one of the ring
nitrogens, which locks the molecule into a single
tautomeric form and removes the source of ambiguity.
The ambident character of imidazoles requires care in
selecting those conditions that will lead to alkylation on the desired nitrogen atom.

By way of illustration, nitration of 2-isopropyl-
imidazole (55) affords the 4- or 5-nitro derivative
(56, 57).  Alkylation with methyl iodide affords
isomer 58.  The same reaction carried out with dimethyl sulfate under neutral or acidic conditions
provides the isomer methylated at the alternate

nitrogen atom.   There is thus obtained the antiprotozoal agent *ipronidazole (59).*[14]

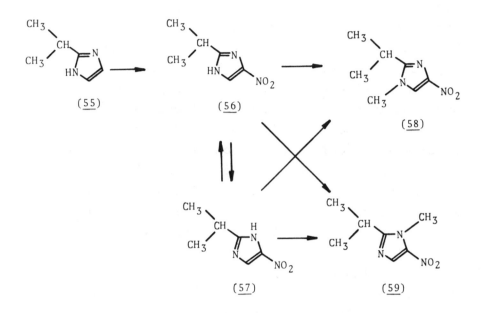

In a similar vein, alkylation of 4-(5)-nitro-
imidazole with N-(2-chloroethyl)morpholine affords a
mixture of N-alkylated imidazoles *(61 and 62).*   The
compound containing the adjacent ring substituents
*(61)* is the antitrichomonal agent *nimorazole.*[15]

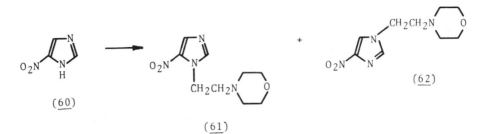

(60)    (61)    (62)

Acetylation of the hydroxymethyl imidazole *63* affords the corresponding ester *(64)*, nitration *(65)* followed by hydrolysis gives intermediate *66*, and reaction of this alcohol with potassium cyanate in hydrogen fluoride gives the carbamate *ronidazole (67)*.[16]

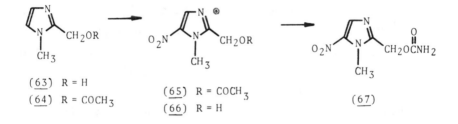

(63) R = H
(64) R = COCH₃

(65) R = COCH₃
(66) R = H

(67)

Treatment of 2-methyl-4-(5)-nitroimidazole at reduced temperatures with N-benzoylaziridine in the presence of boron trifluoride etherate leads regio-specifically to the N-alkylated derivative *(69)*. Hydrolysis of the amide function affords the primary amine *70*. Acylation of this with methylchlorothio-formate affords the antiprotozoal thioncarbamate, *carnidazole (71)*.[17] The same sequence, starting with the C-2 ethyl analogue *(72)* affords *sulnidazole (75)*.[17]

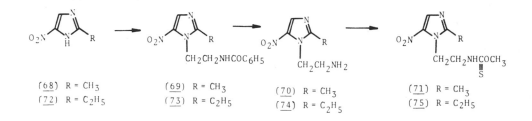

(68) R = CH₃
(72) R = C₂H₅

(69) R = CH₃
(73) R = C₂H₅

(70) R = CH₃
(74) R = C₂H₅

(71) R = CH₃
(75) R = C₂H₅

Hydroxymethylation (formaldehyde) of nitroimidazole *76* affords *77*, which is oxidized to aldehyde
*78*.   To prepare the other fragment for this convergent
synthesis, reaction of epichlorohydrin with morpholine
leads to the aminoepoxide *79*, which is reacted with
hydrazine to afford *80*.   Reaction of this substituted
hydrazine with dimethyl carbonate affords oxazolinone
*81* by sequential ester interchange reactions. Condensation of *81* with aldehyde *78* affords the antitrichomonal agent *moxnidazole (82).*[18]

Nitroimidazoles substituted by an aromatic ring
at the 2-position are also active as antitrichomonal
agents.   Reaction of p-fluorobenzonitrile *(83)* with
saturated ethanolic hydrogen chloride affords iminoether *84*.   Condensation of that intermediate with the
dimethyl acetal from 2-aminoacetaldehyde gives the
imidazole *85*.   Nitration of that heterocycle with
nitric acid in acetic anhydride gives *86*.   Alkylation
with ethylene chlorohydrin, presumably under neutral
conditions, completes the synthesis of the antitrichomonal, *flunidazole (87).*[19]

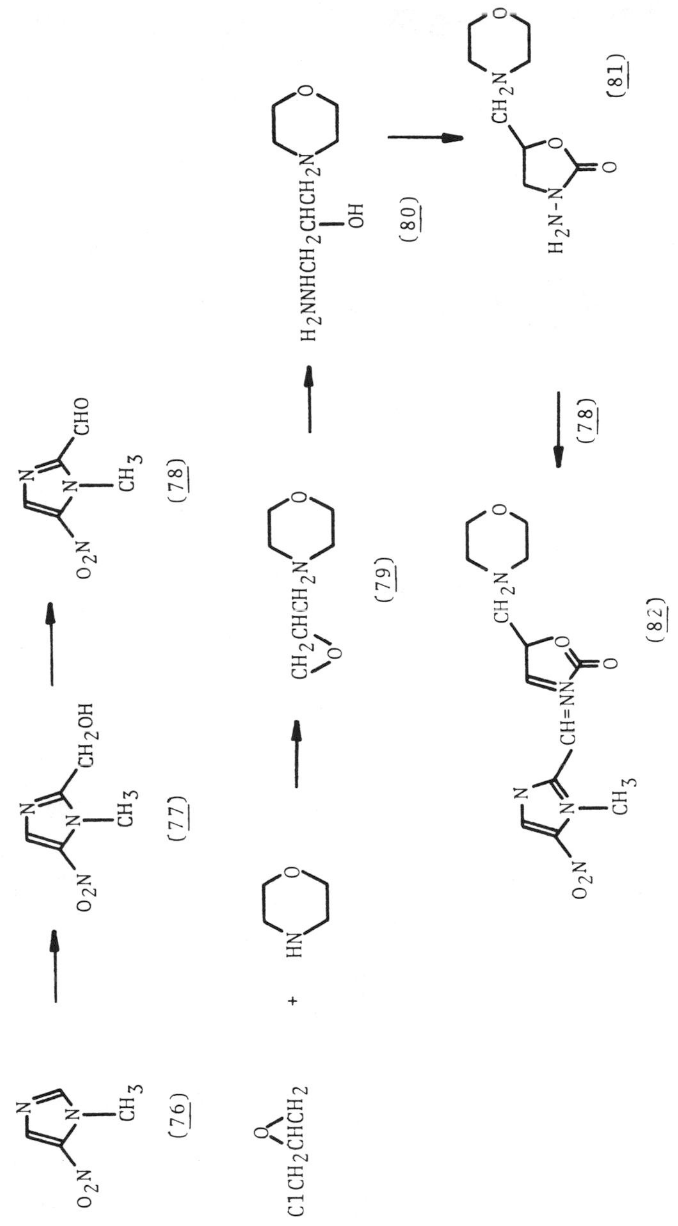

O₂N — imidazole ring — CH₃ **(76)**

+

ClCH₂CHCH₂ (epoxide) / HN–morpholine **(79)**

O₂N — imidazole(CH₂OH)(CH₃) **(77)**

O₂N — imidazole(CHO)(CH₃) **(78)**

CH₂CHCH₂N–morpholine (epoxide) **(79)**

H₂NNHCH₂CHCH₂N–morpholine, OH **(80)**

morpholine–NCH₂– oxazolidinone, H₂N–N **(81)**

morpholine–NCH₂– oxazolidinone, CH=NN–imidazole(CH₃)(O₂N) **(82)**

**(78)**

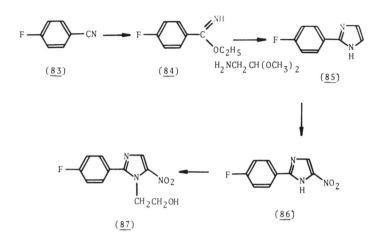

Imidazoles devoid of the nitro group no longer
show useful antiprotozoal activity, however, several

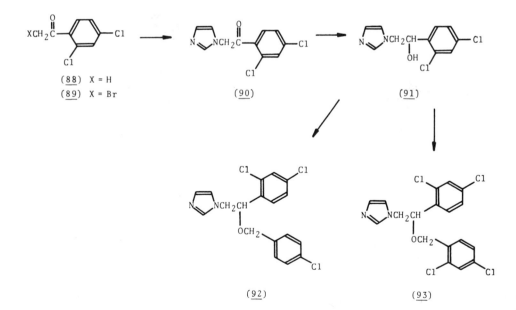

such compounds have proven to be efficacious as
antifungal agents.  Alkylation of imidazole with
bromoketone 89 prepared from 2,4-dichloroacetophenone
(89) affords the displacement product 90.  Reduction
of the carbonyl group with sodium borohydride gives
the corresponding alcohol 91.  Alkylation of the
alkoxide from that alcohol with 4-chlorobenzyl chloride
leads to *econazole (92)*[20]; alkylation with 2,4-di-
chlorobenzyl chloride gives *miconazole (93)*.[20]

    *Ethonam (99)*, an imidazole derivative with a
very different substitution pattern, is also reported
to possess antifungal activity.  To prepare it,
alkylation of aminotetralin 94 with methylchloro-
acetate gives the glycine derivative 95.  Heating
with formic acid then affords the amide 96; this
compound is then reacted with ethyl formate to yield
hydroxymethylene ester 97.  Reaction with isothio-
cyanic acid gives the imidazole-2-thiol 98.  (The

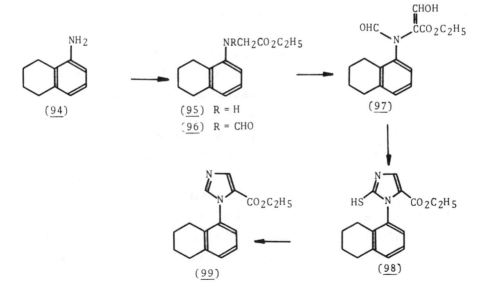

sequence may involve first hydrolysis of the formamido
group, followed by addition of the amine to isothio-
cyanic acid; cyclization of the thiourea nitrogen
with the formyl function would complete formation of
the heterocycle.) Desulfurization by means of Raney
nickel finishes the synthesis of *ethonam* (*99*).[21]

Not a hormone in the true sense of the word,
histamine (*100*) does act as a potent mediator, leading
to a host of biological responses. Many of the
symptoms attributed to allergies owe their manifes-
tations to exaggerated reaction to endogenous histamine released in response to an external stimulus.
Secretion of gastric acid is another process under the
control of histamine. It was hypothesized quite some
time ago that pathological conditions traceable to
excess histamine secretion or exaggerated sensitivity
to that base could be treated by compounds that
antagonized the response to histamine by competition
for its receptor sites. The benzhydryl type antihistaminic compounds for the treatment of allergic
diseases represent such competitive inhibitors.

It was noted, however, that a subset of responses
known to be triggered by histamine failed to be
blocked by the classical antihistaminic drugs. This,
as well as further sophisticated pharmacological
work, led to the classification of histamine receptors
as $H_1$ and $H_2$. To simplify grossly, the $H_1$ receptor
controls the responses familiar to every hayfever
sufferer; these effects can be alleviated readily by
classicial antihistamines. The latter interestingly
bear little or no structural similarity to histamine

itself.  The $H_2$ receptor on the other hand controls
secretion of acid in the stomach; classicial antihistamines have no effect on histamine-induced gastric
acid secretion.  Excess gastric acid secretion is
believed by many to be intimately involved in the
etiology of ulcers and exacerbation of preexisting
ulcers; thus, compounds that can act as selective
antagonists to the $H_2$ receptor are of considerable
potential therapeutic significance.

The $H_1$ antagonists were developed serendipitously
in the course of random screening.  On the other
hand, development of the $H_2$ antagonists started from
the premise that one of the best ways to produce an
antagonist is to investigate compounds that bear some
structural elements of the native agonists.  Pre-
cedence for this came from comparison of the structure
of β-adrenergic agonists and their blockers.  Systema-
tic modification of the histamine molecule achieved
its first success toward the preparation of an $H_2$
antagonist with *burimamide (107)*.[22]  Esterification of
diamino acid *101* leads to *102*.  Reduction with sodium
amalgam serves to convert the ester to a carbinol
*(103)*, and treatment of that aminoalcohol with
ammonium isothiocyanate affords the imidazothione *105*,
probably by the intermediacy of thiourea *104*.  (Strict
accounting of oxidation states seems to demand
oxidation of the carbinol to an aldehyde in the course
of this reaction.)  Reduction of the thione with iron
powder in acid probably proceeds via the enol form to
afford the desired imidazole *(106)*.[23]  Condensation

with methyl isothiocyanate completes the synthesis of
*burimamide (107)*.

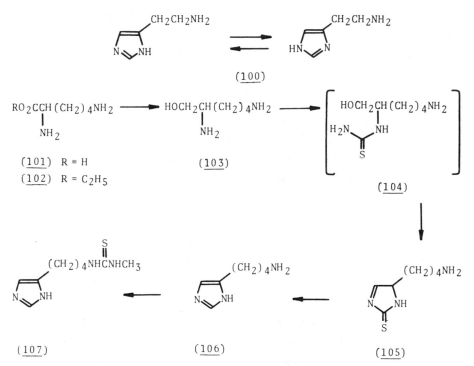

Further exploration of the histamine molecule revealed
that addition of a methyl group to the 4-position led
to an agonist with appreciably increased selectivity
for the $H_2$ receptor.[24] Application of that principle
to the prototype antagonist, as well as bioisosteric
replacement of one of the side chain methylene groups
by sulfur, affords *metiamide (111)*.[25] Reduction of
the imidazole carboxylic ester *108* gives the corresponding carbinol *(109)*. Reaction of that with 2-
mercaptoethylamine, as its hydrochloride, leads to
intermediate *110*. In the strongly acid medium, the

amine is completely protonated; this allows the thiol
to express its nucleophilicity without competition
and the acid also activates the alcoholic function
toward displacement. Finally, condensation of the
amine with methyl isothiocyanate gives *metiamide*
*(111).*  Side effects observed in some of the clinical
trials with this agent were attributed to the presence
of the thiourea function in the molecule.  A system-
atic search for a functional group isoelectronic with
thioureas revealed that cyanoguanides were biologically equivalent, and this substitution avoided the
side effects of the former.  In one of the schemes
for preparing the desired product, primary amine *110*
is reacted with complex nitrile *112*.  The resulting

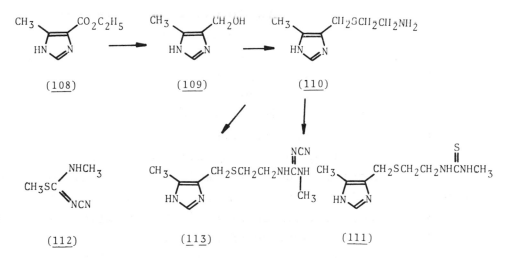

addition-elimination sequence affords the highly
successful agent for the treatment of ulcers,
*cimetidine (113).*[25]

Imidazole provides the nucleus for the antineoplastic agent *dacarbazine (116)*. Diazotization of
the commercially available aminoamide *114* with nitrous
acid gives diazonium salt *115*. Reaction of this salt
with dimethylamine under anhydrous conditions leads
to *dacarbazine (116)*.[26]

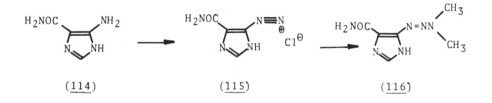

(114)                    (115)                    (116)

The diaryl indole, *indoxole (117*, see Chapter
11) represents a unique nonsteroidal antiinflammatory
agent in that it lacks the labile acidic proton
usually found in this class of drugs. Commercialization
of indoxole was precluded by its marked photosensiti-
zing side effect.  Subsequent work from another
laboratory showed that biological activity was
retained when the indole nucleus was replaced by
imidazole.  Condensation of 4,4'-dimethoxybenzil with
ammonium acetate and the ethyl hemiacetal of trifluoro-
acetaldehyde affords the aniinflammatory agent
*flumizole (120)* in a single step.[27]  The reaction can
be rationalized by assuming either initial formation
of a carbinolamine followed by condensation with one
of the aryl carbonyls, or, alternately, by formation
of an imine with one of the carbonyls followed by
attack on the hemiacetal.  Repetition of the process
and tautomerization will lead to the imidazole ring.

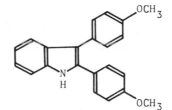

(117)

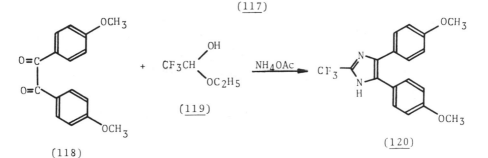

(118)                 (119)                            (120)

The pharmacology of both the endogenous amines
and drugs that act on the sympathetic nervous system
can be best explained by assuming that responses are
mediated by two different types of receptors.   The
existence of $\alpha$- and $\beta$-adrenergic receptors has by
now received considerable experimental backing.   (It
might be added as an aside that there is considerable
evidence that these two classes of receptors can be
further subdivided into $\beta_1$ and $\beta_2$ and possibly $\alpha_1$ and
$\alpha_2$ receptors.)   It is an interesting fact that with
few exceptions, drugs that act on the $\beta$-adrenergic
system all possess some chemical elements of the
endogenous agonist epinephrine.

In contrast to this, there are no such structural
constraints on $\alpha$-adrenergic agonists or antagonists.
Some of the most active $\alpha$-sympathomimetic agents in
fact contain an imidazoline moiety as part of the
pharmacophore.   The appropriate ring system can be

formed by a variety of methods.  One of the more
common involves condensation of a compound containing
a carbon atom at the acid oxidation level (nitrile,
imino ether) with ethylenediamine.  Thus, reaction of
the benzothiophenoacetonitrile derivative *121* with
ethylenediamine gives the adrenergic α-agonist *metizoline (122)*.[28]  As expected the α-adrenergic activity
of *122* is expressed as vasoconstriction.  The compound
is used topically as a nasal decongestant, acting on
the mucosal vasculature.

     In a similar vein, condensation of carboxylic
acid *123* with ethylenediamine leads to *domazoline
(124)*.[29]

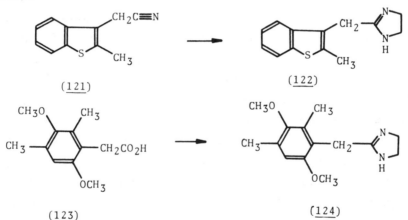

formed by a variety of methods.

Interposition of an oxygen atom between the
aromatic ring and the imidazoline-bearing side chain
leads to a compound reported to show antidepressant
activity.  Its preparation begins with alkylation of
phenol *125* with chloroacetonitrile to afford intermediate *126*.  Condensation of that nitrile with the

mono-p-toluenesulfonamide from ethylenediamine affords
the antidepressant imidazoline, *fenmetozole (127)*.[30]

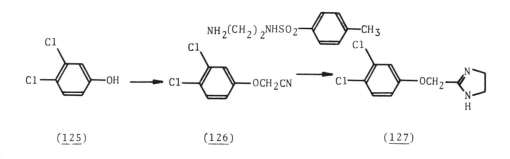

(125)                    (126)                    (127)

    Preparation of a rather more complex imidazoline
drug starts with the alkylation of the carbanion from
p-chlorophenylacetonitrile *(128)* with 2-bromopyridine.
Reaction of the product *(129)* with ethylenediamine
serves to form the imidazoline ring *(130)*.  Air
oxidation then affords the tertiary carbinol by
attack at the highly activated, multiply benzylic
carbon.  There is thus obtained the antidepressant
*dazadrol (131)*.[31]

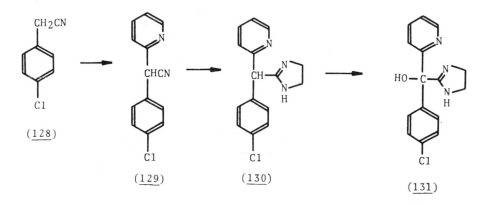

(128)              (129)        (130)              (131)

Replacement of hydrogen by fluorine in biologically active compounds often leads to marked increases
in potency.  Although much work has gone into incorporation of fluorine in various drug series, compounds
in which all the protons are replaced by that halogen
atom are rare.  One such relatively simple molecule
in which only the active hydrogens remain shows
sedative activity. Condensation of the imine from
hexafluoroacetone (132) with sodium cyanide leads to
a trimer which incorporates the cyanide (135). The
sequence can be rationalized by assuming, as the
first step, addition of cyanide to the imine function
to form an aminonitrile (133).  Reaction of the amine
function with a second molecule of imine leads to the
aminal 134.  Cyclization, followed by reaction of the
newly formed imine function with a third molecule of
133, gives the observed product as its sodium salt
(135).  Acidification (136), followed by hydrolytic

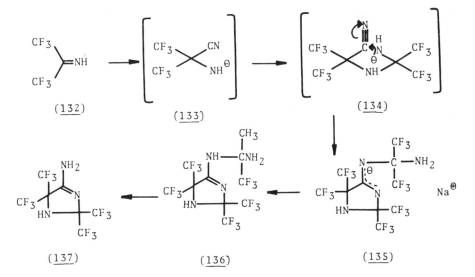

removal of the exocyclic aminal in strong acid, affords the sedative *midaflur (137)*.[32]

CNS activity apparently is retained when the heterocycle is changed to an imidazolidinone. Alkylation of the anion from the imidazolidinone *138* with dimethylaminoethyl chloride affords *imidoline (139)*,[33] a compound with tranquilizer activity.

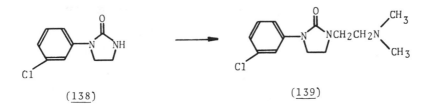

(138)                                    (139)

The imidazole ring system provides the nucleus for two diuretic agents with structures unusual for that activity.  Reaction of the N-cyanoaniline *140* (obtainable from the aniline *(139)* and cyanogen bromide) with N-methylchloroacetamide leads to the heterocycle *142*.  The sequence can be rationalized by

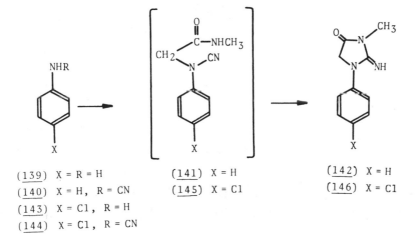

(139) X = R = H              (141) X = H              (142) X = H
(140) X = H, R = CN          (145) X = Cl             (146) X = Cl
(143) X = Cl, R = H
(144) X = Cl, R = CN

assuming N-alkylation of the aniline as the first
step (141). Cyclization of that hypothetical intermediate gives *azolimine* (142).[34] The same sequence
starting with p-chloroaniline (143) affords
*clazolimine* (146).[34]

Formal interchange of the carbonyl and imino
groups and replacement of the methyl group by acetonitrile interestingly affords a compound with antiinflammatory and presumably no diuretic activity.
Reaction of p-chlorophenylisocyanate (147, obtained
from 143 and phosgene) with iminodiacetonitrile (148)
gives the expected urea 149. Simple heating of that
intermediate leads to condensation of the aniline
with a nitrile group and formation of *nimazone*
(150).[35,36] It is of interest that this agent is
distantly related to the arylacetic acid antiinflammatory agent by a formal hydrolytic step.

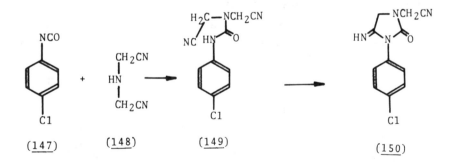

Hydantoins are well-known anticonvulsant agents
and as such have found extensive use in the treatment
of epilepsy. Replacement of one of the carbonyl
groups by thiocarbonyl is consistent with anticonvulsant activity. Thus, condensation of the ethyl ester

of leucine (151) with allyl isothiocyanate gives the
thiourea 152.  Cyclization of that intermediate
affords albutoin (153).[37]

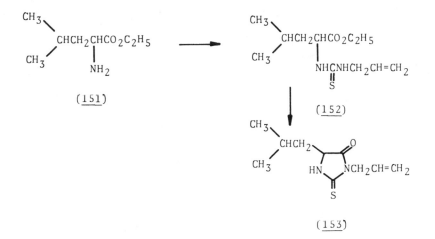

(151)

(152)

(153)

4.  DERIVATIVES OF PYRAZOLE

Pyrazolones rank among some of the more venerable
nonsteroidal antiinflammatory agents.  The activity
of antipyrine (154) was discovered not too long after
that of aspirin.  The preparation of a plethora of
analogues of that compound, all bearing additional
substitution at the 4-position, was described in some
detail in the earlier volume.

The pyrazolone ring is apparently sufficiently
nucleophilic to undergo Mannich reaction.  Thus,
condensation of antipyrine with formaldehyde and the
substituted morpholine 155 affords directly the
antiinflammatory agent morazone (156).[38]  It is of
interest that 155 has biological activity in its own
right; this amphetamine derivative, phenmetrazine,

not surprisingly, shows CNS stimulant and appetite-
suppressing activity.[39]

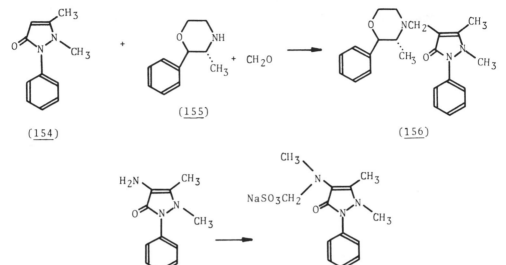

(155)

(154)

(156)

(157)

(158)

Many of the modifications of the pyrazolone
antiinflammatory agents are intended to increase the
limited hydrophilicity of the parent molecules.
Reaction of *aminopyrine (157)* with formaldehyde and
sodium hydrogen sulfite affords *dipyrone (158)*.  The
first step can be rationalized as an Eschweiler-Clark
type N-methylation reaction, with bisulfite acting as
the reducing agent.  The resulting mono N-methyl
analogue of *157* then apparently forms the sulfite
adduct of the carbinolamine of formaldehyde.


5.   DERIVATIVES OF OXAZOLE AND ISOXAZOLE
As has been noted previously, the benzene ring of the
phenylalkanoic acid antiinflammatory agents can be

replaced by a variety of other aryl groups.  However,
each of these subclasses does seem to have its own
specific SAR.  In those cases where the aryl group is
phenyl, optimal activity is obtained with a 2-arylated
propionic acid; acetic acids are suitable for other
classes.  In the case at hand a terminally substituted
propionic acid was chosen for further development.
Acylation of aminoketone *159* with the half acid
chloride-ethyl ester of succinic acid affords the
amide *160*. Cyclization by means of phosphorous oxychloride serves to form the oxazole ring.  Saponification of the ester gives the antiinflammatory
agent *oxaprozin (162)*.[40]

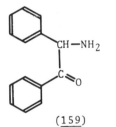

(159)

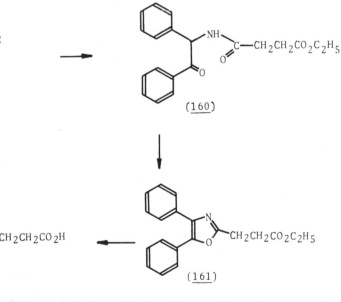

(160)

(162)          (161)

Amphetamine and its derivatives have been much
used--and abused--as weight-reducing agents.  As a
consequence of the CNS-stimulating activity shown by

these agents, they are fairly efficient in suppressing
symptoms of hunger.  Much ingenuity has been exercised
towards incorporating the phenylethylamine moiety in
various molecules, in attempts to dissociate the
anorexic activity of amphetamine from its other
effects on the CNS.  Never completely successful,
this work has led to some molecules that look quite
unlike the lead compound.  In one study, reduction of
the cyanohydrin from benzaldehyde (163) with lithium
aluminum hydride affords the corresponding aminoalcohol 164.  Reaction of this intermediate with
cyanogen bromide in the presence of sodium acetate
leads initially to the N-cyano intermediate 165.
Acetate is a sufficiently strong base to catalyze the
cyclization of the hydroxyl group onto the nitrile.
The initially formed iminooxazolidine then rearranges
to the more stable aminooxazoline (167) which is

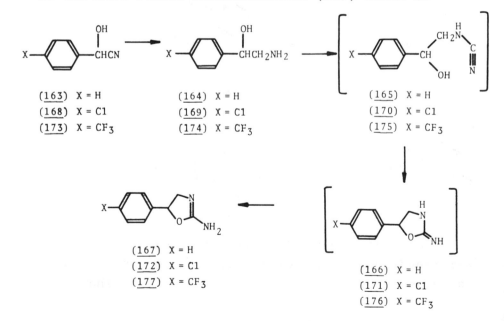

(163) X = H      (164) X = H      (165) X = H
(168) X = Cl     (169) X = Cl     (170) X = Cl
(173) X = CF₃    (174) X = CF₃    (175) X = CF₃

(167) X = H
(172) X = Cl
(177) X = CF₃

(166) X = H
(171) X = Cl
(176) X = CF₃

known as *aminorex (167)*.[41] The same sequence starting
from the cyanohydrins of p-chlorobenzaldehyde and
p-trifluoromethylbenzaldehyde affords, respectively,
*clominorex (172)*[41] and *fluminorex (177)*.[41]

Formal oxidation of the methylene group in
*aminorex* and dialkylation of the amine affords a
compound with antidepressant activity.  This activity
is also not totally unexpected in a compound related,
although very distantly, to amphetamine.  Condensation
of the alkoxide obtained from treatment of ethyl
mandelate *(178)* with N,N-dimethylcyanamide can be
envisioned to form initially the adduct *179*.  Cyclization of the anion onto the ester group then serves
to form the oxazolinone ring.  There is thus obtained
the antidepressant *thozalinone (180)*.[42]

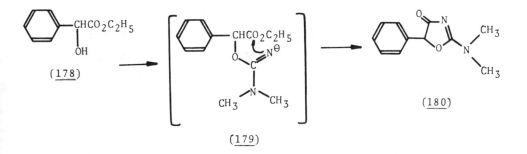

*Phenylephrine (181)* is a well-known α-sympatho-
mimetic agent. As a consequence of this activity, the
drug is used extensively for those conditions requiring
a vasoconstricting agent.  Modification of the functionality so as to include the aliphatic oxygen and
basic nitrogen in an oxazolidine ring is compatible
with this biological activity.  Condensation of

norphenylephrine *(182)* with cycloheptanone results in
formation of the cyclic carbinolamine derivative
*ciclafrine (183)*.[43]

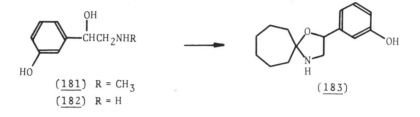

(181)  R = CH_3
(182)  R = H

(183)

Hydrazides of isonicotinic acid, *isoniazid* for
example, were among the first compounds to be used as
antidepressant drugs.  It is generally accepted that
these agents owe their action to increased brain
levels of neurotransmitter amines by inhibition of
the enzyme monoamine oxidase (MAO).  The pyridine
ring present in these molecules can, interestingly,
be replaced by an isoxazole moiety.  Thus, interchange of the isoxazole ester *184* with benzylhydrazine
affords directly the MAO-inhibiting antidepressant
*isocarboxazid (186)*.[44]

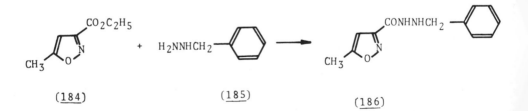

(184)                        (185)

(186)

## 6. DERIVATIVES OF THIAZOLE

The intensive research on β-adrenergic blocking
agents has been discussed in some detail in Chapter
5. As noted there, interposition of an oxymethylene
moiety between the aromatic ring and the aminoalcohol
side chain of sympathomimetic agents is often compatible with antagonist activity. More recently it has
been found that replacement of the aromatic ring in
sympathomimetic amines or their antagonists by a
heterocycle often gives active compounds (see also
*timolol*, below). In the preparation of one example,
displacement of halogen on 2-bromothiazole *(187)* by
means of the alkoxide from glycerol acetonide (188)
affords the ether *189*. Hydrolysis of the acetonide
leads to the glycol *190*. Reaction with an equivalent
of methanesulfonyl chloride gives the mesylate *(191)*.
(Although the terminal mesylate predominates, some
secondary ester is probably formed as well; this is

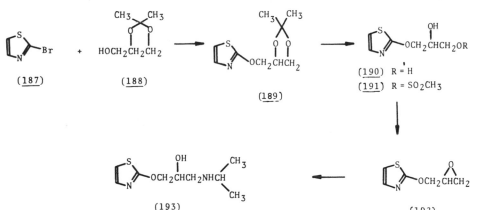

not separated since it serves just as well for the
subsequent reaction.)  Exposure of the hydroxymesylate
to sodium methoxide results in formation of the
epoxide by internal displacement (192).  Opening of
the oxirane by means of isopropylamine affords finally
tazolol (193).[45]  This compound, unexpectedly, does
not show the properties of a classical β-adrenergic
blocking agent; tazolol retains sufficient intrinsic
sympathomimetic activity to be described as a cardiotonic agent.

As noted above, nitrofurans and nitroimidazoles
have proven useful moieties for the preparation of
antibacterial and antiprotozoal agents.  It is thus
of note that nitrothiazoles have also been used
successfully in the preparation of antiparasitic
agents.  Condensation of 6-nitro-2-aminothiazole
(194, available from nitration of aminothiazole) with
ethylisocyanate yields the antiprotozoal agent
nithiazole (195).[46]  In a similar vein, condensation

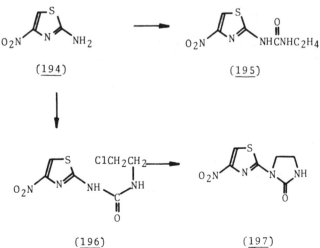

of *194* with 2-chloroethylisocyanate leads to the
chloroethylurea *196*.   Treatment with base serves to
form the pendant imidazolinone ring.   There is thus
obtained the antischistosomal compound *niridazole*
*(197)*.[47]
     The thiazole ring has been found to be an
occasional surrogate for a phenyl ring in certain
antiinflammatory agents.   Note that the side chain is
restricted to a simple acetic acid in this series.
Reaction of p-chloro-2-mercaptoacetophenone *(198)*
with ethyl cyanoacetate in the presence of base
affords thiazole *200*. The reaction may involve an
adduct such as the iminothioether *199* as an intermediate.   Saponification of the ester moiety of *200*
then gives the antiinflammatory agent *fenclozic acid*
*(201)*.[48]

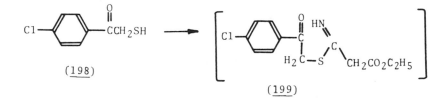

(198)

(199)

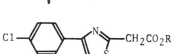

(200)  R = C2H5
(201)  R = H

A distantly related acid with a more highly
functionalized ring shows choleretic rather than
antiinflammatory activity.  That is, the compound is
useful in those conditions in which the flow of bile
is to be increased.  Construction of the thiazolone
ring is accomplished by a method analogous to that
used above to build the thiazole ring.  Thus, condensation of ethyl mercaptoacetate with ethyl cyanoacetate
leads to the thiazolinone (203); an intermediate such
as 202, involving addition of mercaptide to the
nitrile function, can be reasonably invoked.
Methylation of 203 with methyl sulfate proceeds on
nitrogen with the concomitant shift of the double
bond to give 204.  Bromination of the active methylene
(205) followed by displacement of halogen by piperidine
affords the choleretic *piprozolin* (206).[49]

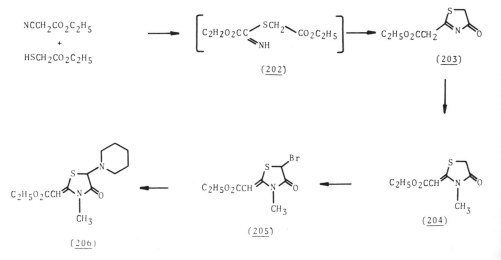

### 7.  MISCELLANEOUS FIVE-MEMBERED HETEROCYCLES
Acylation with 3-chloropropionyl chloride of the

amidoxime *207* from 2-ethylphenylacetonitrile gives
the corresponding N-acylated derivative *208*.   This
cyclizes to the oxadizole *(209)* on heating.
Displacement of chlorine with diethylamine affords
the muscle relaxant-analgesic agent *proxazole (210)*.[50]

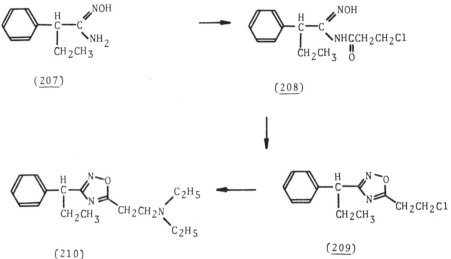

(207)

(208)

(210)

(209)

Thiadiazoles have proven of some utility as
aromatic nuclei for medicinal agents.   For example,
the previous volume detailed the preparation of a
series of *"azolamide"* diuretic agents based on this
class of heterocycle.   It is thus of note that the
1,2,5-thiadiazole ring provides the nucleus for a
clinically useful agent for treatment of hypertension
which operates by an entirely different mechanism,
β-adrenergic blockade.   In its preparation, reaction
of the amide-nitrile *211* with sulfur monochloride
leads directly to the substituted thiadiazole *212*.[51]

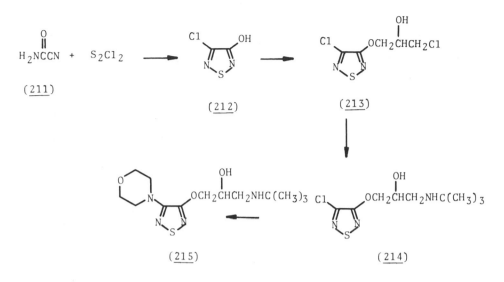

Condensation of that intermediate with epichlorohydrin
in the presence of a catalytic amount of piperidine
affords the chlorohydrin *213*, admixed with some
epoxide.   Reaction with tertiary butylamine completes
construction of the propanolamine side chain.
Displacement of the remaining halogen atom of *214*
with morpholine under more strenuous conditions
affords *timolol (215).*[52]

   A somewhat different scheme is used to gain
entry to the alternate symmetrical 1,3,4-thiadiazole
ring system.   Reaction of thiosemicarbazide with
isovaleric acid affords the ring system *(217)* in one
step.   The reaction may be rationalized by positing
acylation to intermediate *216* as the first step.
Sulfonylation of the amino group of *217* with p-
methoxybenzenesulfonyl chloride affords the oral
hypoglycemic agent *isobuzole (218).*[53]   Careful
examination of the structure will reveal elements of

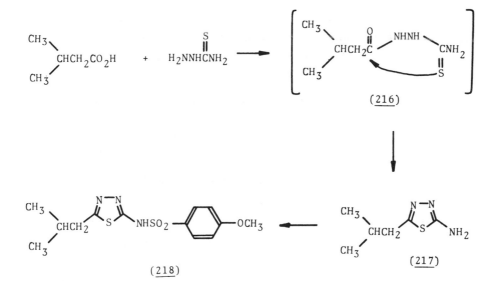

(216)

(218)                                                    (217)

the sulfonylurea functionality often associated with that activity.

## REFERENCES

1.  W. Herz and J. L. Rogers, *J. Am. Chem. Soc.*, *73*, 4921 (1951).

2.  J. R. Carson, D. N. McKinstry and S. Wong, *J. Med. Chem.*, *14*, 646 (1971).

3.  G. Lambelin, J. Roba, C. Gillet and N. P. Buu-Hoi, German Patent 2,261,965 (1973); *Chem. Abstr.*, *79*: 78604a (1973).

4.  W. G. Frankenburg and A. A. Vaitekunas, *J. Am. Chem. Soc.*, *79*, 149 (1957).

5.  C. D. Lunsford, A. D. Cale, Jr., J. W. Ward, B.

V. Franko and H. Jenkins, *J. Med. Chem.*, *7*, 302 (1964).

6.  C. L. Miller and R. A. Hall, U. S. Patent 3,183,245 (1965).

7.  Anon., British Patent 1,106,007 (1968); *Chem. Abstr.*, *68*: 86809e (1968).

8.  C. A. Johnson, U. S. Patent 3,253,987 (1966); *Chem. Abstr.*, *65*: 4332c (1966).

9.  F. F. Ebetino, British Patent 1,016,840 (1966); *Chem. Abstr.*, *64*: 11215c (1966).

10. J. G. Michels, U. S. Patent 2,927,110 (1960).

11. A. Fujita, M. Nakata, S. Minami and H. Takamatsu, *Yakugaku Zasshi*, *86*, 1014 (1966).

12. W. R. Sherman and D. E. Dickson, *J. Org. Chem.*, *27*, 1351 (1962).

13. H. R. Snyder, Jr., C. S. Davis, R. K. Bickerton and R. P. Halliday, *J. Med. Chem.*, *10*, 807 (1967).

14. K. Butler, H. L. Howes, J. E. Lynch and D. K. Pirie, *J. Med. Chem.*, *10*, 891 (1967).

15. P. N. Giraldi, V. Mariotti, G. Namini, G. P. Tosolini, E. Dradi, W. Logemann, I. de Carnevi and G. Monti, *Arzneimittelforsch.*, *20*, 52 (1970).

16. Anon., Netherlands Patent 6,609,552 (1967); *Chem. Abstr.*, *67*: 54123u (1967).

17. J. Heeres, J. H. Mostmans and R. Maes, German Patent 2,429,755 (1975); *Chem. Abstr.*, *82*: 156309m (1975).

18. C. Rufer, H.J. Kessler and E. Schroder, *J. Med. Chem.*, *14*, 94 (1971).

19. Anon., Netherlands Patent 6,413,814 (1965); *Chem. Abstr.*, *63*: 18097b (1965).

20. E. F. Godefroi, J. Heeres, J. Van Cutsem and
    P. A. J. Janssen, *J. Med. Chem.*, *12*, 784 (1969).

21. E. F. Godefroi, J. Van Cutsem, C. A. M. Van Der
    Eycken and P. A. J. Janssen, *J. Med. Chem.*, *10*,
    1160 (1967).

22. J. W. Black, W. A. M. Duncan, C. J. Durant, C.
    R. Ganellin and E. M. Parsons, *Nature*, *236*, 385
    (1972).

23. S. Akabori and T. Kaneko, J. Chem. Soc., Japan,
    53, 207 (1932); *Chem. Abstr.*, *27:* 293 (1933).

24. G. J. Durant, J. C. Emmett, C. R. Ganellin, A.
    M. Roe and R. A. Slater, *J. Med. Chem.*, *19*,
    923 (1976).

25. G. J. Durant, J. C. Emmett, C. R. Ganellin, P.
    D. Miles, M. E. Parsons, H. D. Prain and G. R.
    White, *J. Med. Chem.*, *20*, 901 (1977).

26. Y. F. Shealy, C. A. Krauth and J. A. Montgomery,
    *J. Org. Chem.*, *27*, 2150 (1962).

27. J. G. Lombardino, German Patent 2,155,558 (1972);
    *Chem. Abstr.*, *77:* 101607 (1972).

28. Anon., French Patent M1614 (1963); *Chem. Abstr.*,
    *58:* 12574e (1964).

29. Anon., French Patent 1,353,049 (1964); *Chem.
    Abstr.*, *61:* 4146c (1964).

30. M. Julia, Bull. *Soc. Chim. Fr.*, *1365* (1956).

31. L. A. Walter, German Patent 1,905,353 (1969);
    *Chem. Abstr.*, *72:* 317904 (1970).

32. W. J. Middleton and W. J. Krespan, *J. Org. Chem.*,
    *35*, 1480 (1970).

33. W. B. Wright, Jr., and H. J. Brabander, Belgian Patent 623,942 (1962); *Chem. Abstr.*, *60:* 14513e (1964).

34. J. W. Hanifin, Jr., R. Z. Gussin and E. Cohen, German Patent 2,251,354 (1973); *Chem. Abstr.*, *79:* 18717e (1973).

35. F. K. Kirchner and A. W. Zalay, U. S. Patent 3,429,911 (1969); *Chem. Abstr.*, *70:* 96783b (1969).

36. J. Perronnet and J.P. Demonte, *Bull. Soc. Chim. Fr.*, *1168* (1970).

37. S. Oba, Y. Koseki and K. Fukawa, J. Soc. Sci. Phot. Japan, 13, 33 (1951); *Chem. Abstr.*, *46:* 3885e (1952).

38. O. Hengen, H. Siemer and A. Doppstadt, *Arzneimittelforsch.*, *8*, *421* (1958).

39. F. H. Clarke, *J. Org. Chem.*, *27*, 3251 (1962).

40. Anon., French Patent 2,001,036 (1969); *Chem. Abstr.*, *72:* 66930w (1970).

41. G. I. Poos, J. R. Carson, J. D. Rosenau, A. P. Roszkowski, N. M. Kelley and J. McGowin, *J. Med. Chem.*, *6*, 266 (1963).

42. R. A. Hardy, C. F. Howell and C. Q. Quinones, U. S. Patent 3,037,990 (1962).

43. G. Satzinger and M. Herrmann, German Patent 2,336,746 (1975); *Chem. Abstr.*, *83:* 10047 (1975).

44. T. S. Gardner, E. Wenis and J. Lee, *J. Med. Chem.*, *2*, 133 (1970).

45. A. P. Roszkowski, A. M. Strosberg, L. M. Miller, J. A. Edwards, B. Berkoz, G. S. Lewis, O. Halpern and J. H. Fried, *Experientia*, *28*, 1336 (1972).

46.  R. C. O'Neill, A. J. Basso and K. Pfister, U. S. Patent 2,755,285 (1956); *Chem. Abstr.*, *51:* 2873a (1957).

47.  C. R. Lambert, M. Wilhelm, H. Striebel, F. Kradolfer and P. Schmidt, *Experientia*, *20*, 452 (1964).

48.  Anon., Netherlands Patent 6,614,130 (1967); *Chem. Abstr.*, *68:* 68976g (1968).

49.  G. Satzinger, Ann., 665, 150 (1963).

50.  Anon., British Patent 924,608 (1963); *Chem. Abstr.*, *59:* 6415h (1963).

51.  L. M. Weinstock, P. Davis, B. Handelsman and R. Tull, *Tetrahedron Lett.*, 1263 (1966).

52.  B. K. Wasson, W. K. Gibson, R. S. Stuart, H. W. R. Williams and C. H. Yates, *J. Med. Chem.*, *15*, 651 (1972).

53.  F. L. Chubb and J. Nissenbaum, *Can. J. Chem.*, *37*, 1121 (1959).

# 9

# Six-Membered Ring Heterocycles

The six-membered ring heterocycles are of exceptional importance in the context of willingly self administered organic substances. One need only mention glucose and nicotine to make this point. The biological acceptability, within reasonable limits, of these materials is paralleled by the availability of a substantial number of drugs.

Substitution of a pyridine ring for a benzene ring often is compatible with retention of biological activity and occasionally this moiety is an essential part of the pharmacophore. Such substitution of =N for CH= is an example of the common medicinal chemical strategy known as bioisosterism.

### 1. PYRIDINES

The aliphatic hydrogens of α-picoline (1) are relatively acidic, so that treatment with phenyl lithium

produces the carbanion which can add to chloral,
forming 2.  Acid hydrolysis leads to unsaturated acid
3, which is sequentially reduced to acid 4, Fischer-

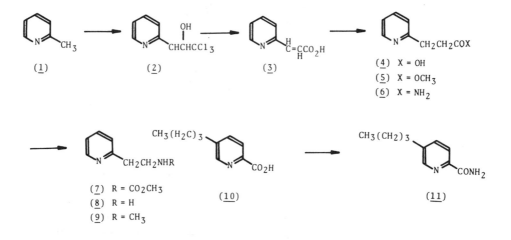

esterified to 5 and transamidated to 6.  Hofmann
rearrangement with NaOBr followed by methanol gives
carbamate 7, which is hydrolyzed to 8 and monomethy-
lated.  This fairly lengthy process affords the
vasodilator, *betahistine (9)*.[1]

As the result of a screening program examining
microbial fermentation products for pharmacological
activity (other than antibiotic activity), *fusaric
acid (10)* was isolated from *Fusarium oxysporum*
following the discovery that extracts were potent
inhibitors of dopamine β-hydroxylase, and thus inter-
fered with the biosynthesis *in vivo* of the pressor
neurohormone, norepinephrine.  To refine this lead,
amidation of *10 via* the acid chloride was carried out

to give the antihypertensive analogue *bupicomide*
*(11)*.[2]

Reaction of ethyl picolinate *(12)* with dimsyl
sodium (from dimethylsulfoxide and sodium hydride)
produces *oxisuran (13)*, an antineoplastic agent.[3]

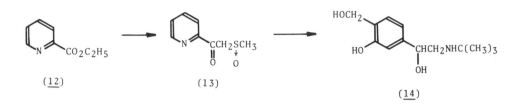

(12)                        (13)

(14)

An adrenergic $\beta_2$-receptor agonist related concept-
ually to *salbutamol (14)* can be made by substituting
a pyridine ring for the benzene.  In this case synthesis starts by hydroxymethylation and formation of
the o-benzylether of 3-hydroxypyridine *(15)* to give
*16*.  Manganese dioxide perferentially oxidizes the
sterically more accessible primary alcohol group to
the aldehyde, and subsequent aldol condensation with
nitromethane produces nitrocarbinol *17*.  Catalytic
reduction with Raney nickel gives amine *18* which
reacts in turn with t-butyl bromide to give amine *19*.
Hydrogenolysis of the protecting benzyl moiety finishes
the synthesis of the bronchodilator, *pirbuterol*
*(20)*.[4]

Substantial interest in the pharmacological
properties of the nonsteroidal antiinflammatory
agents related to *mefenamic* and *flufenamic acid* led
to examination of a series of aminopyridines instead

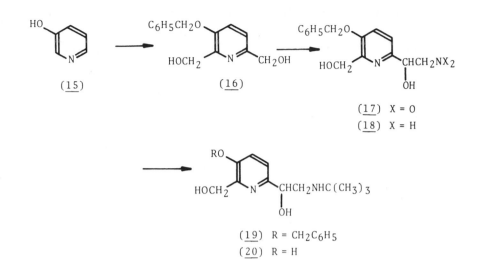

of anthranilates. Thermal displacement of the halogen of 2-chloronicotinate derivatives *(21)* with the
requisite anilines *(22 or 23)* led to antiinflammatory
agents *flunixin (24)*[5] and *clonixin (25)*,[6] respectively.

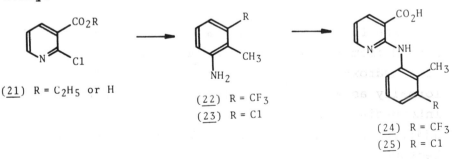

The glyceryl ester of *clonixin, clonixeril (28)*,
is also an antiinflammatory agent. It was prepared

*via* a somewhat roundabout method. *Clonixin (25)* was
reacted with chloroacetonitrile and triethylamine to
give *26*. Heating *26* with potassium carbonate and
glycerol acetonide displaced the activating group to
produce ester *27* which was deblocked in acetic acid
to produce *clonixeril*.[7]

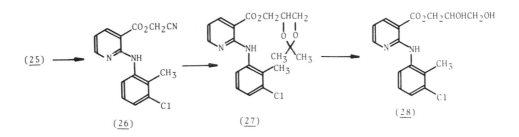

Interestingly, a substance somewhat closely
related to *flunixin*, *triflocin (30)*, is a diuretic
rather than an antiinflammatory agent. It can be
prepared by nucleophilic aromatic displacement on 4-
chloronicotinic acid *(29)* with m-trifluoromethyl-
aniline.[8]

The topical antifungal agent *ciclopirox (32)* was
formed from 2-pyrone *31* by an azaphilone reaction
with hydroxylamine.[9] This may be viewed at least
formally as an ester (lactone)-amide exchange to an
intermediate oximinoester, which ring-closes *via* an
addition-elimination sequence to expel the original
lactone ring oxygen in favor of the hydroxylamine
nitrogen. Lactones which readily convert to lactams
in this manner are known as azaphilones.

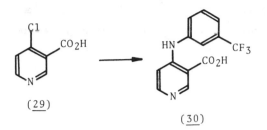

(29)

(30)

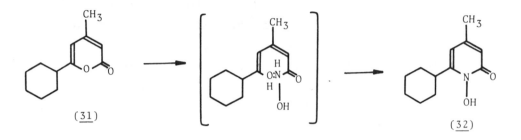

(31)

(32)

A 1,4-dihydropyridine having coronary vasodilatory activity and, therefore, intended for relief of the intense chest pains of angina pectoris is *nifedipine* (34). Using a portion of the classical Hantzsch pyridine synthesis, condensation of two moles of

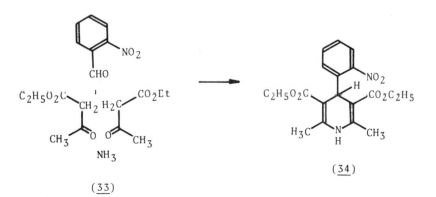

(33)

(34)

ethyl acetoacetate and one each of ammonia and
2-nitrobenzaldehyde (collectively *33*) leads to
*nifedipine*.[10] In the classical Hantzsch process, an
oxidative step is needed to produce the pyridine ring
system.

### 2. PIPERIDINES

Perhaps following up the rigid analogue concept, an
epinephrine analogue with a cyclized side chain is
the $\beta_2$agonist/bronchodilator, *rimiterol* (*38*). Reaction
of 3,4-dimethoxybenzaldehyde (*35*) with 2-pyridyl
lithium gives carbinol *36*. Oxidation with permanganate
and ether cleavage with HBr produces catechol *37*.
Hydrogenation with a palladium catalyst in acid
medium leads to *rimiterol* by reduction of both the
pyridine ring and the ketone function.[11]

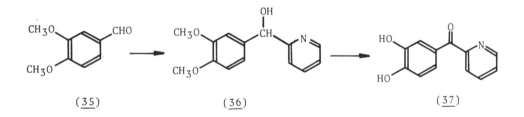

(35)              (36)              (37)

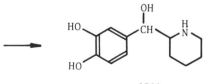

(38)

Propiophenone *(39)* does not easily form ketals
directly.  A solution for this difficulty involves
conversion to the *gem*-dichloride *(40)* with $PCl_5$ and
solvolysis to the ketal *(41)* using sodium methoxide.
Acid-catalyzed ketal exchange with piperidine glycol
*42* leads to the parenteral anesthetic, *etoxadrol*
*(43)*.[12]  Repetition of the same steps starting with
benzophenone led to *dioxadrol (44)*, which is described
as an antidepressant agent.[12]

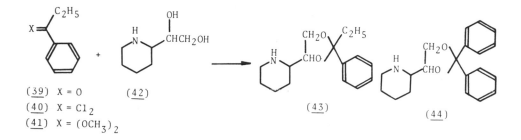

(39) X = O          (42)
(40) X = Cl$_2$
(41) X = $(OCH_3)_2$

(43)

(44)

In the course of an investigation aimed at
refining hypotensive leads, 4-benzylpyridine *(45)* was
reduced with a platinum catalyst in acidic medium to
the corresponding piperidine, and this was alkylated
with dimethylaminoethyl chloride to give *46*.  This

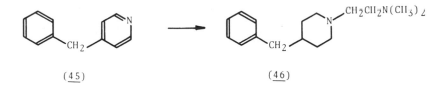

(45)                              (46)

product, *pimetine*, is primarily of interest as a
hypolipidemic agent.[13]

Possibly patterned after the clinically useful
p-fluorobutyrophenone *haloperidol*, *lenperone (49)* too
is a potentially useful tranquilizer.  The synthesis
proceeds from ketone *47* by alkylation with halide *48*
followed by deketalization.[14]

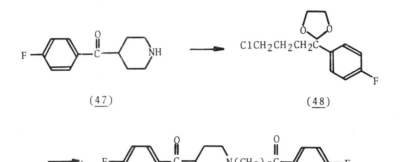

(47)                                        (48)

(49)

The reader will recall that many sulfonylurea
derivatives are oral hypoglycemic agents and therefore useful oral antidiabetic drugs in adult-onset
diabetes.  One more complex than most is *gliamilide*
*(54)*.  Piperidine derivative *50*, prepared by reduction
of the corresponding pyridine, undergoes amide exchange
to *51* on heating in pyridine with sulfamide ($H_2NSO_2NH_2$).
Reaction with hydrazine and HCl removes the phthaloyl
protecting group, and acylation of the liberated
amino function with 2-methoxynicotinyl chloride gave
sulfonylurea *52*.  When this was reacted with the

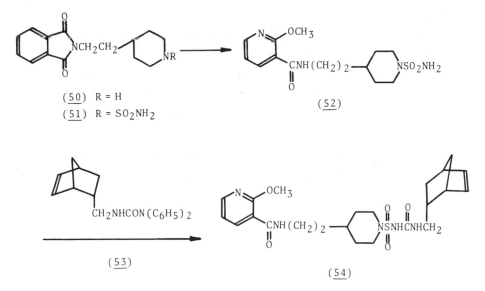

(50) R = H

(51) R = SO$_2$NH$_2$

(52)

(53)

(54)

bicyclic *endo*-diphenyl urea *53*, amide exchange took place with expulsion of the better leaving group in this case, diphenylamine. There was thus obtained *gliamilide (54)*.[15]

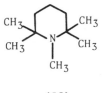

(55)

A number of years ago, pentamethylpiperidine *55* was found to be a rather potent, though not very specific, ganglionic blocking agent. This finding was of particular interest, as it was at that time believed that a quaternary ammonium function was a

minimal structural feature for such drugs.  In refining 55 as a lead, triacetone amine (56, synthesized from acetone, ammonia and calcium chloride) was
reduced with sodium borohydride and N-alkylated to
give 57.  Cyanoethylation with acrylonitrile (with
the aid of sodium t-butoxide) led to nitrile 58.
Reduction with lithium aluminum hydride produced the
primary amine and Eschweiler-Clark methylation ($CH_2O$
and $HCO_2H$) completed the synthesis of pemerid (59),
an antitussive agent.[16]  This activity is incidentally
unrelated to ganglionic blockade.

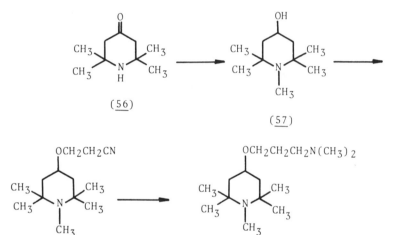

Yet another (see lenperone) butyrophenone related
to haloperidol is pipamperone (64).  N-benzyl-4-
piperidone (60) has a venerable history as starting
material for both central analgesics and CNS drugs.
This synthon has been used by the Janssen group as a
building block for numerous such drugs.  Reaction of

60 with KCN and piperidine HCl, leads to the aminonitrile (61). The reaction probably represents
cyanation of the intermediate imine. Hydrolysis with
hot 90% sulfuric acid hydrates the nitrile to the
carboxamide (62) and catalytic reduction deblocks the
amine to give 63. Alkylation with p-fluorophenyl-3-
chloropropyl ketone using a catalytic amount of KI
completes the synthesis.[17]

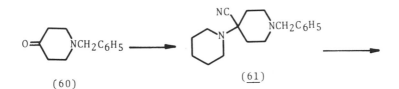

(60)                          (61)

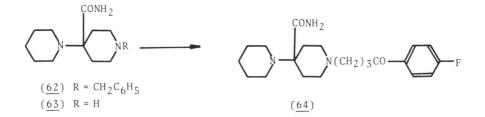

(62) R = CH$_2$C$_6$H$_5$
(63) R = H                          (64)

An interesting reaction ensues when the intermediate synthetic precursor (65) to synthon 60 is
heated with phenylenediamine. The reaction can be
rationalized as involving initial enamine-imine formation (66), followed by intramolecular attack on the
ester carbonyl groups resulting in carbamate formation
(67), which carbamate undergoes intramolecular trans-
amidation to give urea 68. Other scenarios can be
proposed and defended, but the net result is formation

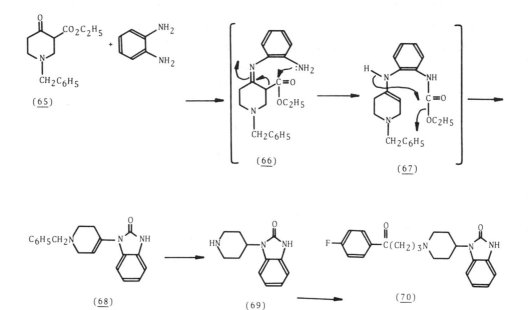

of complex urea derivative *68*, which readily undergoes
catalytic reduction to *69*, a versatile intermediate
for the preparation of a variety of potential drugs.
For example, alkylation with the requisite *haloperidol*
fragment led to the tranquilizer, *benperidol (70)*.[18]
Minor variants led to the tranquilizers *oxiperomide*
*(71)*,[19] *pimozide (72)*,[20] and *clopimozide (73)*,[21] and
the analgesic, *benztriamide (74)*.[22]

Another fruitful investigation was based upon
the cyanohydrin of ketone *60*. This substance *(75)*
undergoes hydride reduction to the corresponding
aminoalcohol, which forms cyclic carbamate *76* on

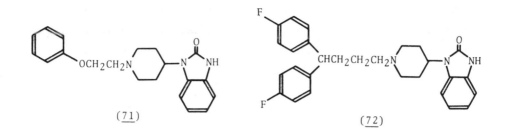

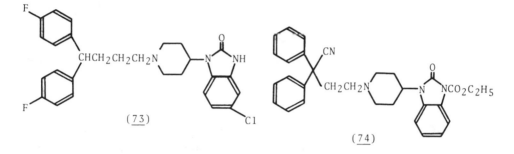

heating with diethylcarbonate. Hydrogenolysis of the
N-benzyl group and alkylation of the liberated amino
group with phenethyl chloride gives *fenspiride (77)*,
an blocking bronchodilator.[23]

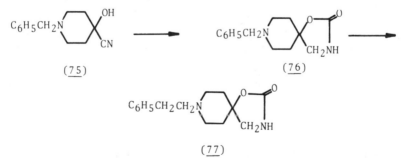

Imidazolone analogues are available, for example,
starting with piperidone *60* and reacting this with
KCN and aniline followed by hydration to amide *78* in

90% sulfuric acid.   Heating *78* with formamide results
in the desired imidazolone formation (*79*).  Catalytic
hydrogenolysis (*80*) and suitable alkylation of this

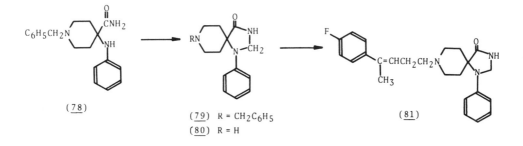

(*78*)

(*79*)  R = CH$_2$C$_6$H$_5$
(*80*)  R = H

(*81*)

secondary amine gives the tranquilizer, *spiriline*
(*81*).[24]  The closely related tranquilizers *fluspiriline*
(*82*)[25] and *fluspiperone* (*83*) are made in the same
general way.

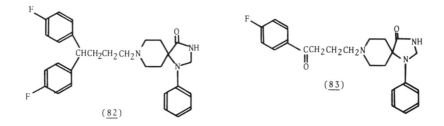

(*82*)

(*83*)

When piperidone *60* is condensed with phenylacetonitrile, using sodium methoxide, *84* results.
Catalytic reduction unexpectedly is nonselective, not
only reducing the olefinic linkage, but also removing

the benzyl protecting group.  The product (85) has to
be rebenzylated to 86 before cyanoethylation to 87
can be carried out.  Hydrolysis of 87 with strong
acid stopped at the glutarimide stage with the production of benzetimide (88), an orally active anticholinergic agent.[26]

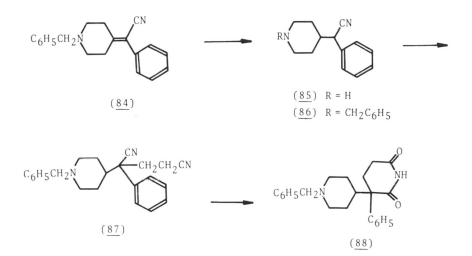

(84)

(85)  R = H
(86)  R = CH₂C₆H₅

(87)

(88)

The action of phenyl Grignard reagent on piperidone 60 followed by dehydration and deblocking leads
to intermediate 89. When this is reacted with complex
halide 90, fenpipalone (91), an antiinflammatory
agent, results.[27]  The requisite halide (90) is made
by treatment of hydroxy pyrrolidine 94 with phosgene.
The reaction may proceed via N-acylation to 93 which
would undergo ring opening as shown with chloride ion
to give 92, which would then cyclize as indicated to
give 90.  Such dealkylation of tertiary amines by
acyl halides is a well-established reaction.  An

alternate and perhaps equally credible intermediate
in this particular case would be bicyclo carbamate
95, which would be formed whether either O- or
N-acylation were the first event.

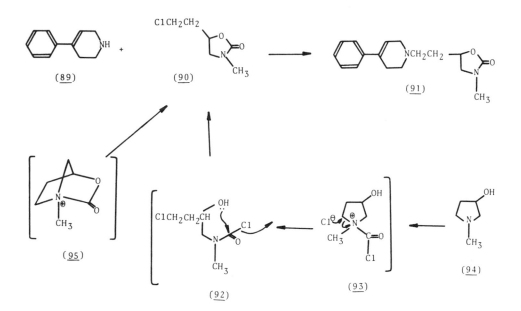

A number of substituted β-aminoacetates inhibit
the enzyme cholinesterase.  The main function of this
enzyme is to hydrolyze acetyl choline and thereby
terminate the action of that substrate as a neurotransmitter.  Such inhibition is functionally equivalent to the administration of exogenous acetylcholine.
Direct administration of the neurotransmitter substance itself is not a useful therapeutic procedure
due to rapid drug destruction and unacceptable side

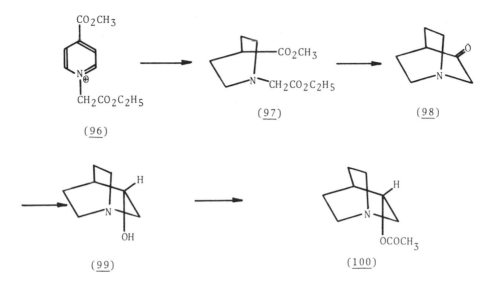

(96)          (97)          (98)

(99)                    (100)

effects. *Aceclidine (100)* was synthesized based upon
these considerations. When glycine analogue *96* is
catalytically reduced, *cis*-diester *97* is produced.
Dieckmann condensation and saponification-decarboxy-
lation then leads to bicyclopiperidone *98*.[28]
Borohydride reduction gives alcohol *99*.[29] Acetylation
completes the synthesis of *aceclidine (100)*, a cholinergic agent.[30]

    Glutarimides may be regarded as oxidized piperi-
dines, and many drugs containing this moiety are
sedatives and anticonvulsants. A spiro derivative,
*alonimid (105)* is such a sedative-hypnotic agent. It
can be prepared by K t-butoxide catalyzed biscyano-
ethylation of phenylacetonitrile, leading to *101*.
Alkaline hydrolysis produces tricarboxylic acid *102*
which is smoothly converted to the glutaric acid
anhydride *(103)* with acetic anhydride. Friedel-Crafts

cyclization leads to the 6-membered ring, with concomitant anhydride reorganization to give *104*.  The

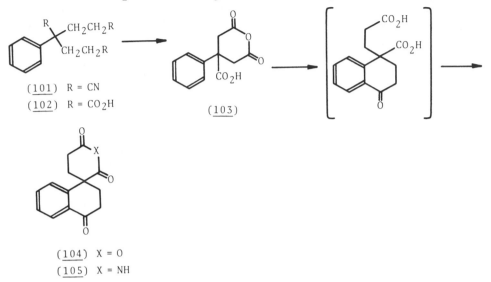

(<u>101</u>)  R = CN
(<u>102</u>)  R = CO$_2$H

(<u>103</u>)

(<u>104</u>)  X = O
(<u>105</u>)  X = NH

azaphilone character of *104* is taken advantage of as
reaction with ammonia produces the desired spiroimide
*105*.[31]   Interest in compounds of this generic type
has cooled considerably in the wake of the *thalidomide*
tragedy.

Homophthalimides have an active methylene group,
and this property is retained by the octahydroisoquino-
line derivative *106*.  Base-catalyzed benzylidine
condensation with benzaldehyde gives *tesimide (107)*,
an antiinflammatory agent.[32]  The imine proton may be
sufficiently acidic for this drug to be classed among
the acidic nonsteroidal antiinflammatory agents.

As a means of introducing both rigidity and
asymmetry for receptor discrimination, bicycloimides
are potentially interesting pharmacological tools.

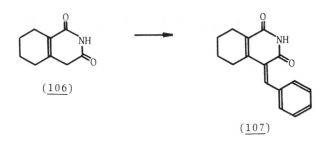

(106)

(107)

One such agent is prepared by NBS and peroxide
bromination of ethyl 4-chlorophenylacetate *(108)* to
give *109*.  This is converted by sodium hydride to the
benzylic carbene, which is inserted into the double
bond of ethyl acrylate to give *cis*-cyclopropane *110*.
Partial saponification cleaves the less hindered
ester moiety to give *111*.  This is next converted to
the alkoxyimide *(112)* on reaction with diethyl carbonate and diammonium phosphate.  Stronger base (NaOEt)
effects displacement to the imide *(113)*, *cyproximide*,
which has tranquilizing properties.[33]

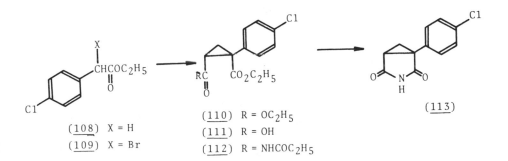

(108) X = H
(109) X = Br

(110) R = OC₂H₅
(111) R = OH
(112) R = NHCOC₂H₅

(113)

### 3. PIPERAZINES AND PYRAZINES

The classical synthetic method for constructing
2-aminopyrazines is illustrated by the synthesis of
*ampyzine (117)*, a CNS stimulant. Condensation of
aminomalonamide and glyoxal leads to pyrazine *114*.
Hydrolysis to the acid and decarboxylation gives
2-hydroxypyrazine *(115)*. Reaction with $PCl_5$ produces
chloride *116*, and heating with dimethylamine completes
the synthesis of *117*.[34]

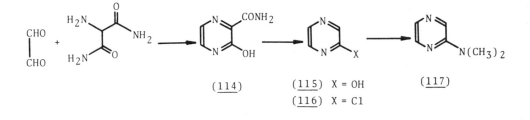

(114)          (115) X = OH          (117)
               (116) X = Cl

Methyl groups are introduced into the aromatic
rings of pyrazines by varying the starting materials.
For example, use of biacetyl and alanylamide produces
trimethyl hydroxypyrazine *118*. Chlorination and
thermal displacement with dimethylamine gives *triampyzine (119)*, an anticholinergic agent intended to
inhibit gastric secretion to control some kinds of
peptic ulcer.[35]

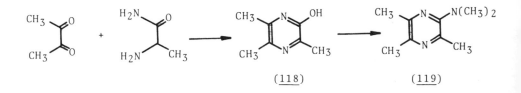

(118)                    (119)

It has been discovered that direct chlorination of pyrazines can be accomplished and this has also been used to make candidate drugs. For example, when 2-methylpyrazine *(120)* is heated with chlorine in carbon tetrachloride, a mixture of the 3-chloro *(121)* and the 6-chloro derivatives result. After separation, *121* is heated with piperidine to give *modaline (122)*, an antidepressant.[36]

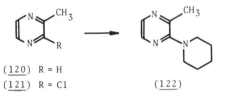

(120) R = H
(121) R = Cl
(122)

When piperazine *(123)* is reacted with two molar equivalents of 3-bromoacetyl chloride, the antineoplastic agent *pipobroman (124)* results.[37] This material is probably an alkylating agent. Exchange of the leaving groups by mesylate moieties is compatible with bioactivity. This has been accomplished by reaction of *124* with silver methanesulfonate to give *piposulfan (125)*, also an antineoplastic agent.[38]

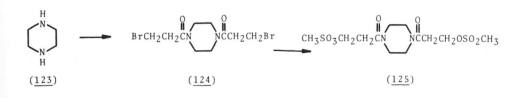

(123)　　　　　　(124)　　　　　　(125)

Azaperone *(128)* is yet another of the tranquilizers related to *haloperidol.* Nucleophilic
aromatic displacement of 2-chloropyridine by piperazine leads to amine *126* which is then alkylated in
turn by 4-chloro-p-fluorobuterophenone *(127)* to give
*azaperone (128)*, which is said to be active by topical
administration.[39]

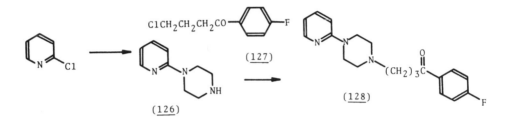

Alkylation of 1-(2-pyrimidyl)piperazine *(129)*
with 3-chloro-1-cyanopropane gives nitrile *130*, which
is reduced with LAH and then acylated with spiro-
glutaric anhydride *131* to synthesize the tranquilizer
*buspirone (132).*[40]

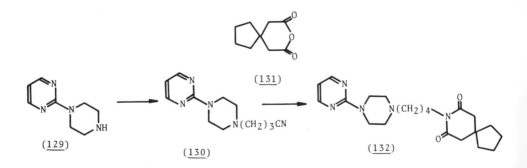

Alkylation of piperazine with the amide formed
by reaction of chloroacetyl chloride with pyrrolidine
gives amide *133*.  Acylation with 3,4,5-trimethoxy-
cinnamoyl chloride completes the synthesis of the
peripheral vasodilator, *cinepazide (134)*.[41]

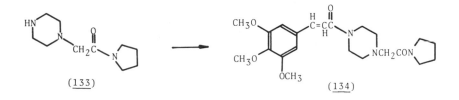

(133)                                    (134)

To round out this group of drugs in which the
piperazine ring appears to serve primarily as a basic
spacer unit, or a conformationally restricted ethylenediamine unit, reaction of N-phenylpiperazine *(135)*
with acrylonitrile produces nitrile *136*.  Conversion

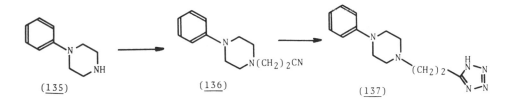

(135)                    (136)                    (137)

of the nitrile moiety to a tetrazole ring *via* a
1,3-dipolar addition process by sodium azide under
ammonium chloride catalysis produces *zolterine (137)*,
an antihypertensive by virtue of its antiadrenergic/
vasodilator activity.[42]  The tetrazole moiety is an

isoelectronic replacement for a carboxylic acid
moeity in a number of drugs.

### 4.   PYRIMIDINES

Two antibacterial agents related structurally to
*trimethoprim (138)* are *diaveridine (141)* and
*ormetoprim (146)*.   *Diaveridine* has been synthesized
by a minor variant of the trimethoprim route[43] in
which veratric aldehyde *(139)* is sequentially condensed
with β-ethoxypropionitrile (to *140*) and then guanidine
to give *141*.[44]  *Ormetoprim* may be made analogously or

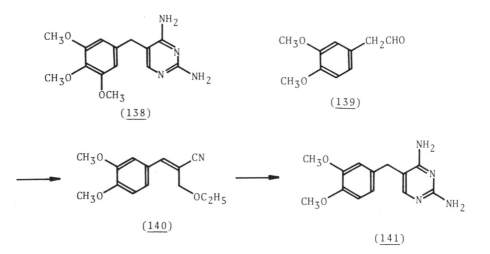

(138)

(139)

(140)

(141)

by benzylic bromination (NBS and peroxide) of acetyl-
pyrimidine *142* to give *143*, which alkylates
3,4-dimethoxytoluene to give substituted thymine *144*
when treated with mercuric chloride in nitrobenzene.
The amino groups are restored in the classic fashion
by conversion of *144* to chloride *145* with POCl$_3$, and

then displacement with ammonia to yield *146*.[45]
*Ormetoprim* (146) is a coccidiostat as well as an
antibacterial agent.

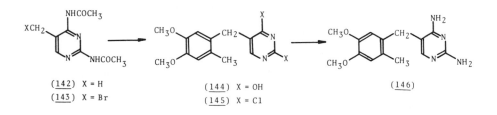

(142) X = H
(143) X = Br

(144) X = OH
(145) X = Cl

(146)

Following the success of *pyrantel* (*147*) as an
anthelmentic[46] a search was undertaken for an analogue
that would have activity against adult whipworms as
well.  This effort was successful with the synthesis
of tetrahydropyrimidine *150*, the anthelminitic,
*oxantel*.[47]  The C-methyl group of *149* is sufficiently
activated that heating together with 3-hydroxybenz-
aldehyde (*148*) in the presence of ethyl formate as a
water scavenger produces *oxantel* directly.

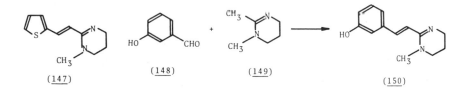

(147)

(148)          (149)

(150)

Convulsive disorders are still a serious therapeutic problem and new agents are being actively
sought.  Classical therapy was based upon the barbi-
turates that are no longer in favor because of their
many side effects and their suicide potential.
Interestingly, a seemingly minor structural variation
of phenobarbital (*151*, shown as its sodium salt)
leads to an anticonvulsant of increased potency and
which has less hypnotic activity.  In this case,
sodium phenobarbital serves as its own base (so the
yield is limited to 50%) and reacts readily with
chloromethylmethyl ether to produce *eterobarb* (*152*).[48]

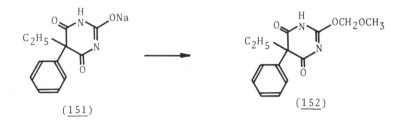

(151)                                   (152)

## 5.  MISCELLANEOUS STRUCTURES

As befits their chemical heterogenecity, the miscellaneous group of drugs in this section belong to a
wide range of pharmacological classes as well.

A pyridazine has found use as an antihypertensive agent.  When levulinic acid is reacted with
hydrazine, *153* results.  This is aromatized to
pyridazine *154* when reacted with bromine in acetic
acid.  One presumes a spontaneous dehydrobromination

converts the intermediate to *154*.  Oxidation to the
acid *(155)* is accomplished with potassium dichromate,
and this is esterified to *156* under Fischer conditions.
Conversion to chloro derivative *157* (with POCl$_3$) is
followed by displacement with hydrazine to give *158*.
The synthesis of blood pressure-lowering *hydracarbazine*
*(159)* is then completed by aminolysis with ammonia.[49]

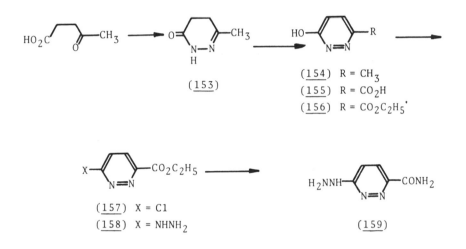

(153)

(154)  R = CH$_3$
(155)  R = CO$_2$H
(156)  R = CO$_2$C$_2$H$_5$

(157)  X = Cl
(158)  X = NHNH$_2$

(159)

The triazinedione, *triazuril (163)* is active as
a poultry coccidiostat.  Diazonium salt *160*, prepared
from the appropriate aniline, is coupled with the
active methylene group of N-carbethoxycyanoacetamide
to give *161*.  Hydrolysis of the cyano group is accompanied by cyclization, and the resulting acid *(162)*
is decarboxylated to *triazuril (163)* on heating.[50]

A morpholine derivative is active as a muscle
relaxant.  To prepare it, reaction of arylphenethanol-
amine derivative *164* with sodium hydride and ethyl

chloroacetate leads to *flumetramide (165)*.[51]

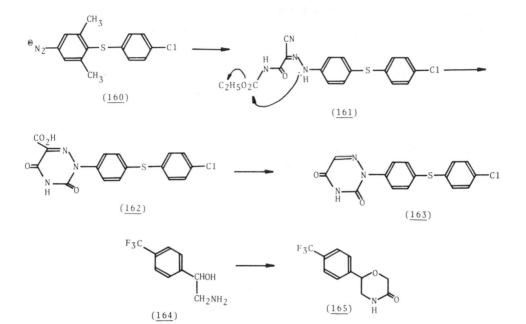

The carbonyl group of compounds related to *165* can be removed with retention of significant pharmacological activity. This can, of course, be done by lithium aluminum hydride reduction[52] or by, in at least one significant case, reaction of aryloxyepoxide *166* with 2-aminoethylbisulfate to give the antidepressant agent, *viloxazine (167)*.[53]

The sultam, *sulthiame (170)*, shows anticonvulsant activity. p-Aminobenzenesulfonamide can be alkylated by ω-chlorobutylsulfonyl chloride *(168)* in

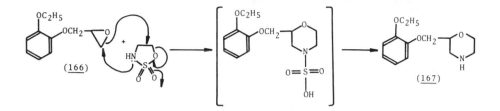

base *via* presumed intermediate *169*, which spontaneously cyclizes to give *sulthiame (170)*.[54]

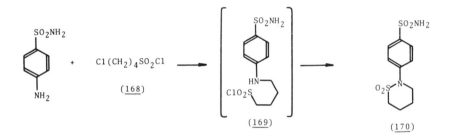

Reaction of 2,6-dimethylaniline with thiophosgene produces isothiocyanate *171*. When the latter is treated with 3-aminopropanol, thiourea *172* is formed, and this, when treated with hot concentrated hydrochloric acid, cyclizes to *xylazine (173)*, an analgetic and muscle relaxant.[55]

A great many quaternary amines are active anticholinergic agents. One such parasympathetic blocking agent is made easily by reacting hyoscyamine with 4-butoxybenzylbromide to produce *butropium bromide* (*174*).[56]

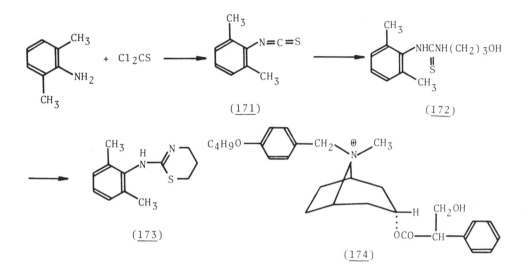

(171)          (172)

(173)

(174)

## REFERENCES

1.  L. A. Walter, W. H. Hunt and R. J. Fosbinder, *J. Am. Chem. Soc.*, *63*, 2771 (1941).

2.  K. Shimizu, R. Ushijima and K. Sugiura, German Patent 2,217,084 (1972); *Chem. Abstr.*, *78:* 29778f (1973).

3.  G. C. Morrison and J. Shavel, Jr., German Patent 1,955,682 (1970); *Chem. Abstr.*, *73:* 35225m (1970).

4.  W. E. Barth, German Patent 2,204,195 (1972); *Chem. Abstr.*, *77:* 151968n (1972).

5. M. H. Sherlock, U. S. Patent 3,839,344 (1974); *Chem. Abstr.*, *82:* 16705n (1975).

6. Anon., Dutch Patent 6,603,357 (1967); *Chem. Abstr.*, *68:* 59439g (1968).

7. M. H. Sherlock, South African Patent 68 02185 (1968); *Chem. Abstr.*, *70:* 96640c (1969); Swiss Patent 534,129 (1973); *Chem. Abstr.*, *79:* 18582g (1973).

8. D. Evans, K. S. Hallwood, C. H. Cashin and H. Jackson, *J. Med. Chem.*, *10*, 428 (1967).

9. W. Dittmar, E. Druckrey and H. Urbach, *J. Med. Chem.*, *17*, 753 (1974); W. Dittmar and G. Lohaus, *Arzneimittelforschung 23*, 670 (1973); German Patent 2,214,608 (1973); *Chem. Abstr.*, *79:* 146419w (1973).

10. F. Bossert and W. Vater, South African Patent 68 01482 (1968); *Chem. Abstr.*, *70:* 96641d (1969).

11. G. H. Sankey and K. D. E. Whiting, *J. Heterocycl. Chem.*, *9*, 1049 (1972).

12. W. R. Hardie, J. Hidalgo and I. F. Halvorstadt, *J. Med. Chem.*, *9*, 127 (1966).

13. A. P. Gray, W. L. Archer, E. R. Spinner and C. J. Cavallito, *J. Am. Chem. Soc.*, *79*, 3805 (1957).

14. J. W. Ward and C. A. Leonard, French Patent 2,227,868 (1974); *Chem. Abstr.*, *82:* 170720v (1975).

15. R. Sarges, *J. Med. Chem.*, *19*, 695 (1976).

16. W. B. Lutz, S. Lazarus and R. I. Meltzer, *J. Org. Chem.*, *27*, 1695 (1962); N. P. Sanzari and J. F. Emele, U. S. Patent 3,755,586 (1973); *Chem. Abstr.*, *80:* 19550c (1974).

17. C. Van der Westeringh, P. Van Daele, B. Hermans,
    C. Van der Eycken, J. Boey and P. A. J. Janssen,
    *J. Med. Chem.*, *7*, 619 (1964).

18. Anon., Belgian Patent 626,307 (1963); *Chem.*
    *Abstr.*, *60:* 10690c (1964).

19. P. A. J. Janssen, U. S. Patent, 3,225,052
    (1965); *Chem. Abstr.*, *64:* 8194b (1966).

20. P. A. J. Janssen, W. Soudijn, I. Van Wijngaarden
    and A. Dreese, *Arzneimittelforschung*, *18*, 282
    (1968).

21. P. A. J. Janssen, C. J. E. Niemegeers, K. H. L.
    Schellekens, F. M. Lenaerts and A. Wanquier,
    *Arzneimittelforschung*, *25*, 1287 (1975).

22. Anon., Belgian Patent 633,495 (1963); *Chem.*
    *Abstr.*, *61:* 1871c (1964).

23. Anon., Dutch Patent 6,504,602 (1965); *Chem.*
    *Abstr.*, *64:* 12679d (1966).

24. Anon., Belgian Patent 633,914 (1963); *Chem.*
    *Abstr.*, *60:* 15882d (1964).

25. P. A. J. Janssen, U. S. Patent 3,238,216 (1966);
    *Chem. Abstr.*, *65:* 8924d (1966).

26. B. Hermans, P. Van Daele, C. Van der Westeringh,
    C. Van der Eycken, J. Boly, J. Dockx and P. A.
    J. Janssen, *J. Med. Chem.*, *11*, 797 (1968).

27. C. D. Lunsford and W. J. Welstead, South African
    Patent 67 03,192 (1968); *Chem. Abstr.*, *70:*
    96,785d (1969).

28. E. E. Mikhlina and M. V. Rubtsov, *Zhur. Obschei*
    *Khim*, *30*, 163 (1960).

29. L. H. Sternbach and S. Kaiser, *J. Am. Chem.*
    *Soc.*, *74*, 2215 (1952).

30. C. A. Grob, A. Kaiser and E. Renk, *Helv. Chim. Acta*, *40*, 2170 (1957).

31. G. N. Walker, U. S. Patent 3,379,731 (1968); *Chem. Abstr.*, *69*: 96497r (1968).

32. H. Zinnes, J. Shavel, Jr., N. A. Lindo and G. Di Pasquale, U. S. Patent 2,634,415 (1972); *Chem. Abstr.*, *76*: 72421e (1972).

33. E. N. Greenblatt and S. R. Safir, U. S. Patent 3,344,026 (1967); *Chem. Abstr.*, *68*: 29443m (1968).

34. G. W. H. Cheeseman, *J. Chem. Soc.*, 242 (1960); F. H. Muehlmann and A. R. Day, *J. Am. Chem. Soc.*, *78*, 242 (1956).

35. Anon., British Patent 1,031,915 (1966); *Chem. Abstr.*, *65*: 5471g (1966).

36. W. B. Lutz, S. Lazarus, S. Klutchko and R. I. Meltzer, *J. Org. Chem.*, *29*, 415 (1964); M. Gainer, M. Kokorudz and W. A. Langdon, *ibid.*, *26*, 2360 (1961).

37. S. Groszkowski, *Roczniki Chem.*, *38*, 229 (1964).

38. B. Horrom and J. A. Carbon, German Patent 1,177,162 (1964); *Chem. Abstr.*, *61*: 13329a (1964).

39. W. Sondijn and I. Van Wijngaarden, *J. Labeled Compounds*, *4*, 159 (1968).

40. H. C. Ferguson, Y.H. Wu, J. W. Rayburn, L. E. Allen and J. W. Kissel, *J. Med. Chem.*, *15*, 477 (1972).

41. C. Fauran and M. Turin, *Chim. Ther.*, *4*, 290 (1969).

42.  W. G. Stryker and S. Hayao, Belgian Patent
     661,396 (1965); *Chem. Abstr.*, *63:* 18114e (1965).
43.  D. Lednicer and L. A. Mitscher, Organic Chemistry
     of Drug Synthesis, Vol. I, p. 263 (1977).
44.  P. Steinbuck, R. Baltzly and H. M. Hood, *J. Org.
     Chem.*, *28*, 1983 (1963).
45.  Anon., Netherlands Application 6,514,743 (1966);
     *Chem. Abstr.*, *65:* 10598c (1966).
46.  Lednicer and L. A. Mitscher, Organic Chemistry
     of Drug Synthesis, Vol. I, p. 266267, Formula
     94, (1977).
47.  J. W. McFarland and H. L. Howes, Jr., *J. Med.
     Chem.*, *15*, *365 (1972).*
48.  *C. M. Samour, J. F. Reinhard and J. A. Vida, J.
     Med. Chem.*, *14*, 187 (1971).
49.  D. Libermann and A. Rouaix, *Bull. Soc. Chim.
     Fr.*, 1793 (1959).
50.  M. W. Miller, German Patent 2,149,645 (1972);
     *Chem. Abstr.*, *77:* 164712z (1972).
51.  W. F. Gannon and G. I. Poos, U. S. Patent
     3,308,121 (1967); *Chem. Abstr.*, *67:* 32693c
     (1967).
52.  K. B. Mallion, R. W. Turner and A. H. Todd,
     British Patent 1,138,405 (1969); *Chem. Abstr.*,
     *70:* 96804j (1969).
53.  S. A. Lee, British Patent 1,260,886 (1972);
     *Chem. Abstr.*, *76:* 99684e (1972).
54.  B. Helferich and R. Behnisch, U. S. Patent
     2,916,489 (1959).
55.  O. Behner, H. Henecka, F. Hoffmeister, H.
     Kreiskott, W. Meiser, H. W. Schubert and W.

Wirth, Belgian Patent 634,552 (1964); *Chem. Abstr.*, *61*: 4369b (1964).

56. S. Tanaka and K. Hashimoto, German Patent 1,950,378 (1970); *Chem. Abstr.*, *73*: 98,819d (1970).

# 10

# Compounds Related to Morphine

The development of the first effective analgesic
drug, opium, was almost certainly adventitious, and
occurred in prehistoric times. The use of the dried
exudate from slitting the immature capsule of the
opium poppy, *Papaver somniferum*, as an analgesic,
sedative and euphoriant, has a long folkloric history.
Isolation of the principal active component *morphine*
*(1)* as a pure crystalline compound represented one
of the early landmarks in organic chemistry.

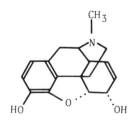

(1)

The history of this class of analgesics might
have stopped there were it not for the manifold
ancillary activities shown by that molecule.  Although
still one of the most widely used agents for treatment
of severe pain, *morphine* is a drug that must be used
with caution.  Side effects include respiratory
depression, induction of constipation, and sometimes
marked sedation.  The one property that most severely
limits use of this drug is its propensity to induce
physical dependence in patients subjected to more
than casual exposure.

1.  Compounds Derived from Morphine
Attempts to modify the molecule so as to maximize
analgesic activity at the expense of side effects
date back almost a full century.  It is ironic that
*heroin* (diacetyl morphine) was in fact prepared in
the course of one such program.  Although early
efforts concentrated on modification of the natural
product, the growth of synthetic organic chemistry
has led more recently to the preparation of molecules
that represent much more deep seated changes in
structure.  The concept of molecular dissection has
been used widely in the design of such lead compounds.
Some of the more recent molecules inspired by morphine
do in fact show promise of providing analgesia with
significantly reduced side effects so that compounds
are now available that show a much reduced tendency
to induce physical dependence, *i.e.*, addiction
liability.

It has long been a puzzle to medicinal chemists

why a natural product that has no evolutionary association with *Homo sapiens* should show such profound
biological activity.  The puzzle was, if anything,
intensified by reports of the occurrence of receptors
for morphine and related opioids in mammalian brains.
Receptors for various endogenous hormones and other
chemical transmitters have been recognized for some
time; it was, however, unexpected to find a specific
receptor for an exogenous chemical that plays no
known role in the normal biochemical functioning of a
mammal.

The identification of the morphine receptor
spurred an effort in many laboratories to find an
endogenous agonist for which that receptor was normally
intended.[1]  Ultimately, a pair of pentapeptides that
bound quite tightly to opiate receptors were isolated
from mammalian brains.  These peptides, called
*enkephalins* (2, 3), show many of the activities of
synthetic opiates in isolated organ systems.  They do
in fact show analgesic activity when injected directly
into the brain.  It is thought that lack of activity
by other routes of administration is due to their
rapid inactivation by peptide cleaving enzymes.

HTyr-Gly-Gly-Phe-MetOH
met-enkephalin
(2)

HTyr-Gly-Gly-Phe-LeuOH
leu-enkephalin
(3)

Fragments of the peptide hormone β-lipotropin
have been found to show similar binding to opiate
receptors.  These molecules, the *endorphins*, show
profound CNS activity in experimental animals.  It is
of interest that one of these, β-endorphin, incorporates in its chain the exact sequence of amino acids
that constitutes methionine enkaphalin.

Although these findings are too recent to have
had an impact on the design of analgesics, it has
already been noted that when properly folded,
molecular models of the enkaphalins show a good
topographical correspondence with molecules such as
morphine. Unless this topographic relationship is
fortuitous, this has the most profound future impli-
cations for the rational design of analgesic drugs.

*Morphine* and related opiates are known to suppress
the cough reflex; these compounds have thus been used
extensively in antitussive preparations.  Since this
activity is not directly related to the analgesic
potency, the ideal agent is one that has much reduced
analgesic activity and thus, presumably, lower addiction potential.  The weak analgesic *codeine (4)* is

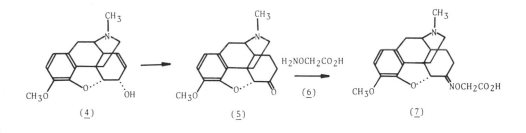

still used in many such preparations, and a variety
of analogues have been prepared as substitutes. For
example, condensation of *dihydrocodeinone (5)* (available in several steps from 4) with hydroxylamine
derivative 6 affords the antitussive agent *codoxime*
*(7)*.[2]

Replacement of the N-methyl group of morphine by
an allyl moiety leads to a narcotic antagonist. That
is, the resulting drug, *nalorphine*, not only shows
little analgesic activity but will in fact block most
of the actions of morphine. Presumably, it binds to
the opiate receptor but has little intrinsic agonist
activity. Incorporation of a new hydroxyl group at
the 14-position in morphine has been found empirically
to potentiate greatly the activity of morphine.
Combination of these two modifications in a single
drug gives a very potent narcotic antagonist, *naloxone*
*(8)*. It is possible, by suitable modification of
various structural features in narcotic analgesic
molecules, to devise compounds, which show both
agonist and antagonist activities; it has been found
both in experimental animals and in man that such
mixed agonists-antagonists afford analgesics with
much reduced addiction liability. The work that
follows apparently was aimed at building agonist
activity into the *naloxone* structure.

The starting material for these 14-hydroxy compounds is the opium alkaloid *thebaine (9)*. Although
present in only small amounts in the alkaloid fraction
from *Papaver somniferum*, it constitutes the major
component (as much as 26% of the dried latex) from a

related poppy, *Papaver bracteatum*.[3]  Reaction of *9*
with hydrogen peroxide leads to intermediate *11*.  The
oxidation may be visualized as a 1,4-oxidation process
of the diene system to afford an intermediate such as
*10*.  Successive reduction of the double bond (*12*) and
demethylation affords *oxymorphone* (*13*).[4]  This molecule
is then protected as the diacetate; N-demethylation
followed by saponification affords the key intermediate
*14*.[5]

Alkylation of the secondary amine in *14* with
1-bromo-3-methyl-2-butene leads to the mixed analgesic
agonist-antagonist *nalmexone* (*15*).[6]  In a somewhat
more elaborate scheme, the carbonyl group in *14* is
first protected as its cyclic ethylene ketal (16).
Alkylation with cyclopropylcarbonyl chloride affords
the O,N-diacylated product (*17*); treatment with
lithium aluminum hydride results in reductive cleavage
of the O-acyl group and reduction of the amide carbonyl
to a methylene group (*19*).  Hydrolysis of the acetal
then affords the mixed analgesic/antagonist *naltrexone*
(*21*).[7]  Acylation of *14* with cyclobutylcarbonyl
chloride followed by the same series of transformations as above leads to intermediate *22*.  Reduction
of the carbonyl group in that molecule with sodium
borohydride gives the analgesic agonist/antagonist
*nalbuphine* (*23*).[7]

An indication that the SAR of the narcotic
antagonists was more complex than had been anticipated
came from the observation of the tremendous increase
in milligram potency obtained by fusing an additional
bicyclic ring onto the basic morphine structure. The

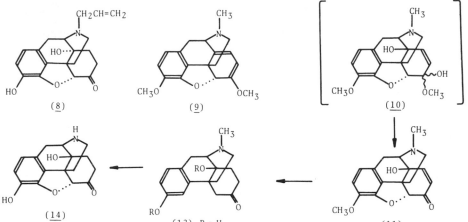

(8)

(9)

(10)

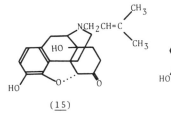

(14)

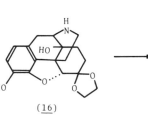

(12) R = H
(13) R = CH₃CO

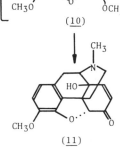

(11)

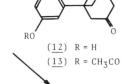

(15)

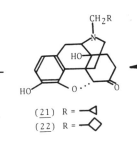

(16)

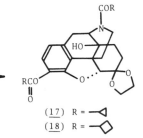

(17) R = △
(18) R = ◻

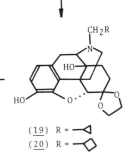

(19) R = △
(20) R = ◻

(21) R = △
(22) R = ◻

(23)

320

resulting molecule, **etorphine** (26) shows three orders
of magnitude greater potency than morphine; this
could be interpreted as a better or tighter fit to
the receptor.  Synthesis of this molecule also takes
advantage of the diene function found in thebaine.
Thus, Diels-Alder condensation of 9 with methyl vinyl
ketone affords the bicyclic adduct 24.  The new ring
is formed by approach of the dienophile from the face
containing the nitrogen bridge, since this is in fact
the least hindered side of the molecule (9a).  Reaction
of the side chain ketone with propylmagnesium bromide
then leads to intermediate 25; demethylation of the
phenolic ether affords etorphine (26).[8]

   In this series, too, replacement of the N-methyl
by a group such as cyclopropylmethyl leads to a
compound with reduced abuse potential by virtue of
mixed agonist-antagonist action.  To accomplish this,
reduction of 24 followed by reaction with tertiary
butylmagnesium chloride gives the tertiary carbinol
27.  The N-methyl group is then removed by the classic
von Braun procedure.  Thus, reaction with cyanogen
bromide leads to the N-cyano derivative (28); hydrolysis affords the secondary amine 29.  (One of the
more efficient demethylation procedures, such as
reaction with ethyl chloroformate would presumably be
used today.) Acylation with cyclopropylcarbonyl
chloride then leads to the amide 30.  Reduction with
lithium aluminum hydride (31) followed by demethylation of the phenolic ether affords buprenorphine
(32).[9]

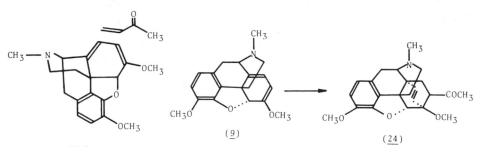

(9a)

(9)

(24)

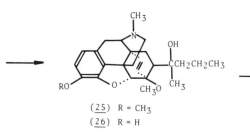

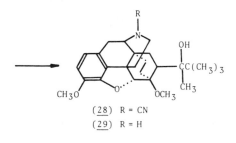

(25) R = CH₃
(26) R = H

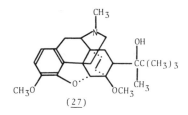

(27)

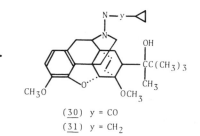

(28) R = CN
(29) R = H

(30) y = CO
(31) y = CH₂

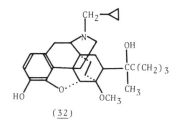

(32)

### 2. Morphinans

In the course of earlier work it had been ascertained that the furan oxygen of morphine was not essential to analgesic activity.[10] This observation led to the preparation of a considerable number of quite potent deoxy analogues of morphine, since these compounds were relatively easily accessible by totally synthetic routes. Combination of this deoxy nucleus (called *morphinan*) with the tertiary hydroxyl found in molecules such as *naloxone* has led to quite potent analgesics; appropriate modification of the substituent on nitrogen then has led to mixed agonists-antagonists. These compounds, too, show much reduced addiction liability. For example, alkylation of the anion from tetralone *33* with 1,4-dibromobutane gives the spiro ketone *34*. Condensation of the carbonyl group with the anion obtained on treatment of acetonitrile with butyl lithium leads to the carbinol *35*; the cyano group is then reduced to the primary amine *(36)* by means of lithium aluminum hydride. Treatment of *36* with acid leads to the corresponding tertiary benzylic carbonium ion; this undergoes Wagner-Meerwein rearrangement and proton loss to give the phenanthrene derivative *37*, a key intermediate in this series.[11] Several schemes have been developed for proceeding from this point; however, some relatively direct routes suffer from lack of regiospecificity. For example, internal cyclization of epoxide *38* affords both the desired ring system *(45)* and its isomer *(39)*.[12] In one regiospecific route, amine *37* is

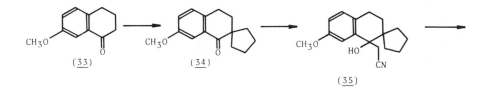

(33)  (34)  (35)

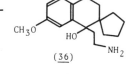

(36)

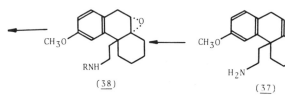

(37)  (38)

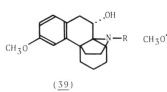

(39)

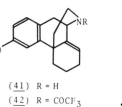

(41) R = H
(42) R = COCF₃

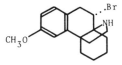

(40)

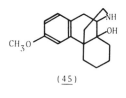

(45)

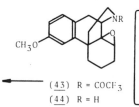

(43) R = COCF₃
(44) R = H

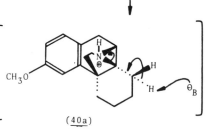

(40a)

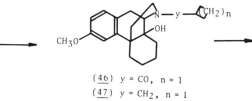

(46) y = CO, n = 1
(47) y = CH₂, n = 1
(48) y = CO, n = 0
(49) y = CH₂, n = 0

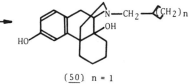

(50) n = 1
(51) n = 0

324

treated with bromine to afford the bicyclic bromo-
amine *40*. The reaction can be rationalized by
assuming initial bromonium ion formation on the
underside of the molecule; opening of the ring by the
amine will lead to the observed product as its hydrobromide salt. Reaction of *40* with sodium bicarbonate
results in the rearrangement to the desired skeleton.
The inorganic base is not in this case the reagent;
rather, it is likely that once *40* is present as the
free base, it undergoes the internal displacement *via*
the aziridinium ion. Following protection of the
amine as the trifluoroacetamide *(42)*, the double bond
is oxidized to give mainly the β-epoxide *(43)*.
Hydrolysis of the amide linkage *(44)* followed by
treatment with lithium aluminum hydride affords the
desired aminoalcohol *45*. Both the regio and stereochemistry of this last reaction follow from the
diaxial opening of oxiranes. Acylation of this
intermediate with cyclobutylcarbonyl chloride gives
the corresponding amide *(46)*. Reduction of the amide
*(47)* followed by O-demethylation affords *butorphanol*
*(50)*.[13] The same sequence on *45* starting with cyclopropyl carbonyl chloride leads to *oxilorphan (51)*.[14]

### 3. Benzomorphans
Further dissection of the morphine molecule showed
that potent analgesics could be obtained even when
one of the carbocyclic rings was omitted. One such
compound, *pentazocine (52)*, has found considerable
use as an analgesic in the clinic. There is considerable evidence to indicate this drug has much less

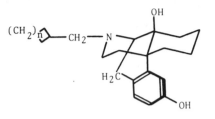

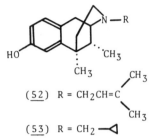

(52) R = CH₂CH=C⟨CH₃/CH₃

(53) R = CH₂ ◁

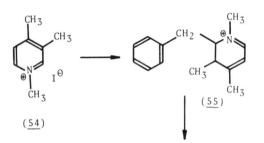

(54)

(55)

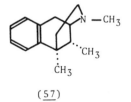

(57)

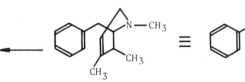

(56)

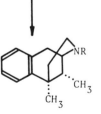

(58) R = CN
(59) R = H

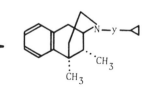

(60) R = CO
(61) R = CH₂

addiction potential than does morphine.  The
corresponding cyclopropylmethyl analogue *cyclazocine*
*(53)*, perhaps as a consequence of its greater balance
of antagonist activity, has proven to be quite hallucinogenic.

Omission of the phenolic group from *cyclazocine*
results in a molecule which retains analgesic activity.
In a classical application of the Grewe synthesis,[15]
the methylated pyridinium salt *54* is condensed with
benzylmagnesium bromide.  There is thus obtained the
dihydropyridine *55*.  Treatment of that intermediate
with sodium borohydride results in reduction of the
iminium function to afford the tetrahydro derivative
*56*.  Cyclization of *56* on treatment with acid leads
to the desired benzomorphan nucleus. The *cis* compound
*(57)* is separated from the mixture of isomers and
demethylated by the cyanogen bromide procedure *(58,*
*59)*. Acylation with cyclopropylcarbonyl chloride (to
*60*) followed by reduction of the resulting amide
yields *volazocine (61)*.[14]

Oxidation of the benzylic methylene group in
*cyclazocine* to a ketone is also consistent with
analgesic activity.  Acetylation of benzomorphan *62*
affords the diacetate *63*.  Selective hydrolysis of
the phenolic acetate *(64)* followed by methylation of
the thus uncovered phenol affords intermediate *65*.
The remaining acetate is then hydrolyzed *(66)*.
Oxidation of that compound with chromium trioxide in
sulfuric acid leads cleanly to the desired ketone
*(67)*. Treatment with hydrobromic acid serves to
demethylate the phenolic ether function *(68)*.  Direct

alkylation of the secondary amine with cyclopropylmethyl bromide gives *ketazocine (69)*.[16]

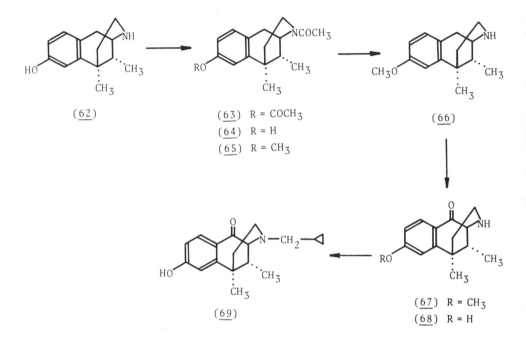

(62)

(63) R = COCH₃
(64) R = H
(65) R = CH₃

(66)

(67) R = CH₃
(68) R = H

(69)

## 4.   Phenylpiperidines

Extensive molecular dissection of the morphine molecule over the past several decades led to a host of
molecules which showed narcotic analgesic activity
even though they possessed but faint suggestion of
the structural features present in morphine itself.
Thus, both cyclic molecules such as *meperidine (70)*
and *alphaprodine (71)*, and acyclic compounds such as
*methadone (72)* were found to be effective analgesics.
Common features of these compounds were formalized by
the Beckett-Casy rule, which states as minimal required
structural features: (a) an aromatic ring attached to

(b) a quaternary center, and finally (c) the presence
of nitrogen at a distance equivalent to two carbon
atoms from the quaternary center (73).  Although
sufficient exceptions have recently been found to
suggest that this is an oversimplification, it is of
historical importance because of its guiding influence
on analgesic research over a considerable span of
time.

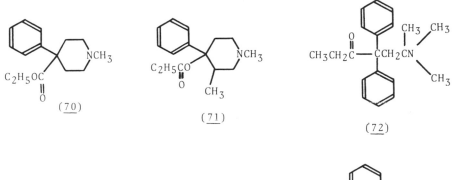

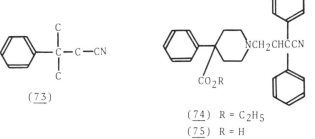

(74)  R = C₂H₅
(75)  R = H

It will be recalled that a common side effect of
*morphine* is the induction of constipation.  This
property of the drug has often been exploited in the
design of preparations used to control diarrhea.

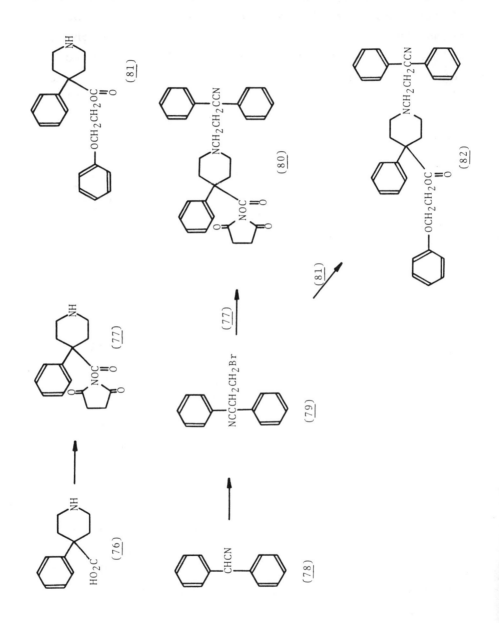

There has also been some work devoted to the preparation of a compound that would show greater selectivity toward activity on the gut and away from activity over the CNS. *Diphenoxylate (74)*[17] has been used extensively in humans for just this purpose; although the drug shows some selectivity, it is far from free of narcotic effects. (The curious will note the compound follows the Beckett rule both in the piperidine and side chain moieties.) Treatment of *74* with potassium tertiary butoxide in DMSO results in saponification to the free acid *difenoxin (75)*.[18]

Certain esters have often been employed in attempts to confer organ selectivity to molecules possessing carboxyl functions. Thus, for example, treatment of piperidinecarboxylic acid *76* with N-hydroxysuccinimide and DCC affords the ester *77*. In a convergent synthesis, the anion from diphenylaceto-nitrile *(78)* is alkylated with dibromoethane to afford the bromide *79*. Alkylation of the piperidine derivative *77* with that halide *79* gives the anti-diarrheal agent *difenoximide (80)*. The same sequence starting with the phenoxyethyl ester *81* gives *fetoxylate (82)*.[20]

Derivatives of 4-phenyl-4-hydroxypiperidine, which may be formally regarded as reversed meperidines, have yielded a series of potent antipsychotic drugs such as *haloperidol (83)* and *bromoperidol (84)*. Retention of carbon at the 4-position interestingly leads to a molecule with quite different activity. The starting material for this molecule could be synthesized by first preparing the amide *(86)* from

the benzyl *(85)* derivative of meperidine.  Reduction
of the amide would then afford the primary amine
*(87)*.  Acetylation *(88)* followed by removal of the
benzyl group would afford the key intermediate *(89)*.
Alkylation with 4-chloro-p-fluorophenylbutyrophenone
affords *aceperone (90)*.[21]  This compound exhibits
vasodilator and antihypertensive activity.

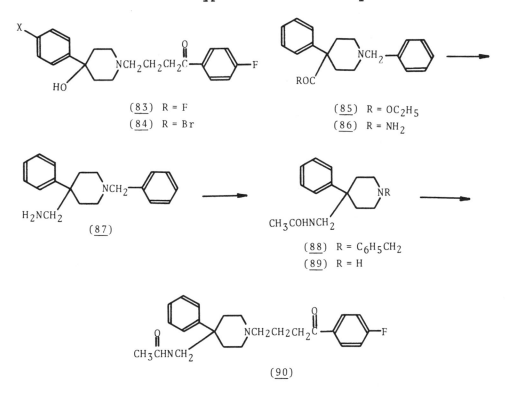

(83) R = F
(84) R = Br

(85) R = OC$_2$H$_5$
(86) R = NH$_2$

(87)

(88) R = C$_6$H$_5$CH$_2$
(89) R = H

(90)

Alkylation of diphenylpiperidinols with bis(p-
fluorophenyl)butyl side chains has also led to antipsychotic compounds.  For example, reductive cyclization of the acylation product *(91)* from fluorobenzene

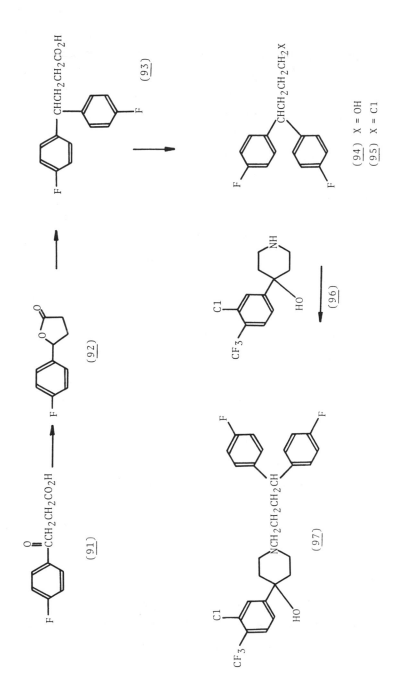

(91)

(92)

(93)

(94) X = OH
(95) X = Cl

(96)

(97)

and succinic anhydride gives the corresponding butyrolactone *92*.   Treatment with fluorobenzene in the
presence of a Friedel-Crafts catalyst leads to the
diarylated acid *93*.   The carboxyl group is then
reduced to the corresponding carbinol *94* by means of
lithium aluminum hydride, and this is converted to
the chloro compound *95* with thionyl chloride.
Alkylation of piperidine *96* with that halide gives
the neuroleptic compound *penfluridol (97)*.[22]

The use of phenylpiperidinols rather than the
meperidine-related piperidines as the basic component
in antidiarrheal compounds results in retention of
activity.   The fact that the base is not directly
related to a narcotic presumably leads to greater
selectivity of action on the gut.   Ring scission of
butyrolactone *98* (obtainable by alkylation of a
diphenylacetate ester with ethylene oxide) with
hydrogen bromide gives the bromo acid *99*.   This is
then converted to the dimethylamide by successive
treatment with thionyl chloride and dimethylamine.
The initial product from this reaction *(100)* is not
observed as it undergoes spontaneous internal displacement to the cyclic imino ether salt *101*.   Treatment
of *101* with amine *102* proceeds at the activated ether
carbon to give *fluperamide (103)*;[23] the same reaction
with amine *103* affords the antidiarrheal agent
*loperamide (105)*.[23]

Incorporation of additional basic centers into
the phenylpiperidinol nucleus leads to a molecule
that shows local anesthetic rather than CNS activity.
Condensation of the protected piperidone *106* with

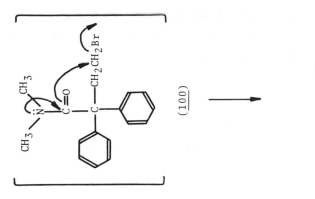

(98)

(99)

(100)

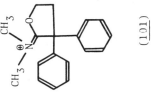

(101)

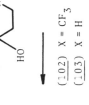

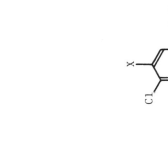

(102) X = CF$_3$
(103) X = H

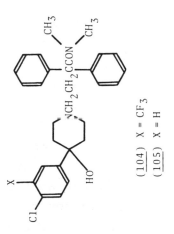

(104) X = CF$_3$
(105) X = H

335

phenylmagnesium bromide affords the desired piperidinol *(107)*.   Alkylation of the carbinol by means of
2-chlorotriethylamine gives the corresponding basic
ether *(108)*.   Hydrolysis of the carbamate protecting
group *(109)*, followed by alkylation of the resulting
secondary amine with N-(chloroethyl)aniline affords
the local anesthetic, *diamocaine (110)*.[24]

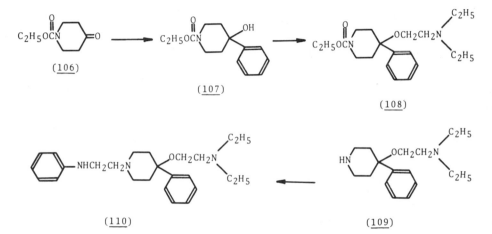

The piperidines discussed thus far contained a
single polar substituent on the heterocyclic ring.
Except for the last entry, the compounds all showed
activity on the CNS or closely related systems.   It
is thus somewhat surprising to find that simple
addition of an aroyl group leads to a compound that
shows antiinflammatory activity.   The seemingly
complex molecule can in fact be obtained in two steps
from simple starting materials.[25]   Thus, Mannich
reaction of p-fluoroacetophenone with paraformaldehyde
and methylamine affords condensation product *111*.
Treatment with aqueous base leads to cyclization by

internal aldol condensation. There is thus obtained
the nonsteroidal antiinflammatory agent *flazalone*
*(112)*.[26]

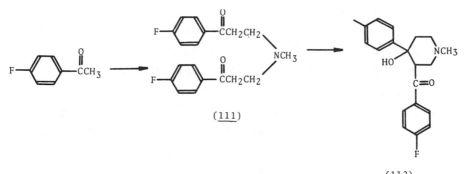

(111)

(112)

## REFERENCES

1.  J. Hughes, T. W. Smith, H. W. Kosterlitz, L. A.
    Fothergill, B. A. Morgan and H. R. Morris,
    *Nature*, *258*, 577 (1975).

2.  J. Fishman, U. S. Patent 3,152,042 (1964); *Chem.
    Abstr.*, *61:* 16111f (1964).

3.  N. Sharghi and L. Lalezari, *Nature*, *213*, 1244
    (1967).

4.  U. Weiss, *J. Am. Chem. Soc.*, *77*, 5891 (1955).

5.  For more detailed discussion, see D. Lednicer
    and L. A. Mitscher, Organic Chemistry of Drug
    Synthesis, Vol. I, 290 (1975).

6.  Anon., French Patent, M6358 (1968); *Chem. Abstr.*,
    *74:* 141,577h (1971).

7. H. Blumberg, I. J. Pachter and Z. Matossian, U. S. Patent 3,332,950 (1967); *Chem. Abstr.*, *67*: 100301 (1967).

8. K. W. Bently and D. G. Hardy, *Proc. Chem. Soc.*, 220 (1963).

9. K. W. Bentley, British Patent 1,136,214 (1968); *Chem. Abstr.*, *70*: 78218b (1969).

10. D. Lednicer and L. A. Mitscher, Organic Chemistry of Drug Synthesis, Vol. I, 292 (1975).

11. I. Monkovic, H. Wong, B. Belleau, I. J. Pachter and Y. G. Perron, *Can. J. Chem.*, *53*, 2515 (1975).

12. I. Monkovic and T. T. Conway, U. S. Patent 3,775,414 (1973); *Chem. Abstr.*, *80*: 37349 (1974).

13. I. Monkovic, H. Wong, A. W. Pircio, Y. G. Perron, I. J. Pachter and B. Belleau, *Can. J. Chem.*, *53*, 3094 (1975).

14. N. F. Albertson, U. S. Patent 3,382,249 (1968); *Chem. Abstr.*, *69*: 96509w (1968).

15. R. Grewe and A. Mondon, *Chem. Ber.*, *81*, 279 (1948).

16. W. F. Michne and N. F. Albertson, *J. Med. Chem.*, *15*, 1278 (1972).

17. D. Lednicer and L. A. Mitscher, Organic Chemistry of Drug Synthesis, Vol. I, 302 (1975).

18. W. Soudyn and I. Van Wijngaarden, German Patent 1,953,342 (1970); *Chem. Abstr.*, *73*, 38571g (1970).

19. E. M. S. Kreider, German Patent 2,161,865 (1972); *Chem. Abstr.*, *17*: 139818f (1972).

20. P. A. J. Janssen, German Patent, 1,807,691 (1969); *Chem. Abstr.*, *71*: 81194g (1969).

21.  P. A. J. Janssen, Belgian Patent 606,849 (1961);
     *Chem. Abstr.*, *56:* 12861i (1962).

22.  Anon., French Patent 2,161,007 (1973); *Chem.*
     *Abstr.*, *79:* 146,415s (1973).

23.  R. A. Stokbroekx, J. Vandenbenk, A. H. M. T. Van
     Heertum, G. M. L. W. Van Laar, M. J. M. C. Van
     der Aa, W. F. M. Van Beren and P. A. J. Janssen,
     *J. Med. Chem.*, *16*, 782 (1973).

24.  B. Hermans, H. Verhoeven and P. A. J. Janssen,
     *J. Med. Chem.*, *13*, 835 (1970).

25.  J. T. Plati and W. Wenner, U. S. Patent 2,489,669
     (1949); *Chem. Abstr.*, *44*, 2555f (1950).

26.  L. Levy and D. A. McLure, U. S. Patent 3,408,445
     (1968); *Chem. Abstr.*, *70:* 47302 (1969).

## 11

# Five-Membered Heterocycles Fused to One Benzene Ring

1. INDOLES

The classic and most convenient synthesis of the indole moiety is that of Emil Fischer. Recent examples of its use for drug synthesis includes one preparation of the nonsteroidal antiinflammatory agent, *indoxole (2)*.[1] Reaction of ketone *1* with phenylhydrazine in acetic acid leads directly to *indoxole (2)*. Alternately, anisoin *(3)* can be reacted

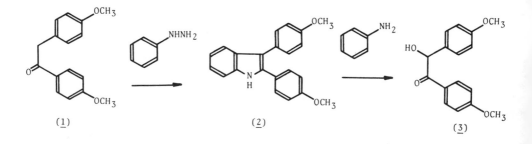

(1)                    (2)                    (3)

340

with aniline by heating in concentrated HCl, proceeding
presumably through direct displacement of OH by
aniline followed by cyclodehydration to 2. A credible
but more involved mechanism can also be written
starting with Schiff's base formation.

A somewhat more complex example of the Fischer
indole synthesis is provided by the tranquilizer,
*milipertine (8)*.[2] It can be prepared by reaction of

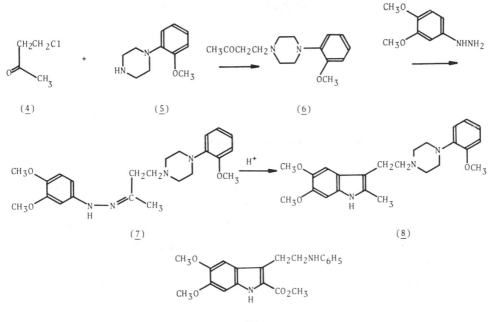

1-chlorobutan-3-one *(4)* with 1-(2-methoxyphenyl)
piperazine *(5)*, which leads to asymmetrical ketone *6*.
Reaction of *6* with 3,4-dimethoxyphenylhydrazine leads
to complex hydrazone *7* which, on treatment with
strong acid, rearranges to *milipertine (8)*. The
course of the last reaction reveals one of the classic

features of the Fischer synthesis-cyclization onto
the more substituted side of the ketone. Another
tranquilizer, *alpertine (9)*, has a rather similar
structure to *8*.

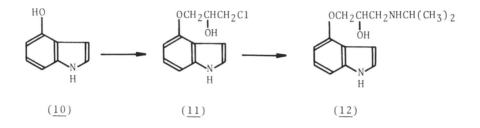

(10)                    (11)                    (12)

   Interest in the psychotropic features of the
mushroom substance, *psilocybine*, led to an exploration
of the chemistry of 4-hydroxyindole *(10)*. The availability of this substance provided a suitable starting
point for the synthesis of *pindolol (12)*, a β-adrenergic
blocking agent.[3] Reaction of *10* with epichlorohydrin
and NaOH led to ether *11* whose halo atom was readily
displaced by isopropylamine to complete the synthesis
of *12*.

   One of the more convenient methods of adding a
twocarbon side chain to the electron-rich 3-position
of indoles is the Speeter-Anthony reaction,[4] illustrated in the synthesis of the antiadrenergic agent,
*solypertine (15)*.[5] In this case, the reaction between
5,6-methylenedioxyindole and oxalyl chloride gives
ketoacid chloride *13*. The sequence then proceeds by
amide formation *(14)* with amine *5*. Reduction with

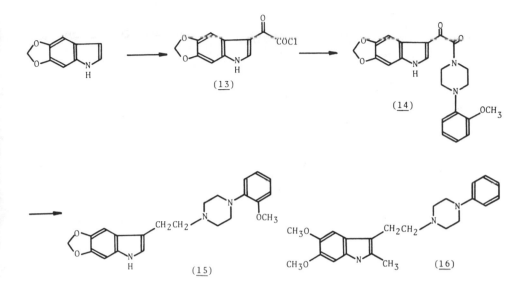

(13)

(14)

(15)

(16)

lithium aluminum hydride reduces both carbonyls to give *solypertine (15)* whose structural relationship to *milipertine (8)* is obvious. Another related drug is *oxypertine (16)*, an antidepressant made by essentially the same route as illustrated for *solypertine*.[5]

Combining the nucleophilicity of the indole 3-position just illustrated and the well-known tendency of C-2 and C-4 vinyl pyridines to add nucleophiles, a convenient synthesis of the tranquilizer *benzindopyrine (19)* was devised.[6] Reaction of N-benzylindole (17) with 4-vinylpyridine (18) in acetic acid produced 19 directly.

Tryptamine and serotonin are naturally occurring indole ethylamino compounds with pronounced pharmaco-

logical activities. They have served as the inspiration for synthesis of numerous analogues.  One such
study involved alkylation of 4-benzamidopyridine *(21)*

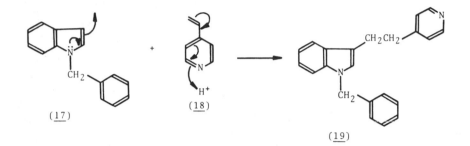

(17)          (18)          (19)

with 2-(3-indolyl)ethylbromide *(20)* to give quaternary
salt *22;* this intermediate was in turn hydrogenated
with a Raney nickel catalyst to give *indoramin (23)*,
which is antihypertensive, apparently because of its
α-adrenergic blocking activity.[7]

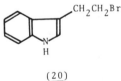
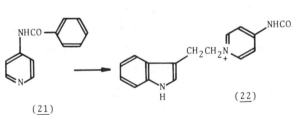

(20)          (21)          (22)

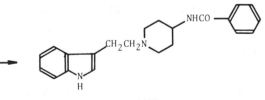

(23)

Because of the resonance stabilization possible
in its deprotonated form, the 5-tetrazolyl moiety is
actually nearly as acidic (pKa ca. 6) as many carboxylic acids.  This has led to its inclusion in many
drug series as a carboxyl surrogate.  Apparently
related in concept to indomethacin (26a), intrazole
(26) is a nonsteroidal antiinflammatory agent which
also inhibits platelet aggregation, and therefore is
of potential value in keeping the contents of the

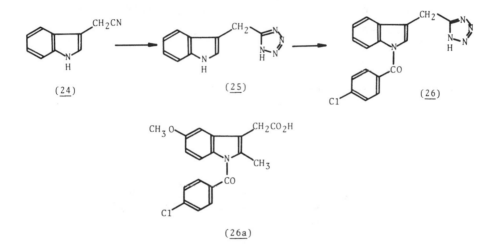

vascular bed free-flowing in certain pathological
conditions.  The synthesis begins with 2-(3-indolyl)-
acetonitrile (24) which is transformed to the tetrazoyl
derivative (25) by 1,3-dipolar reaction with sodium
azide.  The acidic indole NH hydrogen is abstracted
when 25 is treated with two equivalents of sodium

hydride and the salt, when acylated with a single
equivalent of 4-chlorobenzoyl chloride, is smoothly
transformed to *intrazole*.[8] Note that acylation
occurs preferentially at the more nucleophilic (indole)
anion.

When the indole 3-position is already substituted,
electrophilic reagents attack the 2-position instead
often through a 3,3-spiro intermediate. For example,
when 2-(3-indolyl)ethylmercaptan *(27)* reacts with
methyl acetoacetate, the thia-β-carboline analogue *31*
results. It seems plausible that the reaction involves
initial hemithioketal formation *(28)*, followed by
electron release by the indole nitrogen and hydroxide

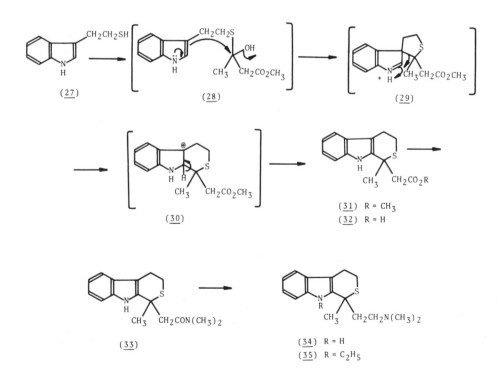

displacement to give *29*.  Compound *29* has interrupted
aromaticity, and a Wagner-Meerwein type rearrangement
would led to carbonium ion *30*, which would eject a
proton to restore indole resonance *(31)*.  In any
case, *31* is the product.  Saponification to the free
acid (*32* is followed by dimethylamide formation *(33)*,
mediated by carboxyl activation *via* mixed anhydride
reaction with ethyl chlorocarbonate. Lithium aluminum
hydride reduction to the tertiary amine *(34)* is
followed by base-mediated N-alkylation with ethyl
bromide to produce *tandamine (35)*, an antidepressant
that inhibits the uptake of norepinephrine into
storage granules.[9]

    *Yohimbine (36)* is a well-known and reasonably
available alkaloid from *Corynanthe yohimbe*, *inter
alia*.  For this reason, and partly because of its
intrinsic pharmacological activity (including reputed
aphrodisiac activity), chemists have frequently
studied its properties.  Oppenauer oxidation is
usually attended by saponification and decarboxylation
in this series, and yohimbone *(37)* is the product.
Wolf-Kischner reduction to *yohimbane (38)*, followed
by sodium hydride mediated alkylation, leads to the
analgesic agent, *mimbane (39)*.[10]

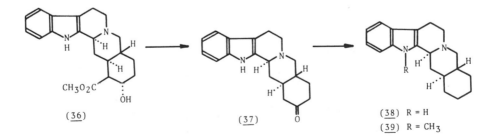

(<u>36</u>)                    (<u>37</u>)                 (<u>38</u>) R = H

                                                       (<u>39</u>) R = CH$_3$

## 2.   REDUCED INDOLES

Although geneologically related to indoles, the
dihydroindoles behave chemically rather like alkyl
anilines.   When diphenylamine reacts with chloro-
propionyl chloride, amide *40* results; this in turn
readily cyclizes to oxindole *41*.   Sodium hydride
followed by 2-chloroethyldimethylamine alkylates the
3-position (possibly through an intermediate
aziridinium ion); partial demethylation is accomplished by refluxing with ethylchlorocarbonate,
followed by hydrolysis of the intermediate carbamate
to give indolinone *42*, the antidepressant *amedalin*.[11]
Repetition of this sequence on the chloropropyl
homologue, followed by reduction of the appropriate
indolinone produces dihydroindole *43*, *daledalin*,
which also has antidepressant activity.[11]

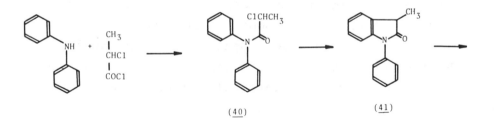

(40)    (41)

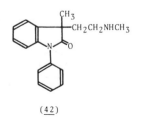

(42)

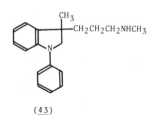

(43)

Hydrazides also containing a metasulfonamide function are known to exhibit diuretic activity. Substitution of an N-aminodihydroindole for the hydrazine is consistent with this activity. Preparation of one such agent is carried out by reaction of 2-methyl-N-aminoindoline *(44)* with 3-sulfamoyl-4-chlorobenzoyl chloride *(45)*, leading to the diuretic *indapamide (46)*.[12]

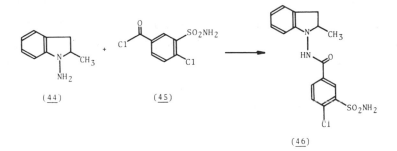

A more highly oxidized indole relative is isatin *(47)*. The ketonic carbonyl group is nonenolizable and has interesting properties. In strong acid it

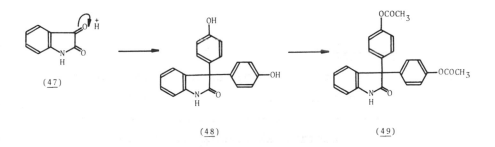

becomes protonated, and the oxygen can be replaced by electron-rich moieties. Almost 100 years ago such a condensation with phenol was discovered to lead to *48*. Acetylation led to *oxyphenisatin (49)* which has carthartic properties.[13]

It is also clearly anticipated that the ketonic moiety will form normal carbonyl derivatives. When isatin *(47)* is treated with sodium hydride and methyl iodide, the acidic hydrogen is alkylated to produce *50*. Then, reaction of the ketone carbonyl with thio-semicarbazine leads to *methisazone (51)*.[14] At the time of its discovery, *methisazone* was one of a very few antiviral leads showing activity in whole animal tests, and led to an extensive exploration of the properties of analogues.

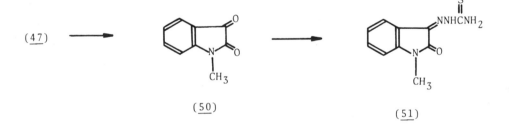

(47)                                     (50)                      (51)

### 3. INDAZOLES

The compounds of medicinal interest in this group so far have all been nonsteroidal antiinflammatory agents or analgesics. The prototype is *benzydamine (55)*.[15] An interesting alternate synthesis of this substance starts by sequential reaction of

N-benzylaniline with phosgene, and then with sodium
azide to produce carbonyl azide 52.   On heating,
nitrogen is evolved and a separable mixture of nitrene
insertion product 53 and the desired ketoindazole 54
results.   The latter reaction appears to be a Curtius-
type rearrangement to produce an N-isocyanate (54a),
which then cyclizes. Alkylation of the enol of 54

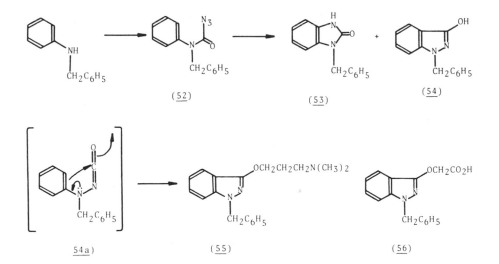

(52)            (53)            (54)

54a)            (55)            (56)

with sodium methoxide and 3-dimethylaminopropyl
chloride gives *benzydamine*.[16]   Alternatively, use of
chloroacetamide in the alkylation step followed by
acid hydrolysis produces *bendazac (56)* instead.[17]
*Bendazac*, an acetic acid derivative, more closely
resembles the classical nonsteroidal antiinflammatory
agents.

     Reduction of the benzene ring is also compatible
with activity in this group.   Reaction of N-methyl-
2-thiocarbamoylcyclohexanone *(57)* with methyl hydrazine

produces the analgesic agent, *tetrydamine (59),*
probably with the intermediacy of alkylhydrazone
*58.*[18]

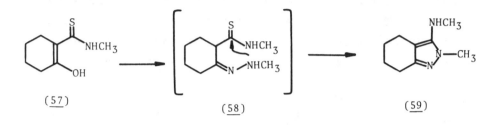

(57)                         (58)                    (59)

### 4.  BENZIMIDAZOLES

The control of worm infestations of domestic animals
(horse, sheep, cattle, pigs) and humans is an important
therapeutic objective for which *thiabendazole (60)*
serves as the prototype of numerous benzimidazole
derivatives.[19]   A widely used synthesis of this
system is illustrated by the preparation of *oxibenda-*
*zole (62).*[20] First, 4-hydroxyacetamide is alkylated
by use of KOH and n-propyl bromide, and the product
is nitrated to give *61.*  The latter compound is

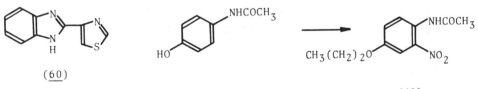

(60)

(61)

hydrolyzed, reduced to the phenylenediamine with
$SnCl_2$, converted to the 2-aminobenzimidazole system

by S-methylthiourea and subsequently acylated by
methylchloroformate to produce *62*.   *Lobendazole*

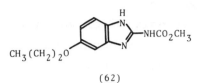

(62)

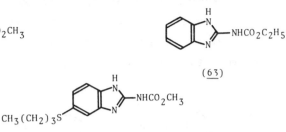

(63)

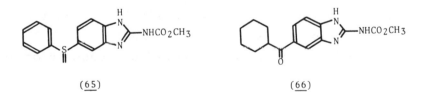

(64)

*(63),*[21] *albendazole (64),*[22] *oxfendazole (65),*[23]
*mebendazole (66),*[24] and *cyclobendazole (67)*[24] are all
made by fairly obvious variants on this basic scheme.
*Cambendazole (69)*, best of 300 antihelmintic agents
in an extensive study, is made by nitration of
*thiabendazole (60)* to 68, followed by catalytic
reduction and acylation with isopropyl chloroformate.[25]

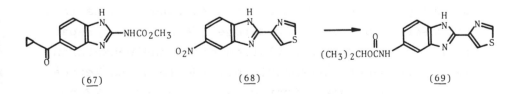

Flubendazole (70) belongs in this chemical class and is synthesized by similar methods but its bioactivity is expressed as an antiprotozoal agent.

At least in one case, a seemingly minor variation in the overall structure, change to the benzimidazolinone system, considerably alters the nature of

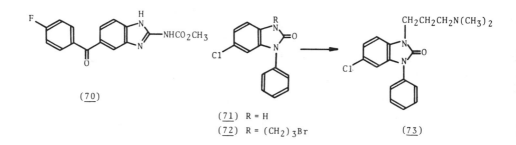

(70)

(71) R = H
(72) R = $(CH_2)_3Br$

(73)

the bioactivity exhibited. Treatment of 4-chloro-N-phenylbenzimidazolinone *(71)* with t-BuOK and 3-bromopropylchloride leads to halide *72*, which itself undergoes halogen displacement on heating with dimethylamine to produce the antidepressant, *clodazon (73)*.[26]

## 5.   MISCELLANEOUS

The pharmacological properties of *khellin (74)* have inspired a continuing interest in analogues. Change of the pyrone ring to a benzofuran ring results in a uricosoric agent, *benzbromarone (78)*. In its preparation, Friedel-Crafts acylation of 2-ethylbenzofuran *(75)* with 4-methoxybenzoyl chloride leads to ketone *76*, which undergoes ether cleavage to phenol *77* on

heating with pyridine hydrochloride; subsequent
bromination produces benzbromarone (78).[27]

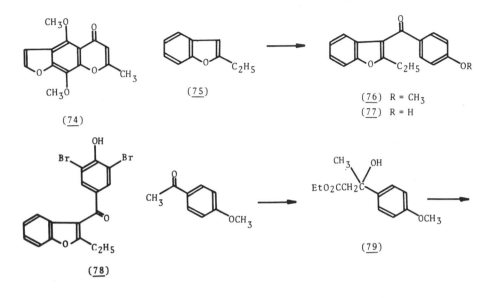

(74)

(75)

(76) R = CH₃
(77) R = H

(78)

(79)

Another khellin-inspired benzofuran is the
cardiotonic and vasodilating agent, benfurodil (84).[28]
The reported synthesis begins by Reformatsky reaction
between zinc, 4-methoxyacetophenone and ethyl bromoacetate to give 79. The alcoholic function is dehydrated with tosic acid, NBS leads to the allylic
bromide (80a) via the Wohl-Ziegler procedure, and
then SN₂ displacement with NaOAc produces acetoxyketone
80b. Treatment with HCl then closes the butenolide
ring to give 81. A Fries rearrangement, followed by
demethylation, acetylation, and then ether formation
with bromoacetone gives 82, which condenses to form
the furan ring on base treatment; then sodium borohydride reduction produces alcohol 83. The synthesis

of *benfurodil* *(84)* is concluded by reaction with
succinic anhydride and pyridine.

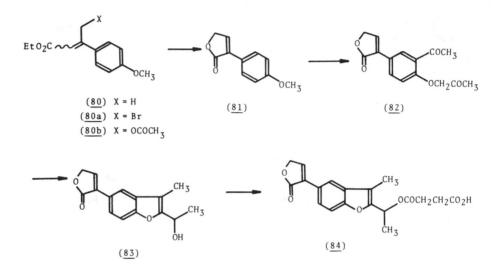

(<u>80</u>) X = H

(<u>80a</u>) X = Br                    (<u>81</u>)                    (<u>82</u>)

(<u>80b</u>) X = OCOCH₃

(<u>83</u>)                    (<u>84</u>)

    Probably inspired by *ibuprofen* and its analogues,
the nonsteroidal antiinflammatory agent *benoxaprofen*

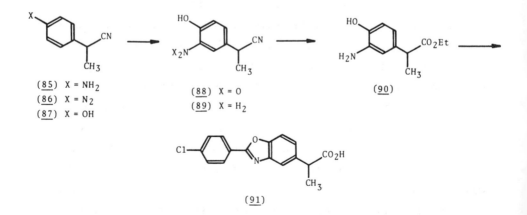

(<u>85</u>) X = NH₂

(<u>86</u>) X = N₂                    (<u>88</u>) X = O                    (<u>90</u>)

(<u>87</u>) X = OH                    (<u>89</u>) X = H₂

(<u>91</u>)

(91) is synthesized by starting with substituted
aniline 85.[29]  A Sandmeyer-type sequence of diazotization (86) and acid hydrolysis leads to phenol 87,
which undergoes nitration (88) and reduction to give
aminophenol 89.  Hydrolysis of the nitrile and
esterification produces ester 90, which is converted
to benoxaprofen (91) by acylation with 4-chlorobenzoyl
chloride, followed by cyclization and then by
saponification of the ethyl ester.

     A catecholamine potentiator that apparently
operates by inhibition of norepinephrine reuptake and
that also inhibits gastric secretion is talopram
(94).  Its specific synthesis is hard to locate, but
a general approach to this class of substance is
available in the literature.[30]  A suitable sequence
would start from gem-dimethylphthalide 92 by reaction
with phenyl Grignard reagent, followed by perchloric

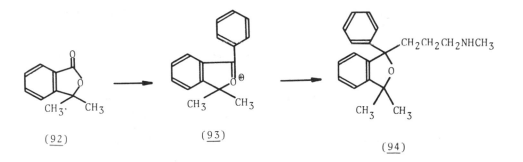

(92)                    (93)                    (94)

acid dehydration of the tertiary carbinol to give
oxonium ion 93.  Reaction of 93 with 3-dimethylamino-
propyl magnesium chloride would lead to the tertiary

amino analogue of *94*.  Demethylation would be accomplished by refluxing with ethyl chlorocarbonate, and the synthesis of *talopram* could be concluded by hydrolysis of the intermediate carbamate.

## REFERENCES

1.  J. Szmuszkovicz, E. M. Glenn, R. V. Heinzleman, J. B. Hester, Jr., and G. A. Youngdale, *J. Med. Chem.*, *9*, 527 (1966).

2.  S. C. Laskowski, French Patent 1,551,082 (1968); *Chem. Abstr.*, *72*: 43,733v (1970).

3.  Anon., Netherlands Application 6,601,040 (1966); *Chem. Abstr.*, *66*: 18,669x (1967).

4.  M. E. Speeter and W. C. Anthony, *J. Am. Chem. Soc.*, *76*, 6209 (1954).

5.  S. Archer, D. W. Wylie, L. S. Harris, T. R. Lewis, J. S. Schulenberg, M. R. Bell, R. K. Kulling and A. Arnold, *J. Am. Chem. Soc.*, *84*, 1306 (1962).

6.  A. P. Gray and W. L. Archer, *J. Am. Chem. Soc.*, *79*, 3554 (1957).

7.  J. L. Archibald and J. L. Jackson, South African Application 6803204 (1969); *Chem. Abstr.*, *72*: 121,363r (1970).

8.  P. F. Juby and T. W. Huidyma, *J. Med. Chem.*, *12*, 396 (1969).

9.  D. A. Demerson, German Patent 2,301,525 (1975); *Chem. Abstr.*, *85*: 103,883z (1976); W. Lippmann and T. A. Pugsley, *Biochem. Pharmacol.*, *25*, 1179 (1976).

10. J. Shavel, Jr., and M. Von Strandtmann, French Patent 1,405,326 (1965); *Chem. Abstr.*, *63:* 13,342a (1965).

11. A. Canas-Rodriguez and P. R. Leeming, *J. Med. Chem.*, *15*, 762 (1972).

12. L. Beregi, P. Hugon and M. Laubie, French Patent 2,003,311 (1969); *Chem. Abstr.*, *72:* 100,500t (1970).

13. A. Baeyer and M. J. Lazarus, *Ber.*, *18*, 2641 (1885).

14. D. J. Bauer and P. W. Sadler, *Brit. J. Pharmacol.*, *15*, 101 (1960).

15. D. Lednicer and L. A. Mitscher, Organic Chemistry of Drug Synthesis, Vol. I, p. 323 (1977).

16. G. Palazzo, G. Corsi, L. Baiocchi and B. Silvesterini, *J. Med. Chem.*, *9*, 38 (1966); L. Baiocchi, G. Corsi and G. Palazzo, *Ann. Chim. (Roma)*, *55*, 116 (1965).

17. G. Palazzo, U. S. Patent 3,470,194 (1969); *Chem. Abstr.*, *72:* 110,697n (1970).

18. G. Massaroli, L. Del Corona and G. Signorelli, *Boll. Chim. Farm.*, *108*, 706 (1969).

19. D. Lednicer and L. A. Mitscher, Organic Chemistry of Drug Synthesis, Vol. I, p. 326 (1977).

20. Anon., British Patent 1,123,317 (1968); *Chem. Abstr.*, *69:* 722k (1968).

21. P. P. Actor and J. F. Pagano, Belgian Patent 66,795 (1966); *Chem. Abstr.*, *65:* 5307g (1966).

22. R. J. Gyurik and V. J. Theodorides, U. S. Patent 3,915,986 (1975); *Chem. Abstr.*, *84:* 31,074r

(1976).

23.   E. P. Averkin, C. C. Beard, C. C. Dvorak, J. A.
      Edwards, J. H. Fried, J. G. Killian, R. A.
      Schlitz, T. P. Kistner, J. H. Druoge, E. T.
      Lyons, M. L. Sharp and R. M. Corwin, *J. Med.
      Chem.*, *18*, 1164 (1975).

24.   J. L. H. Van Gelder, A. H. M. Raeymaekers and L.
      F. C. Roevens, German Patent 2,029,637 (1971);
      *Chem. Abstr.*, *74:* 100,047s (1971).

25.   D. R. Hoff, M. H. Fisher, R. J. Bochis, A. Lusi,
      F. Waksmunski, J. R. Egerton, J. J. Yakstis, A.
      C. Cuckler and W. C. Campbell, *Experientia*, *26*,
      550 (1970).

26.   Anon., Belgian Patent 659,364 (1965); *Chem.
      Abstr.*, *64:* 2,093d (1966).

27.   N. P. BuuHoi, E. Basagni, R. Royer and C.
      Routier, *J. Chem. Soc.*, 625 (1957).

28.   J. Schmidt, M. Susquet, G. Callet, J. Le Meur
      and P. Comoy, *Bull. Soc. Chim. France*, 74
      (1967); J. Schmidt, M. Susquet, P. Comoy, J.
      Bottard, G. Callot, T. Clim and J. Le Meur,
      *ibid.*, 953 (1966).

29.   D. W. Dunwell, D. Evans, T. A. Hicks, C. H.
      Cashin and A. Kitchen, *J. Med. Chem.*, *18*, 53
      (1975).

30.   F. J. McEvoy, R. F. Church, E. N. Greenblatt and
      G. R. Allen, Jr., *J. Med. Chem.*, *15*, 1111 (1972).

# 12

# Six-Membered Heterocycles Fused to One Benzene Ring

The prevalence of heterocyclic rings among drugs and biochemical agents of mammalian origin can lead to the erroneous assumption that the presence of such rings in drugs means that this moiety of necessity constitutes part of the pharmacophore. As was noted in the case of the monocyclic heterocycles, these ring systems, in fact, often merely serve the function of a generalized aromatic system. The SAR of such molecules frequently demonstrates that the heterocyclic ring can be replaced by some other moiety with comparable electron distribution and lipophilicity without loss of biological activity. Sometimes, however, a given heterocyclic system does constitute part of the pharmacophore. Replacement of the particular ring system in such cases leads to loss of the desired biological activity. Recognition of pharmacophoric functions is today still largely an empirical

art, although susceptible to experimental inquiry.
It is expected that art will more closely approach
science with the emergence of a deeper understanding
of the mechanisms of action of drugs on the molecular
level, and the increasing frequency with which
receptors are now being isolated and studied.

### 1.  QUINOLINES

The quinoline antimalarial agents constitute one of
the earliest examples of pharmacophoric heterocyclic
systems.  It was recognized in the 1930's that chloro-
quinolineamines bearing an additional amino group in
the side chain were often endowed with activity
against the plasmodia that cause malaria.[1]  Further
exploration of these molecules led to an agent with
antiamebic activity. Mannich condensation of quinolol
1 with paraformaldehyde and N,N-diethylpropylenediamine
affords the antiamebic agent, *clamoxyquin (3)*.[2]

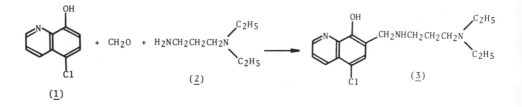

The structures of drugs that have proven clinically useful for treatment of hypertension tend to
fall into discrete classes according to their mode of
action.  It is thus usually a safe assumption that a
drug containing a guanidine function will show the

properties of a peripheral sympathetic blocking
agent; also, phenoxypropanolamines and some phenylethanolamines will be effective by virtue of their
β-adrenergic blocking activity. Experimental agents
on the other hand tend to show much greater structural
diversity; by the same token, it is more difficult to
relate mode of action to structure in these cases.
It is thus of note that a rather simple aminoquinoline
shows hypotensive activity.

The synthesis of this aminoquinoline starts with
one of the standard sequences for preparation of 4-
hydroxyquinolines, i.e., with the formation of the
Shiff base (5) from the appropriately substituted
aniline and diethyl oxaloacetate. Thermal cyclization gives the quinolone (6); this then spontaneously
tautomerizes to the enol form (7). Saponification
followed by decarboxylation gives the desired quinolol
(8). Treatment of 8 with phosphorus oxychloride
leads to replacement of the hydroxyl group by chlorine
(9).[3] Displacement of halogen by ammonia leads to
the corresponding amine, probably by an addition-
elimination mechanism. There is thus obtained
amquinsin (10),[4] a hypotensive agent. Formation of
the Shiff base of amquinsin with veratraldehyde gives
leniquinsin (11),[5] possibly a prodrug.

A related and relatively simple quinoline derivative has been reported to exhibit antidepressant
activity. Its preparation merely involves displacement of halogen in 12 with piperazine to afford
quipazine (13).[6]

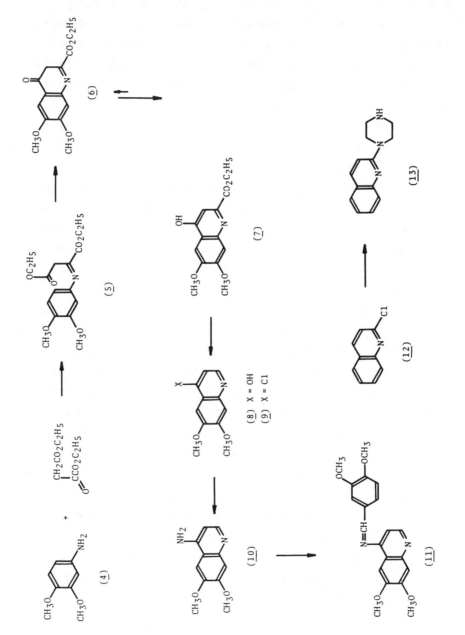

364

Derivatives of phenylethanolamine substituted by
a phenolic hydroxyl on the para position have been
known for some time to exhibit β-adrenergic agonist
activity.  As a consequence of this property, the
compounds have proven useful as bronchodilators for
the treatment of asthma (see Chapter 3).  Since such
sympathomimetic drugs tend to have undesired activity
on the cardiovascular system in addition to the
desired activity on the bronchii, considerable work
has been devoted to the preparation of compounds that
would show selectivity for the adrenergic receptors
($β_2$) that predominate in the lung.  Attachment of the
side chain to a heterocyclic aromatic phenol has been
one avenue that has shown promise for achieving this
selectivity.

Halogenation of the acetyl compound *14* affords
the corresponding chloroketone *(15)*.  (Compound *14* is
obtainable by acylation of the quinolol.  The pyridine
ring is, of course, deactivated in the acidic conditions of the reaction.)  Displacement of halogen by
means of isopropylamine leads to the aminoketone

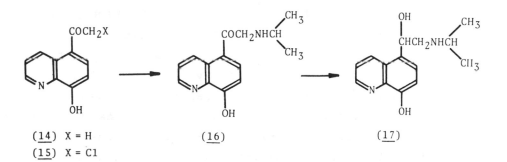

(*14*) X = H
(*15*) X = Cl                    (*16*)                    (*17*)

(16). Reduction of the carbonyl group by means of
sodium borohydride goes in a straightforward manner
to give the aminoalcohol, *quinterenol (17)*.[7] It is a
reasonable assumption that the heterocyclic system in
this case simply serves as a surrogate benzene ring.

Modern methods for raising poultry tend to
concentrate large numbers of birds in a very small
space. Although economically very attractive, the
resulting dense population is an ideal setting for
the extremely fast spread of avian epidemics, particularly those respiratory infections spread by droppings.
The single-celled parasitic coccidia pose a particular
threat to poultry flocks under these conditions.
Considerable work has thus been devoted to the development of poultry coccidiostats. The rapidity with
which these parasites develop resistance to chemotherapeutic agents serves as impetus for the development
of a constant flow of drugs with new structures.

The "quinates" constitute the prototype for the
quinoline poultry coccidiostats; many such agents can
be prepared using the following general synthetic
schemes. For example, alkylation of catechol with
isopropyl bromide affords ether *18*. Nitration perforce
affords derivative *19*. Catalytic reduction of the
nitro group followed by condensation of the resulting
aniline (*20*) with dimethyl ethoxymethylene malonate
(*21*) affords the anil *22*. The reaction is most
reasonably rationalized by assuming a conjugate
addition-elimination sequence. Heating of the last
intermediate in Dowtherm affords the coccidiostat

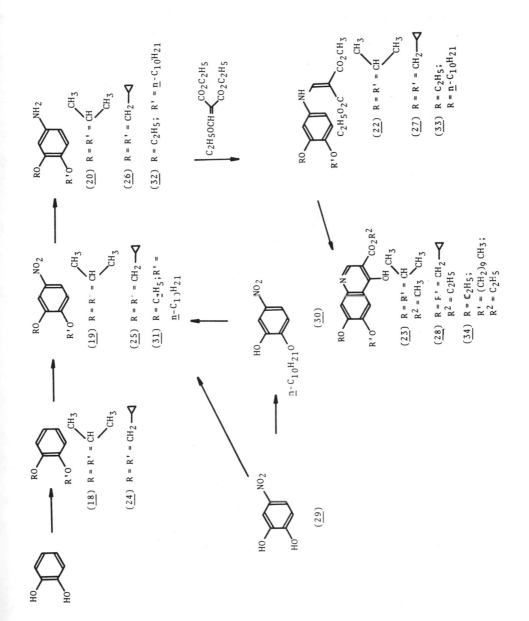

(18) R = R' = CH<CH₃ CH₃

(24) R = R' = CH₂▽

(19) R = R' = CH<CH₃ CH₃

(25) R = R' = CH₂▽

(31) R = C₂H₅; R' = n-C₁₀H₂₁

(20) R = R' = CH<CH₃ CH₃

(26) R = R' = CH₂▽

(32) R = C₂H₅; R' = n-C₁₀H₂₁

(29)

(30)

(22) R = R' = CH<CH₃ CH₃

(27) R = R' = CH₂▽

(33) R = C₂H₅; R = n-C₁₀H₂₁

(23) R = R' = CH<CH₃ CH₃; R² = CH₃

(28) R = R' = CH₂▽; R² = C₂H₅

(34) R = C₂H₅; R' = (CH₂)₉CH₃; R² = C₂H₅

367

*proquinolate (23).*[8] The same sequence using cyclo-propylmethyl bromide as alkylating agent for catechol and, later, diethylmethoxymethylenemalonate affords *cyproquinate (28).*[9]

The synthesis may be varied by reversing the alkylation and nitration steps. Thus for example, intermediate *25* can be obtained by alkylation of nitrocatechol *29*. The difference in reactivity of the two phenolic groups in *29* (<u>meta</u> and <u>para</u> to an electron withdrawing group, respectively) may be used to prepare derivatives carrying different alkyl groups on each of the catechol oxygens. Alkylation of *29* with decyl bromide gives ether *30*; reaction of the remaining phenolic function with ethyl iodide then gives *31*. This intermediate then is converted to *decoquinate (34)*[10] when subjected to the rest of the synthetic sequence.

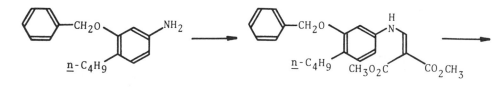

(<u>35</u>)                    (<u>36</u>)

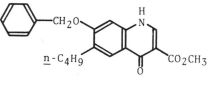

(<u>37</u>)

Replacement of one of the ethereal oxygen atoms by a methylene group is compatible with anticoccidial activity.  For example, condensation of substituted aniline *35* with dimethyl ethoxymethylenemalonate affords aminoacrylate *36*.  Thermal cyclization in diphenyl ether gives *nequinate (37)*.[11]

Replacement of the remaining ether oxygen by basic nitrogen leads to a compound that shows anti-malarial activity.  Nitration of aniline derivative *38* leads to substitution para to the alkyl group. (Protonation of the amine under the reaction conditions leads to deactivation of the position para to that group relative to that para to alkyl.  The position meta to the protonated amine is less deactivated.)

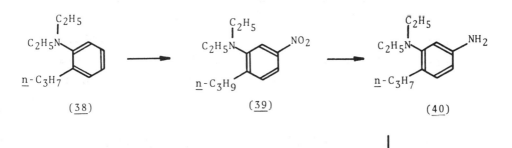

(38)                    (39)                        (40)

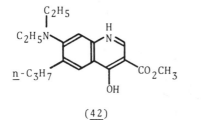

(42)

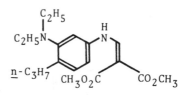

(41)

Reduction of the newly introduced nitro moiety affords
aniline *40*.    This is then subjected to the familiar
condensation-cyclization sequence to give antimalarial
*amquinate (42)*.[12]

Alkylation on nitrogen in this class leads to
compounds with antibacterial activity, apparently due
to inhibition of DNA gyrase. Condensation of aniline
derivative *43* with diethyl ethoxymethylenemalonate,
followed by cyclization of the resulting intermediate
affords the quinoline *44*.   Alkylation with ethyl
iodide by means of sodium hydride in DMF gives the
corresponding N-ethyl compound. (Deprotonation of *44*
leads to an ambident anion; alkylation at nitrogen
may be favored by the greater nucleophilicity and
steric accessibility of that atom.)   Saponification
of the ester affords *oxolinic acid (46)*.[13]   This
compound interestingly again illustrates the inter-
changeability of aromatic rings; the prototype antibacterial agent, *nalidixic acid (47)*,[14] contains a

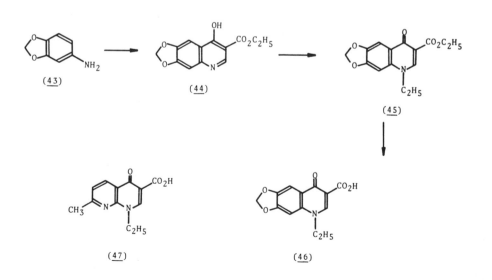

1,8-naphthyridine ring system and can be considered
an azaquinolone.

Reduction of either ring of quinolines greatly
alters biological activity.  Although the agent in
which the carbocyclic ring is reduced can be considered a substituted pyridine, it is included here
because it is prepared by using chemistry more akin
to that of quinolines.  Condensation of the cyclo-
hexanedione derivative 48 with the malondialdehyde
enol ether 49 leads directly to the tetrahydroquinoline 51.  The sequence can be envisaged as involving
first an addition-elimination reaction to afford,
after double bond migration, intermediate 50; aldol
cyclization will then afford the observed product.

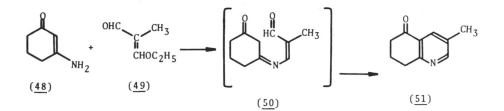

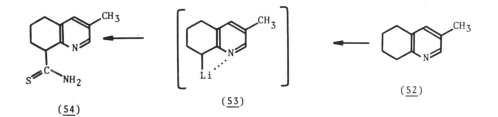

Reduction of the carbonyl group by Wolff-Kishner
reaction gives intermediate 52.[15]  Treatment of that
compound with butyl lithium gives the corresponding

metalated derivative (53); reaction of 53 with tri-
methylsilyl isothiocyanate affords the corresponding
thioamide. There is thus obtained the gastric antisecretory agent *tiquinamide (54)*.[16] This synthetic
sequence is of special interest in that direct chemical
reduction of quinolines usually results in reduction
of the heterocyclic ring.

Reduction of the heterocyclic ring and incorporation of a nitro function affords a compound with
antischistosomal activity, *oxamniquine (60)*. Its
synthesis begins with chlorination of 2,6-dimethyl-
quinoline, which proceeds regiospecifically on the
methyl group adjacent to the ring nitrogen (56).

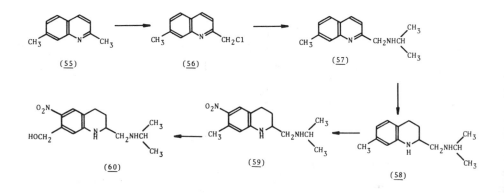

Displacement of halogen by isopropylamine gives
intermediate 57.  High pressure catalytic hydrogenation leads to reduction of the heterocyclic ring
(58), and nitration proceeds <u>para</u> to the NH group
(59). Microbiological oxidation of the methyl group
in that last intermediate using *Aspergillus sclero-
torium* affords *oxamniquine (60).*[17]

## 2.  ISOQUINOLINES

As has been noted elsewhere, blockers of α-adrenergic
receptors often bear little structural resemblance to
the phenylethanolamines which are the endogenous
agonists.  A relatively simple tetrahydroisoquinoline
derivative in fact shows hypotensive activity by
virtue of its α-adrenergic blocking properties.
Alkylation of tetrahydroisoquinoline itself with
bromochloropropane gives intermediate 62.  Displacement
of the halogen with sodium ethylmercaptide gives
thioether 63.  Oxidation of sulfur by means of peracetic acid is stopped at the sulfoxide stage to
afford *esproquin (64).*[18]

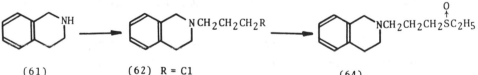

(61)          (62)  R = Cl

              (63)  R = SC₂H₅          (64)

The use of β-adrenergic agonists as bronchodilators is discussed in some detail in Chapter 3.

As mentioned there, requirements for activity include
the phenylethanolamine side chain and a phenolic
hydroxyl group or its equivalent disposed para to the
side chain.  It is of note that the side chain hydroxyl
can be omitted from molecules that contain the full
catechol substitution of epinephrine with retention
of good activity. One such compound, *trimethoquinol*
*(71)*, which in addition contains the side chain
sterically constrained by cyclization to a tetrahydroisoquinoline has proven to be a clinically
useful bronchodilator.  Condensation of trimethoxy-
benzaldehyde with ethyl chloroacetate under Darzens
conditions gives the glycidic ester *66;* this is then
converted to the sodium salt *(67)*.  This salt is then
treated with dopamine *(69)* under conditions which
will cause decarboxylation and rearrangement of *67* to
the corresponding aldehyde *(68)*.  The reaction conditions are coincidentally the same as those of the
Pictet-Spengler synthesis.  Thus, the intermediate
aldehyde reacts with the amine to form carbinolamine
*70* or the corresponding imine.  This then cyclizes to
the tetrahydroisoquinoline, *trimethoquinol (71)*.[19]
Interestingly, only the 1-S isomer is an active
bronchodilator.

Guanidines attached to a group of appropriate
lipophilicity have proven to be useful antihypertensive agents, active by virtue of their peripheral
sympathetic blocking activity.  *Debrisoquine (72)* is
in fact used clinically for that indication.[20]  The
7-bromo analogue *(76)* also shows antihypertensive

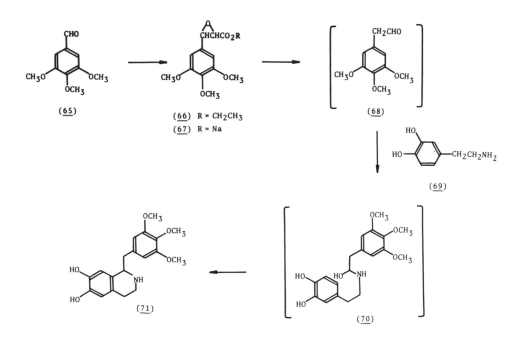

activity, and can be prepared as follows.  Diazotization of the aminodihydroisoquinoline *73*,
followed by conversion of the diazonium salt to the
bromide by heating in the presence of HBr, affords
intermediate *74*.  Reduction of the imine function
with sodium borohydride gives the saturated heterocycle *75*.  Condensation of this secondary amine with
S-methylthiourea affords *guanisoquin (76)*.[21]

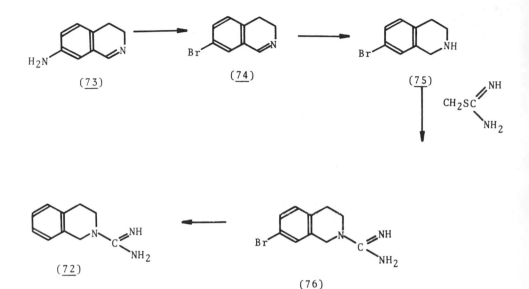

Formation of blood clots is a process necessary for maintenance of the integrity of the circulatory system.  Any break in the system results in clotting to seal off the potential leakage.  The final step in the process involves stabilization of the clot by a protein called fibrin.  A number of pathological conditions result in the formation of clots within the circulatory system in the absence of injury. Such clots--also known as emboli--present a serious hazard by their potential for blocking circulation of blood to vital organs.  The considerable research devoted to agents that will lyse the fibrin in clots has led to the development of the clinically useful agent, *urokinase*.  This drug is a fibrinolytic protein-aceous enzyme isolated from human urine.  The diffi-culty involved in isolation of significant amounts and the antigenicity of urokinase and a related

microbial product, streptokinase, has led to the
search for simple molecules that will accomplish the
same end.  A tetrahydroisoquinoline derivative *(80)*
has shown this activity in animal test systems.  Its
formation involves classical isoquinoline chemistry,
and begins with acylation of two molar equivalents of
phenethylamine *77* with adipic acid to afford the
diamide *78*.  Ring closure of the amide by means of
phosphorus oxychloride gives the usual Bischler-
Napieralski product *79*--although with an intervening
butylene chain.  Reduction of the imine by means of
sodium borohydride affords the fibrinolytic agent,
*bisobrin (80).*[22]

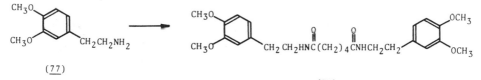

(77)

(78)

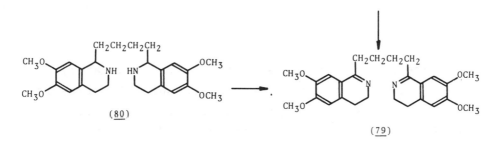

(80)

(79)

Products of Bischler-Napieralski cyclizations
discussed thus far have been reduced in order to
afford the desired biologically active compounds.
Occasionally, the products obtained directly from the

cyclization have biological activity in their own
right.   In one example, acylation of 2-phenethylamine
with p-chlorophenoxyacetyl chloride affords the amide
*83;* then, cyclization by means of phosphorus pentoxide
gives the antiviral agent *famotine (84).*[23]   The same
sequence starting with the p-methoxy acid chloride *85*
gives *memotine (87),* an antiviral agent.[23]

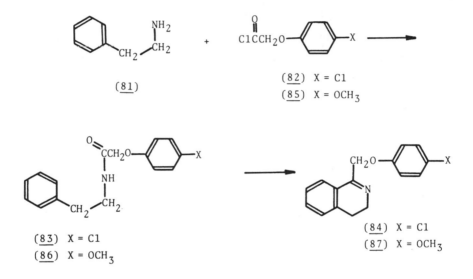

(81)

(82) X = Cl
(85) X = OCH$_3$

(83) X = Cl
(86) X = OCH$_3$

(84) X = Cl
(87) X = OCH$_3$

The majority of nonsteroidal antiinflammatory
agents contain an acidic carboxyl group.  A series of
experimental agents in this class have been prepared
in which the acidic proton is supplied by a highly
enolizable proton from a function such as a β-dicarbonyl
incorporated into a heterocyclic system.  As an
example, an acylated, highly oxidized isoquinoline
moiety can fulfill this function (see also the benzo-
thiazines below).  Toward this end, reaction of

homophthalic acid with ammonia affords the imide *89*;
triethylamine catalyzed condensation of that intermediate with p-chlorophenylisocyanate affords the
corresponding amide.  There is thus obtained the
antiinflammatory agent *tesicam (90)*.[24]

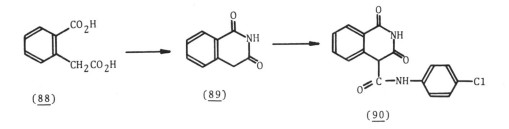

(88)                          (89)

(90)

### 3.  QUINAZOLINES

Quinazolines containing an electron-rich carbocyclic
ring have been associated with smooth muscle relaxant
activity.  The mechanism of action (phosphodiesterase
inhibition, α- adrenergic blockade) and organ selectivity (bronchi, vascular smooth muscle) vary greatly
with substitution on the heterocyclic ring.

Nitration of 3,4-dimethoxypropiophenone *(91)*
affords the nitro derivative *92*, and catalytic reduction leads to the aminoketone *(93)*.  This is then
converted to the corresponding formamide by means of
formic-acetic anhydride.  Treatment with ammonia
completes construction of the quinazoline ring.
There is thus obtained the bronchodilator-cardiotonic
agent, *quazodine (95)*.[25]

In a similar vein, condensation of the substituted
anthranilamide *96* with trimethyl orthoformate affords
directly the quinazolone *98*.  Reaction with phosphorus

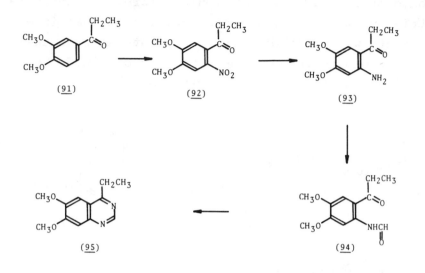

oxychloride converts the carbonyl to the enol chloride
(99).   Displacement of halogen with monosubstituted

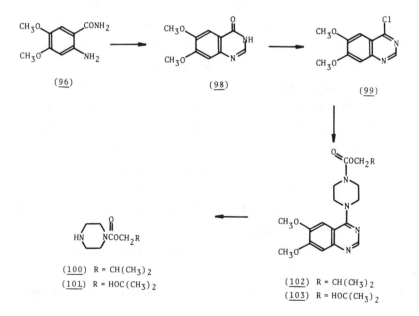

piperazine *100* gives the bronchodilator *piquizil*
(*102*);[26] the same reaction with piperazine *101* leads
to another bronchodilator *hoquizil* (*103*).[27]

A similar scheme is used to construct a quinazoline containing halogen at both positions 2 and 4.
The differences in reactivity of these halides make
available compounds bearing two different amine
substituents. Nitration of aldehyde *104*, followed by
oxidation affords the acid *106*. The acid is then
converted to the primary amide (*107*), and the nitro
group is reduced catalytically to the corresponding

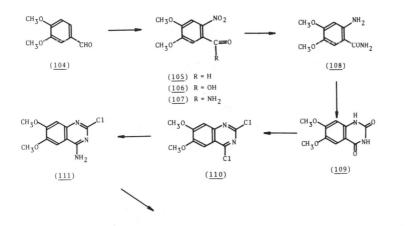

(*105*) R = H
(*106*) R = OH
(*107*) R = $NH_2$

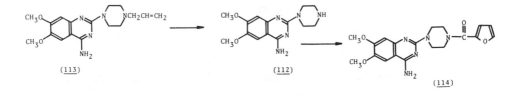

amine *(108)*. Condensation with urea completes construction of the heterocyclic ring *(109)*; this is
converted to the desired dichloride by reaction with
phosphorus oxychloride *(110)*. Reaction with ammonia
in THF at room temperature serves to replace the more
reactive chlorine by a primary amine *(111)*. Displacement of the remaining halogen is achieved with
piperazine under more strenuous conditions *(112)*.
Alkylation of the piperazine nitrogen with allyl
bromide affords the antihypertensive agent *quinazocin*
*(113)*.[27] Acylation at the same position gives the
recently commercialized antihypertensive agent *prazosin*
*(114)*.[28]

The same scheme starting with 3,4,5-trimethoxy-
benzaldehyde *(115)* affords initially dichloroquina-
zoline *116*. Reaction of this intermediate with
ammonia leads to replacement of the amine at the
2-position *(117)*. Displacement of the remaining
chlorine with piperazine carbamate *101* affords the
antihypertensive agent *trimazocin (118)*.[29]

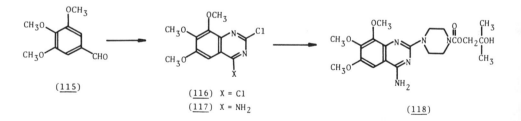

The extensive series of antibacterial agents
consisting of derivatives of 5-nitrofurfural has been
discussed in Chapter 8. It is of interest that a

derivative of nitrofuran in which the carbonyl is at
the acid oxidation stage and incorporated into a
quinazoline also shows antibacterial activity; this
agent, *nifurquinazol (124)*, is prepared as follows.
Treatment of the amide from 5-nitrofuroic acid with
phosphorus oxychloride leads to the corresponding
nitrile *(120)*. This intermediate is then converted
to the iminoether *(121)* with ethanolic hydrogen
chloride.[30] Condensation with anthranilic acid in the
presence of sodium methoxide gives the quinazolone
*122*. The amide function is then converted to the
iminochloride with phosphorus oxychloride *(123)*.
Replacement of halogen by means of diethanolamine
affords *nifurquinazol (124)*.[31]

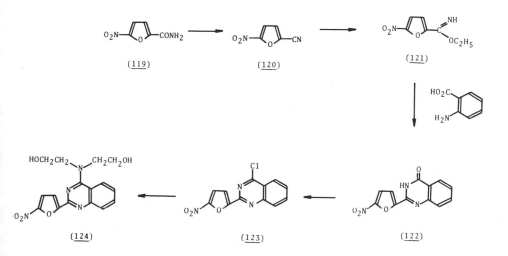

Benzothiadiazines containing halogen and a
sulfonamido group on the carbocyclic ring *(125)* form
a large class of diuretic agents often referred to as

the thiazides; the ring sulfone group can be replaced
by carbonyl with retention of significant biological
activity.[32]   More recently, it has been found that
diuretic activity is retained when one of the ring
nitrogen atoms carries an aryl group.  Toward this
end, the starting aniline *127* is first acetylated
*(128)* by means of acetic anhydride to protect the
primary amine in subsequent steps.  Reaction with
chlorosulfonic acid leads to sulfonyl chloride *129*;
this is converted to the sulfonamide by reaction with
ammonia *(130)*. Oxidation of the methyl group by means
of permanganate cleanly gives the acid *131*; the
acetyl group is then removed by hydrolysis. Treatment
of the resulting anthranilic acid *(132)* with phosgene
then leads to the isatoic anhydride *133*.  Reaction of
that anhydride with ortho-toluidine results in acylation of that aniline by the anthranilic acid *(134)*;
tying up the anthranilic acid up as the anhydride
serves to both activate the carbonyl towards amide
formation and to protect the amine towards self
condensation.  The carbamic acid presumably formed as
an intermediate decarboxylates.  Treatment of the
anthranilamide *134* with acetic anhydride affords
directly quinazolone *135*. (The sequence may be rationalized by assuming acetylation of the aniline as the
first step; formation of an imine between the carbonyl
and amide nitrogen gives the observed product.)
Reduction of the imine function with sodium borohydride in the presence of aluminum chloride gives
the diuretic agent *metolazone* *(136)*.[33]

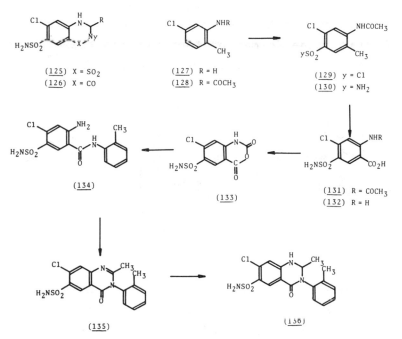

(125) X = SO$_2$
(126) X = CO

(127) R = H
(128) R = COCH$_3$

(129) y = Cl
(130) y = NH$_2$

(134)

(133)

(131) R = COCH$_3$
(132) R = H

(135)

(136)

The majority of nonsteroidal antiinflammatory
agents contain some function which supplies an acidic
proton, be this a carboxyl group or a highly activated
enol system.  A quinazolone devoid of such potential
enolizable protons forms an interesting exception to
this generalization.  (It is tempting in such cases
to speculate that the compound may exert its biological activity by some mechanism distinct from the
rest of the class.)  Alkylation of aminobenzophenone
*137* with isopropyl iodide gives the corresponding
N-alkylated amine *(138)*.  Treatment of that intermediate with urethane in the presence of zinc chloride
serves to form the quinazolone ring.  The reaction
may be rationalized by assuming acylation of the

amine as the first step to form urea *139*.    Intramolecular imine formation then affords the observed
antiinflammatory product, *proquazone (140).*[34]

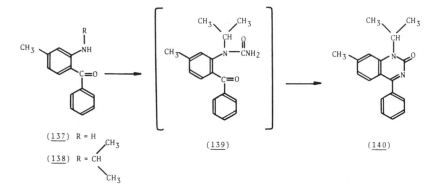

(137) R = H

(138) R = CH⟨CH₃/CH₃⟩

(139)

(140)

A more highly oxidized derivative of quinazoline
forms the heterocyclic moiety of a compound with CNS
activity.   Condensation of the aminopropylpiperazine
*141* with isatoic anhydride gives the anthranilamide
*142*.   Reaction of that amide with phosgene gives
directly the heterocyclic ring.   (The reaction may
proceed by initial formation of the carbamoyl chloride;

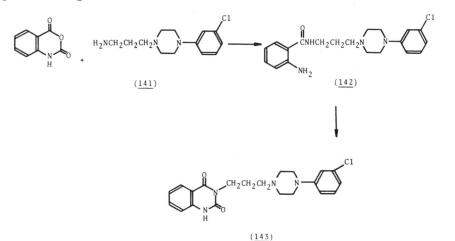

(141)

(142)

(143)

this may then either acylate the amide or alternatively
decompose to an isocyanate.  This last could then add
the amide nitrogen.)  The product of this sequence is
the sedative: tranquilizer *cloperidone (143)*.[35]

### 4.  CINNOLINES AND QUINOXALINES

Replacement of a methine in *oxolinic acid (46)* by
nitrogen is apparently consistent with retention of
antibacterial activity. One approach begins with
reduction of nitroacetophenone *144* to afford the
corresponding aminoketone *(145)*.  Treatment of this
intermediate with nitrous acid leads to the diazonium
salt; the diazonium group condenses with the ketone
methylene group (as its enol form) to lead to the
cyclized product, cinnoline *147*. Bromination proceeds
at the position adjacent the enol grouping *(148)*;

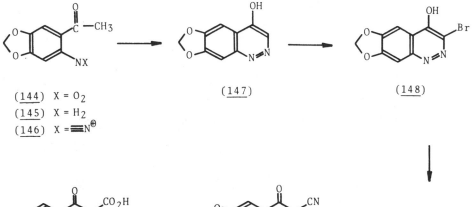

(144)  X = O$_2$
(145)  X = H$_2$
(146)  X = ≡N$^\oplus$

(147)

(148)

(151)

(150)

(149)

then displacement by means of cuprous cyanide (149) followed by alkylation on nitrogen affords cyanoketone 150. Hydrolysis of the nitrile function then gives cinoxacin (151),[36] an antibacterial agent.

The pyrazole derivative phenylbutazone (152) has found extensive clinical use as an antiinflammatory agent. (The acidic proton here is generated by a β-dicarbonyl system.) Incorporation of salient portions of the molecule in a condensed heterocycle yields a compound, cintazone (160), which also exhibits antiinflammatory activity. The synthesis of 160 starts with Grignard addition of methylmagnesium bromide to ortho-aminobenzophenone (153), affording carbinol 154; dehydration gives the corresponding olefin (155). The cinnoline ring is then constructed by a sequence similar to that used above. Thus treatment of the amine with nitrous acid gives the diazonium salt; treatment with mild base (ammonium hydroxide) causes the salt to close to the cinnoline (157). Catalytic reduction in acetic acid affords initially the product (158) of 1,4-addition of hydrogen; this product is in tautomeric equilibrium with cyclic hydrazine 159. Condensation of 159 with diethyl amylmalonate leads to formation of the pyrazolodione ring. There is thus obtained cintazone (160).[37]

Oxidation of 2,3-dimethylquinoxaline (from phenylenediamine and diacetyl) with either peracids or hydrogen peroxide in acetic acid gives the 1,4-dioxide (162).[38] Treatment of this bis-N-oxide with selenium dioxide leads to oxidation of one of the methyl groups to the methyl carbinol and formation of

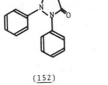

(152)

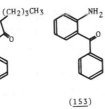

(153)

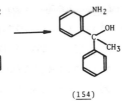

(154)

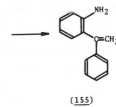

(155)

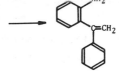

(156)

(157)

(158)

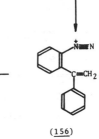

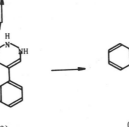

(159)

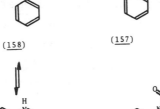

(160)

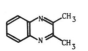

(161)

(162)

(163)

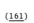

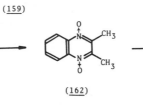

(164)

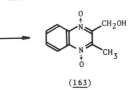

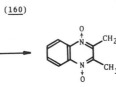

(165)

389

*mediquox (163),*[39] an agent used to treat respiratory
infections of poultry.  Reaction of *162* with selenium
dioxide under more strenuous conditions proceeds to
the aldehyde stage *(164)*.  Condensation of the carbonyl
group with methyl carbazate affords *carbadox (165).*[40]
The biological activity of *carbadox* is similar to
that of *mediquox*.

### 5.  MISCELLANEOUS BENZOHETEROCYCLES

Partial reduction of lactone *166* (using for example
diisobutylaluminum hydride in the cold) affords
lactol *167*.  Condensation with nitromethane leads to
the corresponding alkylated tetrahydrobenzopyran *170*.
The sequence probably starts by aldol reaction of the
hydroxylactone form of the lactol *(168)* with nitromethane to give the vinyl nitro intermediate *169*;

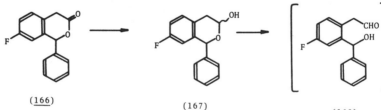

(166)                    (167)                    (168)

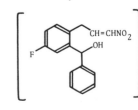

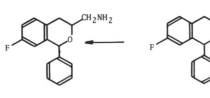

(171)                    (170)                    (169)

intramolecular conjugate addition of the alcohol will
then give the observed product.  Since this last step
is in principle reversible, the reaction is expected
to yield predominantly the thermodynamically favored
bisequatorial cis isomer.  Catalytic reduction of the
nitro group then gives the primary amine anorectic
agent *fenisorex (171).*[41]

Condensation of 2,4-dihydroxypropiophenone *(172)*
with benzoyl chloride and sodium benzoate goes to
afford chromone *174*, probably via ester *173*.  This
procedure is known as the Kostanecki-Robinson reaction.
Methylation *(175)* of the remaining phenolic function
by means of dimethyl sulfate, followed by reaction

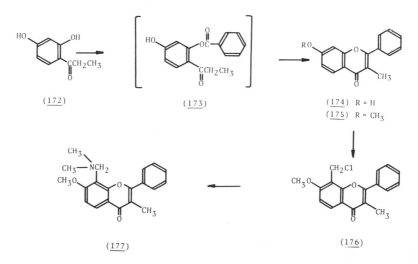

with formaldehyde and hydrogen chloride gives the
chloromethyl intermediate *176*.  Displacement of
chlorine with dimethylamine then affords the respiratory stimulant *dimefline (177).*[42]

Modification of the substitution pattern on the
same chromone gives a compound with smooth muscle
relaxant activity, *flavoxate (184)*.  The synthesis of
this flavone ester is initiated with methylation of
the hydroxypropiophenone *177* to *178* followed by
reduction of the nitro group to yield aniline *179*.
The amine is then used to introduce a nitrile by
diazotization followed by treatment of the diazonium
salt with cuprous cyanide *(180)*; the methyl ether is
then cleaved by means of aluminum chloride. Treatment
of the phenolic ketone *181* with benzoyl chloride and
sodium benzoate serves to build up the chromone ring
*(182)*.  The nitrile is next hydrolyzed to the acid
with sulfuric acid.  Esterification of the carboxyl
as--its acid chloride--with N-(2-hydroxyethyl)piperi-
dine affords *flavoxate (184)*.[43]

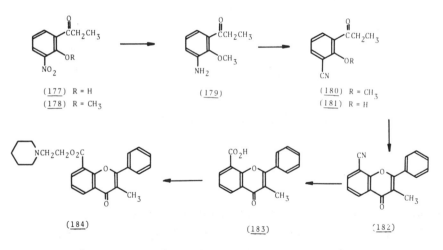

Reaction of salicylamide *185* (obtainable from a
suitable activated derivative of salicylic acid and
N,N-diethylethylenediamine) with ethyl chloroformate

in the cold followed by heating affords the benzoxa-
zinedione _187_.[44]  It is likely that the transformation
proceeds via carbonate _186_; the product, _letimide_
_(187)_, is reported to show analgesic activity.

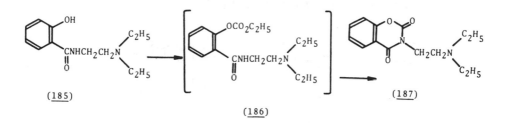

(185)                              (186)                              (187)

Among the heterocyclic systems that have been
used to provide a backbone for acidic, nonsteroidal
antiinflammatory agents are benzo-1,2-thiazine di-
oxides, such as _193-195_.  Entry to the ring system is
gained by an interesting ringenlarging rearrangement.
The necessary intermediate for the expansion reaction
is prepared by alkylation of saccharin _(188)_ with
ethyl bromoacetate to afford the ester _189_.  Treatment
of that with sodium methoxide results in formation of
the anion adjacent to the carbonyl; bond reorganization gives the net result _(190)_ of a ring enlargement.
The driving force for the reaction may well reside in
the fact that the anion of the product is a weaker
base than that of starting material.  Sodium hydroxide
mediated alkylation of the product _(190)_ with methyl
iodide might occur at any one of three sites (O, N or
C) due to the multidentate nature of the anion;
interestingly, the reaction proceeds to give only the
N-methylated product _(192)_.[45]  Amide formation from

*192* by interchange with 2-aminothiazole affords the antiinflammatory agent *sudoxicam (193)*;[46] the same reaction using 2-aminopyridine gives *pyroxicam (194)*.[46] Formation of the amide from *192* and 3-amino5-methyl-isoxazole leads to *isoxicam (195)*.[47]

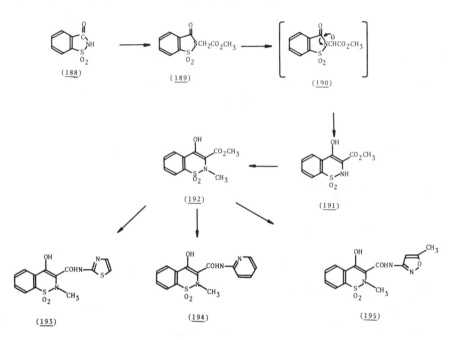

As noted above, a convenient pathway to cinno-lines consists of intramolecular condensation of a diazonium group with a ketonic methyl group, or alternately with a double bond. The analogous reaction with an amide nitrogen leads to 1,2,3-benzotriazines, such as *198*. Reaction of isatoic anhydride with N-aminomorpholine affords the hydrazide *196*; then, treatment with nitrous acid yields initially the diazonium salt *(197)*. Under the reaction conditions

this cyclizes to the triazine *198*, the analgesic
agent *molinazone*.[48] This must be one of the few--if
not the only--compound containing a linear array of
four nitrogens ever to be tried in the clinic.

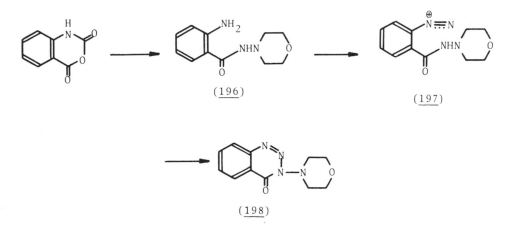

(196)

(197)

(198)

     Changing the substitution pattern on the carbo-
cyclic ring of the benzothiadiazine diuretics is well
known to have a marked effect on the qualitative
biological activity.  Thus, the direct analogue of
the diuretic *chlorothiazide (199)* in which chlorine
replaces one sulfonamide group, *diazoxide (200)*,
shows negligible diuretic activity; instead the
compound is a potent antihypertensive vasodilator.
The same pattern of activity is maintained in a
closely related analogue.  Condensation of amino-
sulfonamide *201* with aldehyde *202* affords the saturated
heterocyclic system *(203)*; oxidation with silver
nitrate leads to the antihypertensive agent *pazoxide
(204)*.[49]

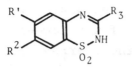

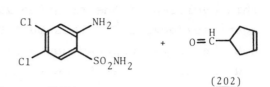

(199) R' = Cl; R$^2$ = SO$_2$NH$_2$; R$^3$ = H       (201)

(200) R' = H; R$^2$ = Cl; R$^3$ = CH$_3$

(202)

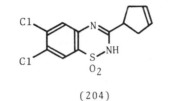

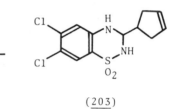

(204)                                    (203)

## REFERENCES

1.  For a fuller discussion, see D. Lednicer and L.
    A. Mitscher, Organic Chemistry of Drug Synthesis,
    Vol. I, p. 341 (1975).

2.  J. H. Burckhalter, W. S. Brinigar and P. E.
    Thompson, *J. Org. Chem.*, *26*, 4070 (1961).

3.  A. R. Surrey and H. F. Hammer, *J. Am. Chem.*
    *Soc.*, *68*, 113 (1946).

4.  F. F. Ebetino and G. C. Wright, French Patent
    1,388,756 (1965); *Chem. Abstr.*, *63*: 589c (1965).

5.  A. Winterstein, U. S. Patent 3,272,806 (1966);
    *Chem. Abstr.*, *65*: 18567 (1966).

6.  R. Rodriguez, German Patent 2,006,638 (1970);
    *Chem. Abstr.*, *73*: 98987g (1970).

7.   Anon., Netherlands Patent, 6,601,980 (1966);
     *Chem. Abstr.*, *66*: 115616k (1967).

8.   E. J. Watson, Jr., Belgian Patent 640,906 (1964);
     *Chem. Abstr.*, *63*: 2962 (1965).

9.   R. H. Mizzoni, F. Goble, J. Szanto, D. C.
     Maplesden, J. E. Brown, J. Boxer and G. De
     Stevens, *Experientia*, *24*, 1188 (1968).

10.  J. J. Ball, M. Davis, J. N. Hodgson, J. M. S.
     Lucas, E. W. Parnell, B. W. Sharp and D.
     Warburton, *Chem. Ind.*, 56 (1970).

11.  Anon., Netherland Application 6,602,994 (1966);
     *Chem. Abstr.*, *68*: 68899j (1968).

12.  R. L. Clark, A. A. Patchett, E. F. Rogers, U. S.
     Patent 3,377,352 (1968); *Chem. Abstr.*, *71*:
     38821x (1969).

13.  D. Kaminsky and R. I. Meltzer, *J. Med. Chem.*,
     *11*, 160 (1968).

14.  D. Lednicer and L. A. Mitscher, Organic Chemistry
     of Drug Synthesis, Vol. I, 492 (1975).

15.  A. C. W. Curran, *J. Chem. Soc.*, *Perkin Trans. I*,
     975 (1976).

16.  A. C. W. Curran and R. G. Shepherd, *J. Chem.
     Soc.*, *Perkin Trans. I*, 983 (1976).

17.  H. C. Richards, South African Patent 6803,636
     (1968); *Chem. Abstr.*, *71*: 30369k (1969).

18.  A. P. Gray and R. H. Shiley, *J. Med. Chem.*, *16*,
     859 (1973).

19.  E. Yamato, M. Hirakura and S. Sugasawa, *Tetrahe-
     dron Suppl.*, *8*, 129 (1966).

20.  D. Lednicer and L. A. Mitscher, Organic Chemistry
     of Drug Synthesis, Vol. I, 351 (1975).

21. R. C. Koch, Belgian Patent 635,308 (1964); *Chem. Abstr.*, *61:* 11978g (1964).

22. J. L. Fliedner, Jr., J. M. Schor, M. J. Myers and I. J. Pachter, *J. Med. Chem.*, *14*, 580 (1971).

23. Anon., Netherlands Application 6,516,328 (1966); *Chem. Abstr.*, *65:* 15351b (1966).

24. S. B. Kadin, South African Patent 68 03,465 (1968); *Chem. Abstr.*, *70:* 115025z (1969).

25. J. L. Minielli and H. C. Scarborough, French Patent M3207 (1965); *Chem. Abstr.*, *63:* 13287 (1965).

26. T. H. Cronin and H.J. E. Hess, South African Patent 67 06512 (1968); *Chem. Abstr.*, *70:* 68419 (1969).

27. Anon., British Patent 1,156,973 (1969); *Chem. Abstr.*, *71:* 91519f (1969).

28. T. H. Althuis and H.J. Hess, *J. Med. Chem.*, *20*, 146 (1977).

29. H.J. Hess, German Offen., 2,120,495 (1971); *Chem. Abstr.*, *76:* 127012e (1972).

30. W. R. Sherman and A. von Esh, *J. Med. Chem.*, *8*, 25 (1965).

31. H. A. Burch, *J. Med. Chem.*, *9*, 408 (1966).

32. D. Lednicer and L. A. Mitscher, Organic Chemistry of Drug Synthesis, Vol. I, 354-360 (1975).

33. B. V. Shetty, L. A. Campanella, T. L. Thomas, M. Fedorchuk, T. A. Davidson, L. Michelson, H. Volz, S. E. Zimmerman, E. J. Belair and A. P. Truant, *J. Med. Chem.*, *13*, 886 (1970).

34. H. Ott and M. Denzer, German Patent 1,805,501 (1969); *Chem. Abstr.*, *71:* 30502 (1969).

35.  S. Hayao, H. J. Havera, W. G. Strycker, T. J.
     Leipzig, R. A. Kulp and H. E. Hartzler, *J. Med.
     Chem.*, *8*, 807 (1965).

36.  W. A. White, German Patent 2,065,719 (1975);
     *Chem. Abstr.*, *83:* 58860k (1975).

37.  F. Schatz and T. Wagner-Jauregg, *Helv. Chim.
     Acta*, *51*, 1919 (1968).

38.  J. K. Landquist and G. J. Stacey, *J. Chem. Soc.*,
     2822 (1953).

39.  J. D. Johnston, U. S. Patent 3,344,022 (1967);
     *Chem. Abstr.*, *67:* 111452b (1967).

40.  J. D. Johnston, Belgian Patent 669,353 (1965);
     *Chem. Abstr.*, *65:* 7196e (1966).

41.  M. W. Klohs, F. J. Petracek, J. W. Bolger and N.
     Sugisaka, South African Patent 72 00,748 (1973);
     *Chem. Abstr.*, *79:* 126310a (1973).

42.  P. da Re, L. Verlicchi and I. Setnikar, *Arznei-
     mittelforsch.*, *10*, 800 (1960).

43.  P. Da Re, L. Verlicchi and I. Setnikar, *J. Med.
     Chem.*, *2*, 263 (1960).

44.  H. J. Havera and S. Hayao, South African Patent
     67 07,712 (1968); *Chem. Abstr.*, *70:* 87821k
     (1969).

45.  J. G. Lombardino, E. H. Wiseman and W. M.
     McLamore, J. Med. Chem., 14, 1171 (1971).

46.  J. G. Lombardino and E. H. Wiseman, *J. Med.
     Chem.*, *15*, 849 (1972).

47.  H. Zinnes, M. Schwartz and J. Shavel, Jr.,
     German Patent 2,208,351 (1972); *Chem. Abstr.*,
     *77:* 164722c (1972).

48.  H. Herlinger, S. Petersen, E. Tietze, F. Hoff-
     meister and W. Wirth, German Patent 1,121,055
     (1962); *Chem. Abstr.*, *56*: 15523e (1962).
49.  J. G. Topliss and A. J. Wohl, Swiss Patent
     558,376 (1975); *Chem. Abstr.*, *82*: 156390f (1975).

# 13

# Benzodiazepines

That the benzodiazepines continue to be prominent on the list of the 200 most frequently prescribed drugs in the United States is both a commentary on the nature of our contemporary society and a measure of their acceptance as anxiolytic and tranquilizing substances. Intensively competitive research into new analogues continues and this chapter chronicles some of the more prominent members of this group not detailed in the original volume.

The original entries into this class, such as *chlordiazepoxide (1)*, were N-oxides.[1] Treatment of the N-acetate *(2)* of *chlordiazepoxide* with aqueous acid served to hydrolyze the acylenamine function to liberate the keto analogue *(3)* which has been identified in excreta as an active metabolite of *1*; this minor tranquilizer has been named *demoxepam.*[2]

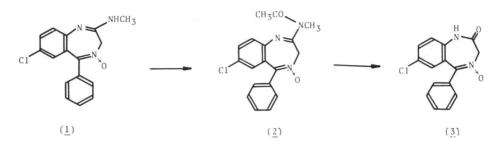

(<u>1</u>)                    (<u>2</u>)                    (<u>3</u>)

It will perhaps be recalled from the earlier
volume that such N-oxides are prone to undergo the
Polonovski rearrangement when treated with acetic
anhydride, and that this was illustrated by the
formation of *oxazepam*.[1] It is not surprising that
the N-methyl analogue *(4)* also undergoes this process,
and hydrolysis of the resulting acetate gives
*temazepam (5)*.[3] Care must be exercised with the
conditions, or the inactive rearrangement product *6*
results.

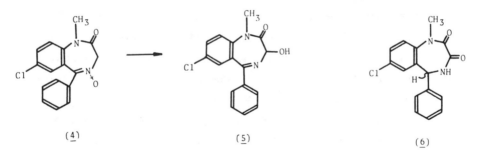

(<u>4</u>)                    (<u>5</u>)                    (<u>6</u>)

The lactam moiety in benzodiazepines is active
toward nucleophiles and numerous analogues have been
made by exploiting this fact. For example, heating
*demoxepam (3)* with N-cyclopropylmethylamine leads to
amidine formation, the minor tranquilizer *cyprazepam*

(7).[4]  On the other hand, treatment of *diazepam (8)*

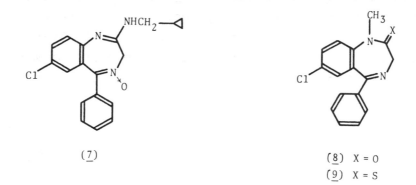

(<u>7</u>)

(<u>8</u>) X = O
(<u>9</u>) X = S

with phosphorus pentasulfide produces the corresponding thionamide, *sulazepam (9)*, also a minor
tranquilizer.[5]  The thionamide moiety is even more

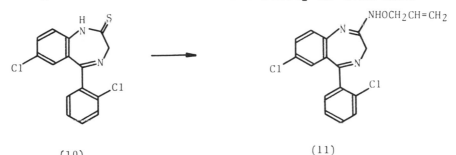

(<u>10</u>)

(<u>11</u>)

prone to aminolytic amidine formation than the lactam
itself.  Reaction of thionamide *10* with O-allyl-
hydroxylamine gave the oximinoether *11, uldazepam.*[6]

An attempt to reduce metabolic N-dealkylation
resulted in the preparation of *fletazepam (16)*, whose
activity is expressed as a muscle relaxant.[7]  Direct
N-alkylation of the amide NH group at a late stage in
the synthesis with trifluoroethyl iodide and NaH went

in poor yield, so the desired alkyl group was introduced at an earlier stage. Alkyation of 4-chloro-
aniline by the trichloromesyl ester of trifluoro-
ethanol (12) produced secondary aniline 13. This
underwent alkylation by aziridine to produce diamine
14. Acylation with 2-fluorobenzoyl chloride produced

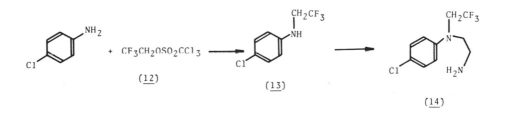

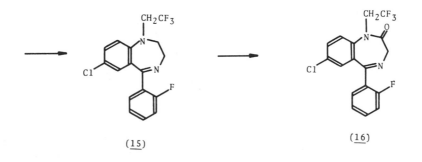

the desired secondary amide which underwent Bischler-
Napieralski cyclodehydration with $POCl_3$ and $P_2O_5$ to
give 15. The lactam moiety was introduced by ruthenium
tetroxide oxidation to give *fletazepam (16)*.
Interestingly, the deoxy analogue minus the fluorine
atom, prepared by a similar route,[7] is also a minor
tranquilizer.

A rather interesting synthesis of the basic ring
system based upon oxidative scission of indole pre-
cursors was used to prepare *prazepam (24)*, a muscle
relaxant.[8]  Starting with indole *17*, N-alkylation to
*18* was accomplished with cyclopropylmethyl bromide
and NaH.  The ester was converted to the amide *(21)*
by the usual sequence and then reduced to primary
amine *22* using lithium aluminum hydride.

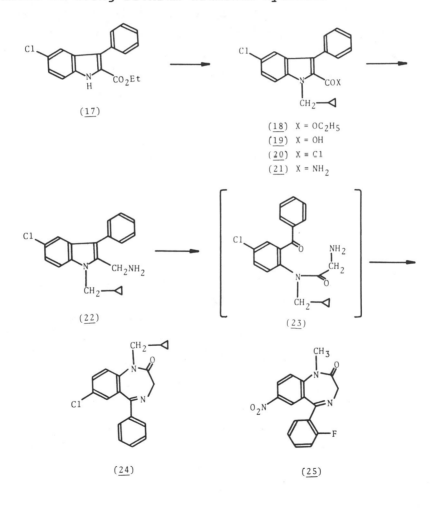

(17)

(18) X = $OC_2H_5$
(19) X = OH
(20) X = Cl
(21) X = $NH_2$

(22)

(23)

(24)

(25)

Oxidation with chromium trioxide in acetic acid
cleaved the indole ring to produce intermediate *23*
which cyclodehydrated to give *prazepam* *(24)*.

Nitration of benzodiazepines takes place at the
electron rich $C_7$ position, and this was used to
prepare *flunitrazepam* *(25)*, a potent hypnotic agent.[9]

It is interesting to note that some 1,5-benzo-
diazepines such as *29* also possess CNS depressant
activity. Treatment of substituted diphenylamine *26*
with methyl malonyl chloride and reduction with Raney
nickel led to orthophenylenediamine analogue *27*.
Sodium alkoxide treatment led to lactam formation
*(28)*, and alkylation in the usual way with NaH and
methyl iodide produced *clobazam* *(29)*.[10]

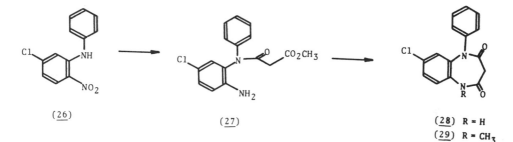

(26)                         (27)                    (28) R = H
                                                     (29) R = CH₃

On the other hand, $MnO_2$ oxidation of lactam *30*
or arylation of secondary lactam *32* with bromobenzene
using Cu powder and potassium acetate both led to
anxiolytic *triflubazam* *(31)*.[11]

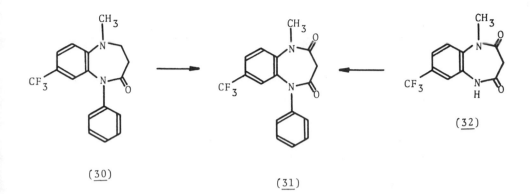

(30)                        (31)                        (32)

## REFERENCES

1.  D. Lednicer and L. A. Mitscher, Organic Chemistry
    of Drug Synthesis, p. 365, 1977.
2.  L. H. Sternbach and E. Reeder, *J. Org. Chem.*,
    *26*, 4936 (1961).
3.  S. C. Bell and S. J. Childress, *J. Org. Chem.*,
    *27*, 1691 (1962).
4.  H. M. Wuest, U. S. Patent 3,138,586 (1964);
    *Chem. Abstr.*, *61*: 7,032f (1964).
5.  G. A. Archer and L. H. Sternbach, *J. Org. Chem.*,
    *29*, 231 (1964).
6.  J. B. Hester, Jr., German Patent 2,005,176
    (1970); *Chem. Abstr.*, *73*: 99,001t (1970).
7.  M. Steinman, J. G. Topliss, R. Alekel, Y.S. Wong
    and E. E. York, *J. Med. Chem.*, *16*, 1354 (1973).
8.  S. Inaba, T. Hirohashi and H. Yamamoto, *Chem.
    Pharm. Bull.*, *17*, 1263 (1969).
9.  L. H. Sternbach, R. I. Fryer, O. Keller, W.
    Metlesics, G. Sach and N. Steiger, *J. Med.*

Chem., 6, 261 (1963).

10.   K.H. Weber, A. Bauer and K.H. Hauptmann, *Ann.*,
      *756*, 128 (1972).

11.   K.H. Weber, H. Merz and K. Ziele, German Patent
      1,934,607 (1970); *Chem. Abstr.*, *72:* 100,771g
      (1970); and K.-H. Weber, K. Minck, A. Bauer and
      H. Merz, German Patent 2,006,601 (1971); *Chem.*
      *Abstr.*, *76:* 3918k (1972).

# 14

# Heterocycles Fused
# to Two Benzene Rings

Pharmacological agents based on dibenzo heterocyclic
compounds had their inception in the formal cyclization
by inclusion of a hetero bridging atom of the two
benzene rings characteristic of diphenylamine and
benzhydryl antihistamines.  As detailed in the earlier
volume, this approach led to the development of the
first of the antipsychotic agents, *chlorpromazine*.
Further modification of the central ring led to
compounds that showed antidepressant rather than
tranquilizing activity.  It might be noted in passing
that it was eventually discovered that the central
ring in antidepressants need not be heterocyclic at
all; some of the more widely used antidepressant drugs
are in fact derivatives of dibenzocycloheptadiene.
Further modification of the dibenzoheterocycles has
not yielded agents with markedly different activities.
The compounds discussed below, with few exceptions,

409

exhibit either antihistaminic or central nervous
system activity.

1.  CENTRAL RING CONTAINING ONE HETEROATOM
Reaction of 2-bromobenzoic acid (1) with chlorosulfonic
acid proceeds to afford the sulfonyl chloride 2;
treatment with dimethylamine leads to the corresponding
sulfonamide (3).  Condensation of bromoacid 3 with
the anion from thiophenol in the presence of copper
powder results in displacement of halogen by sulfur
(4).  Friedel-Crafts cyclization of that sulfide by
means of sulfuric acid gives the desired thioxanthone
(5), which is then reduced to the thioxanthene (6).
Treatment of that intermediate with butyl lithium
serves to form the anion at the methylene group; the
corresponding acyl derivative 7 is obtained by condensation of the anion with methyl acetate.  Mannich
reaction on the ketone with formaldehyde and N-methylpiperazine yields the amino ketone (8). The carbonyl
group is then reduced with sodium borohydride.
Dehydration by means of phosphorus oxychloride in
pyridine gives the major tranquilizer *thiothixene*
(10).[1]  As might be expected, this last reaction
gives a mixture of isomers; the more active Z isomer
is separated from the mixture by fractional crystallization.

The presence of a rather more complex substituent
on the remote piperazine nitrogen atom is consistent
with tranquilizing activity.  The preparation of one
such agent, 16, begins with reaction of thioxanthone
11 (obtained by a sequence analogous to that used to

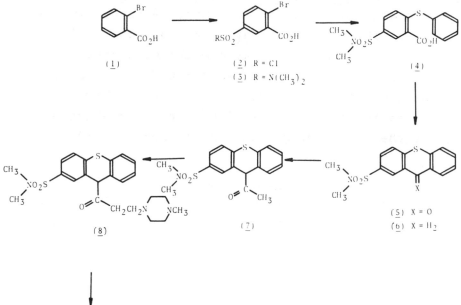

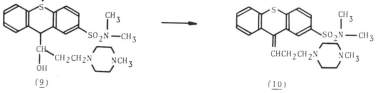

prepare 5) with the Grignard reagent from 3-(tertiary-
amyloxy)propyl bromide to afford alcohol *12*.    Treatment
with hydrogen bromide serves to dehydrate the carbinol,
remove the protecting group from the terminal alcohol,

and finally to convert that alcohol to the corresponding bromide (13). Although this would be expected
as a mixture of isomers, the sharp melting point of
the product suggests it may be homogenous. This
halide is then used to alkylate the monocarbamate
from piperazine, yielding 14. Saponification of the
carbamate affords the secondary amine 15. Michael
condensation of that base with N-methylacrylamide
gives the neuroleptic agent, *clothixamide (16).*[2]

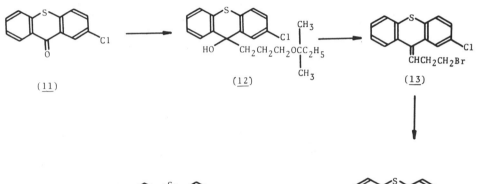

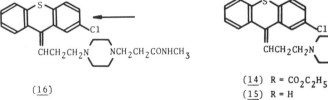

Reduction of the exocylic double bond and inclusion
of the side chain nitrogen in a piperidine ring leads
to a compound (19) which exhibits skeletal muscle
relaxant activity. Its one step synthesis begins
with reaction of thioxanthene (17) with phenyl sodium

to afford the anion at the methylene group of the heterocycle; then, condensation of that anion with piperidine derivative *18* gives directly *methixene* (*19*).[3]

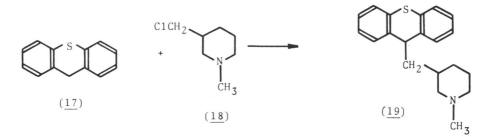

(17)        (18)        (19)

*Lucanthone (20)* constitutes one of the first effective antischistosomal agents. Biological investigation of this agent showed that the active species in man is in fact the hydroxylated metabolic product *hycanthone (21)*. The published synthesis for the latter involves microbial oxidation as the last step.[4] Additional hydroxylated derivatives of *lucanthone* have been investigated. One of these, *becanthone (26)*, made as part of an investigation of antitumor agents, shows activity against schistosomes comparable to that of *hycanthone*. Ullmann reaction of the salt of thiophenol *22* with 2-chlorobenzoic acid in the presence of copper gives the sulfide *23*. Ring closure by means of sulfuric acid gives the corresponding thioxanthone (*24*). Nucleophilic aromatic substitution of the chlorine atom in *24* with aminoalcohol *25* gives *becanthone (26)* directly.[5]

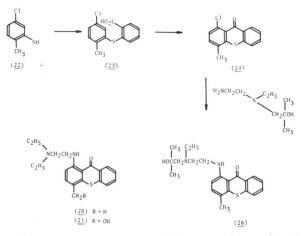

(20) R = H
(21) R = OH

(26)

The thioxanthene tranquilizers described above
may be regarded as phenothiazine analogues in which a
methine group acts as surrogate for nitrogen; that
is, the side chain is attached to $sp_2$ carbon instead
of nitrogen.  It is thus of some interest that further,
rather drastic, modification of the central ring
still gives a compound with tranquilizing activity.
In the case of *clomacran* *(30)*, the side chain is
again attached to carbon, albeit tetrahedral rather
than trigonal carbon.  In addition, the sulfur atom
present in both phenothiazines and thioxanthenes is
replaced by a secondary amine.  This might be interpreted to mean that the nature of the bridge between
the benzene rings is not crucial for biological
activity.  The preparation of *30* begins with reaction
of acridone *27* with the Grignard reagent from 3-chloro-
N,N-dimethylpropylamine to afford tertiary carbinol
*28*; dehydration by means of acid or simply heat gives
the corresponding olefin *(29)*.  Catalytic reduction
completes the synthesis of the tranquilizer, *clomacran*
*(30)*.[6]

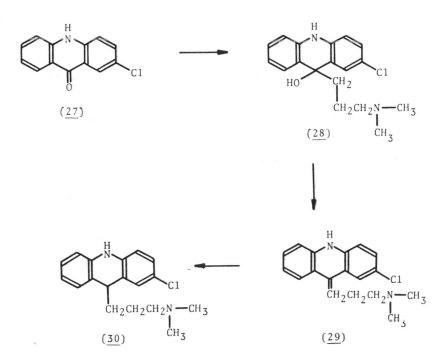

(27)

(28)

(30)

(29)

Nuclei for tricyclic antidepressants and tranquilizers almost invariably contain the three rings
fused in linear array.  It is thus interesting to
note that an angular arrangement of these rings, such

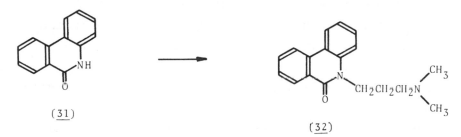

(31)

(32)

as in *fantridone* (32), is consistent with antidepressant activity.  Alkylation of the anion obtained
by treatment of phenathridone (31) with sodium hydride

and 3-chloro-N,N-dimethylpropylamine affords *fantridone* (*32*) directly.[7]

Almost every major structural class discussed to date has featured at least one nonsteroidal anti-inflammatory carboxylic acid.  It is thus perhaps not surprising to find a dibenzoheterocycle serving as the nucleus for one of these agents, *furobufen* (*34*). Straightforward Friedel-Crafts acylation of dibenzo-furan (*33*) with succinic anhydride affords a mixture of 2- and 3-acylated products, with the latter pre-dominating.  The mixture is esterified with methanol, and the methyl ester of the 3-isomer is separated by fractional crystallization.  Hydrolysis back to the acid affords pure *34*.[8]

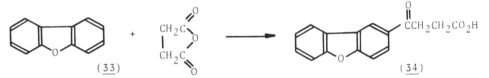

Replacement of sulfur in the phenothiazines by two methylene groups also results in compounds that retain antipsychotic activity; two examples are *carpipramine* (*41*) and *clocapramine* (*44*). Although one might describe this as yet another example of the bioisosteric equivalence of sulfur and ethylene, the observed broad latitude in the nature of the tricyclic system in tranquilizers suggests caution in drawing such a conclusion.  In a convergent synthesis of *41*, reaction of N-benzyl-4-piperidone (*35*) with potassium cyanide and piperidine hydrochloride gives the corres-ponding α-aminonitrile (*36*).  Hydrolysis of the nitrile by means of 90% sulfuric acid gives the amide

*37*; hydrogenolysis of the benzyl protecting group then affords the secondary amine *38*.[9] Alkylation of dibenzazepine *39* with 1-bromo-3-chloropropane gives intermediate *40*. Use of that material to alkylate piperidine *38* affords finally *carpipramine (41)*.[10] The same sequence starting with halogen substituted dibenzazepine *42* leads to the tranquilizer *clocapramine (44)*.[10]

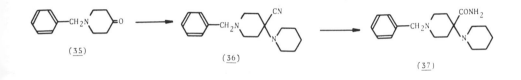

(35)　　　　　(36)　　　　　(37)

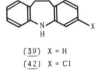

(39) X = H
(42) X = Cl

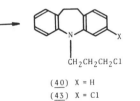

(40) X = H
(43) X = Cl

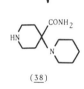

(38)

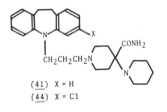

(41) X = H
(44) X = Cl

Many tricyclic tranquilizers and antidepressants
exhibit some measure of anticholinergic activity.
It is of interest to note that attachment of a basic
side chain on carbon of an isomeric dibenzazepine
affords a compound in which anticholinergic activity
predominates, *elantrine (50)*.  Reaction of anthra-
quinone *(45)* with the Grignard reagent from 3-chloro-
N,N-dimethylaminopropane in THF in the cold results
in addition to but one of the carbonyl groups to
yield hydroxyketone *46*.  This is then converted to
oxime *47* in a straightforward manner.  Treatment of
that intermediate with a mixture of phosphoric and
polyphosphoric acids results in net dehydration of

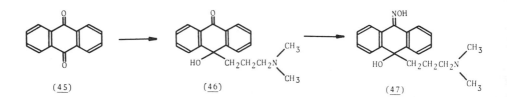

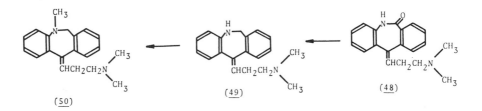

the tertiary carbinol and Beckmann rearrangement of
the oxime to afford the enelactam *48*; the stereochemistry of the product(s) (E,Z) is not specified.
The lactam is then reduced to amine *49* with lithium
aluminum hydride, and the resulting amine is methylated to obtain *elantrine (50)*.[11]

Replacement of the ring nitrogen in *50* by oxygen
yields a molecule that can now again be characterized
as a tranquilizer, although one that shows some
degree of anticholinergic activity. Synthesis of this
agent, *pinoxepin (55)*, begins with the reaction of
1,3-dibromopropane with triphenylphosphine to give the
bromoalkylphosphonium salt *51*.  Displacement of the
remaining bromine by piperazine then leads to the

$$BrCH_2CH_2CH_2Br + (C_6H_5)_3P \longrightarrow Br^{\ominus} (C_6H_5)_3\overset{\oplus}{P}CH_2CH_2CH_2Br \longrightarrow Br^{\ominus} (C_6H_5)_3\overset{\oplus}{P}CH_2CH_2CH_2N\bigcirc NH$$

$$(\underline{51}) \qquad\qquad\qquad (\underline{52})$$

(53)

(54)

(55)

functional phosphonium salt *52*. The latter is then
converted to the corresponding ylide by means of

butyl lithium, and the resulting reactive intermediate
is condensed with ketone *53*.  The product *(54)* in
this case consists largely (4:1) of the Z isomer.
The stereoselectivity may involve complexation of the
betaine intermediate with the heterocyclic oxygen.
Condensation of the terminal secondary amine with
ethylene oxide affords *pinoxepin (55)*. [12]

### 2.   BENZOHETEROCYCLOHEPTADIENES

Both this and the previous volume are of course organ-
ized on the basis of structural classes.  Occasionally, a series of medicinal agents defies attempts at
neat classification by such a scheme. The compounds
that follow could only be called dibenzoheterocycles
by performing the imaginary operation of moving the
hetero atom from the flanking to the central ring of
the molecule.  The chemistry and biological activity
of those molecules does seem to argue for their
inclusion at this juncture.

The first of these compounds, *pizotyline (65)*,
shows activity much akin to related tricyclic depressants such as *imipramine (56)*. [13] One of several
schemes for preparation of the key tricyclic intermediate *63* starts by reaction of 2-chloromethylthio-
phene *57* with triethyl phosphite.  The net transformation (Arbuzov reaction) probably starts with
formation of phosphonium salt *58;* displacement of one
of the ethyoxy groups by chloride at carbon then
leads to loss of ethyl chloride and formation of the
observed phosphonate *59*.  Reaction of the ylide

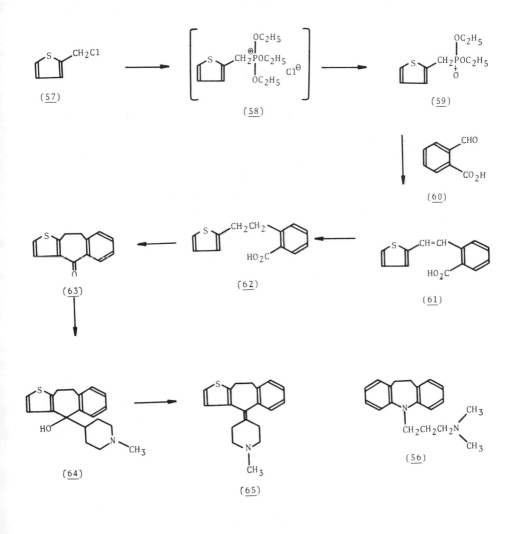

(57)  (58)  (59)  (60)  (63)  (62)  (61)  (64)  (65)  (56)

421

obtained from the last intermediate with hemi phthalal-
dehyde (60) gives the diarylethylene 61.  Reduction
of the double bond (62), followed by Friedel-Crafts
cyclization by means of polyphosphoric acid affords
the requisite ketone 63.  This compound is then condensed with the Grignard reagent from 1-methyl-4-
chloropiperidine, and the resulting carbinol (64) is
dehydrated.  There is thus obtained the antidepressant
agent *pizotyline* (65).[14]

Replacement of the thienyl grouping in 65 by
pyridyl affords *azatadin* (75), a compound in which
antihistaminic rather than antidepressant activity
predominates.  (It is of interest that the equivalent
interchange in the acyclic series affords a pair of
compounds each of which is an antihistamine.)  The
synthesis of the tricyclic system in this case starts
by acylation of the anion from phenylacetonitrile
with ethyl nicotinate to give cyanoketone 66.  Hydrolysis of the nitrile followed by decarboxylation of
the resulting keto-acid gives ketone 67; reduction
then leads to the diarylethane 68.  Functionality is
then introduced into the pyridine ring by the elegant
method introduced by Taylor.[15]  Thus, treatment of 68
with peracid gives N-oxide 69; reaction of that with
phosphorus trichloride leads to the corresponding 2-
chloropyridine (70) with simultaneous loss of the
oxide.  Displacement of halogen with cyanide followed
by hydrolysis of the resulting nitrile (71) gives the
carboxylic acid (72).  Cyclization by means of polyphosphoric acid yields the key tricyclic intermediate
73. The ketone is then condensed with the Grignard

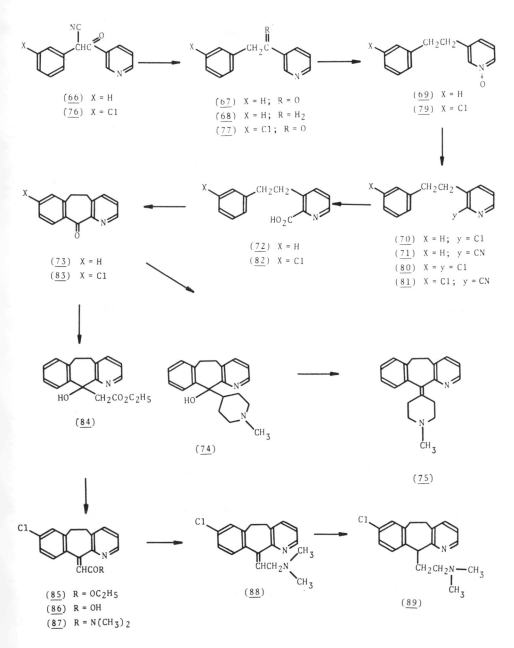

(66) X = H
(76) X = Cl

(67) X = H; R = O
(68) X = H; R = H₂
(77) X = Cl; R = O

(69) X = H
(79) X = Cl

(73) X = H
(83) X = Cl

(72) X = H
(82) X = Cl

(70) X = H; y = Cl
(71) X = H; y = CN
(80) X = y = Cl
(81) X = Cl; y = CN

(84)

(74)

(75)

(85) R = OC₂H₅
(86) R = OH
(87) R = N(CH₃)₂

(88)

(89)

423

reagent from N-methyl-4-chloropiperidine to afford
the carbinol *74*.   Finally, dehydration of this last
intermediate affords the antihistamine *azatadine*
*(75)*.[16]

A similar sequence starting with the acylation
product *(76)* from metachlorophenylacetonitrile gives
the halogenated tricyclic ketone *83*.   Condensation of
that intermediate with ethyl bromoacetate in the
presence of zinc (Reformatsky reaction) gives the
hydroxyester *84*.   This product is then in turn dehydrated under acid conditions *(85)*, saponified to the
corresponding acid *(86)*, and converted to the dimethylamide *(87)* by way of the acid chloride. The amide
function is then reduced to the amine *(88)* with
lithium aluminum hydride; catalytic hydrogenation of
the exocyclic double bond completes the synthesis of
*closiramine* *(89)*.[16]   This compound also exhibits
antihistaminic activity.

## 3.   DERIVATIVES OF DIBENZOLACTAMS

A recurring theme in the present chapter has been the
association of CNS activity with dibenzoheterocycles
that bear a basic chain pendant from the central
ring.   As we have seen, considerable latitude exists
as to the constitution of the central ring.   The
earlier volume in this series described the preparation
of the antidepressant *dibenzepin* *(90)*, in which the
basic function is attached to a lactam nitrogen.[17]
It has been found subsequent to this that attachment
of the basic center in the guise of a piperazine ring

as an amidine derivative again affords a series of compounds with activity on the CNS.

Preparation of the simplest of these examples (95) starts with hydrogenolysis of o-aminobenzoyl-benzoic acid (91) with zinc (activated by copper) in ammonia. Thermal cyclization of the resulting di-phenylmethane (92) gives the desired lactam (93).[18] Treatment of that intermediate with phosphorus oxy-chloride in the presence of N,N-dimethylaniline leads to iminochloride 94. Aminolysis with N-methyl-piperazine affords the hypnotic agent *perlapine* (95).[19]

Replacement of the bridge methylene group in 95 by a secondary amine is consistent with CNS activity, although the compound in this case (99) is described as a sedative agent. The synthetic approach used in this case relies on cyclization of an intermediate in which the piperazine ring is already in place. Thus, reaction of the acid chloride from 96 (available by Ullmann reaction of anthranilic acid on 2,5-dichloro-nitrobenzene) with N-methylpiperazine gives the corresponding amide (97). The nitro group is then reduced to yield aniline 98. Intramolecular dehydra-tion then affords the amidine, *clozapine* (99).[20]

Replacement of the methylene group in 95 by oxygen results in yet another subtle qualitative change in CNS activity. The products of this replace-ment, such as *104* and *111*, are characterized as anxiolytic agents. In the synthesis of *104* we find yet a different approach to the amidine function, beginning with reaction of 2-chloronitrobenzene with

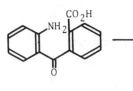 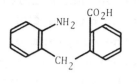 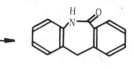

(91)  (92)  (93)

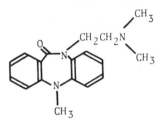 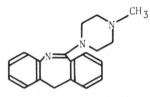 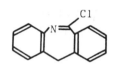

(90)  (95)  (94)

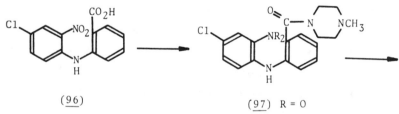

(96)  (97) R = O
(98) R = H

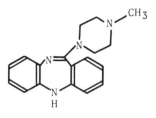

(99)

the anion from p-chlorophenol to afford the product
of aromatic nucleophilic displacement *(100)*; then,
reduction of the nitro group affords the corresponding aniline *(101)*. Treatment of that amine with
phosgene in the presence of excess triethylamine
converts the aniline to the isocyanate *(102)*. Condensation of that intermediate with N-methylpiperazine
affords urea *103*.   Bishler-Napieralski type cyclization
of the urea into the adjacent ring is accomplished
with phosphorus oxychloride. There is thus obtained
*loxapine (104)*.[21]

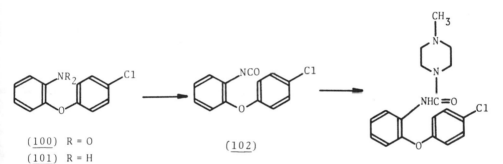

(100) R = O
(101) R = H

(102)

(103)

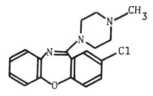

(104)

Another approach to this ring system leaves the
formation of the oxygen bridge to the end.  This
scheme starts by reaction of the dichlorobenzoic acid
*105* with carbonyldiimidazole *(106)* to afford the
reactive intermediate *107*.   Condensation with o-amino-
phenol gives the amide *108*, which is then converted
to the iminochloride with phosphorus pentachloride.
Condensation of *109* with piperazine apparently stops
cleanly at monomer *110*.   Intramolecular Ullmann
condensation in the presence of copper powder leads
to formation of the dibenzoxazepin ring, and thus
*amoxapine (111)*.[22]

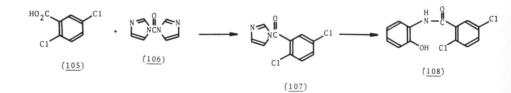

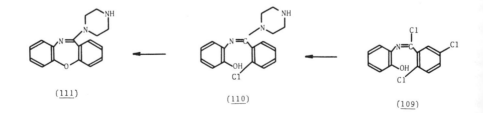

Finally, replacement of the methylene bridge by a sulfur bridge leads to compounds such as *117* and *123* which are major tranquilizers.  Thus, Ullmann condensation of thiosalicylic acid *112* with *ortho-chloronitrobenzene* affords thioether *113*; the nitro group is then reduced to the aniline *(114)*.  Cyclization as above leads to the lactam *115*, which is then converted to the iminochloride derivative *(116)*.  Condensation with N-methylpiperazine affords *clothiapine* *(117)*.[21]  Exactly the same sequence with the methyl substituted thiosalicylic acid derivative *118* leads to *metiapine (123)*.[21]

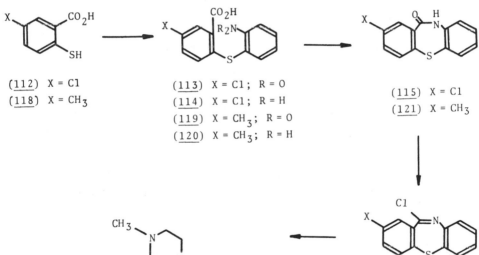

(112) X = Cl
(118) X = CH₃

(113) X = Cl; R = O
(114) X = Cl; R = H
(119) X = CH₃; R = O
(120) X = CH₃; R = H

(115) X = Cl
(121) X = CH₃

(116) X = Cl
(122) X = CH₃

(117) X = Cl
(123) X = CH₃

### 4.   OTHER DIBENZOHETEROCYCLES

Historically, research in industrial medicinal
chemistry has occurred in waves.  The discovery of
some novel structure with unique biological activity
has often occasioned intensive work in numerous
laboratories on the preparation and evaluation of
analogues.  Each such wave recedes when it is realized
that further modification of the molecule is reaching
the point of diminishing returns.  At this juncture,
the structure is often represented in the clinic by
several commercialized drugs; it is judged unlikely
that further work will produce a patentably novel
compound that could make significant inroads on the
market for drugs already available.

Nowhere, perhaps, is this phenomenon better
illustrated than in the phenothiazine class.  The
earlier volume devoted a full chapter to the discussion of this important structural class, which was
represented by both major tranquilizers and antihistamines. The lone phenothiazine below, *flutiazin*
*(130)*, in fact fails to show the activities characteristic of its class.  Instead, the ring system is
used as the aromatic nucleus for a nonsteroidal
antiinflammatory agent.  Preparation of *130* starts
with formylation of the rather complex aniline *123*.
Reaction with alcoholic sodium hydroxide results in
net overall transformation to the phenothiazine by
the Smiles rearrangement.  The sequence begins with
formation of the anion on the amide nitrogen; addition
to the carbon bearing sulfur affords the corresponding
transient spiro intermediate *126*.  Rearomatization

affords thiophenoxide *127;* this then attacks the
adjacent ring and the resulting negative charge on
the ring carbon adjacent to nitrogen is then dis-
charged by expulsion of the nitro group as the nitrite
anion.   The formyl group on what is essentially a
diphenylamine is sufficiently labile so that it too
comes off under the reaction conditions.   There is
thus obtained the phenothiazine carboxylic ester *129.*
Saponification of the ester completes the synthesis
of the veterinary antiinflammatory agent *flutiazin
(130).*[23]

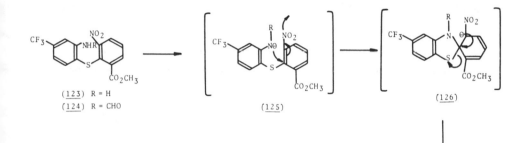

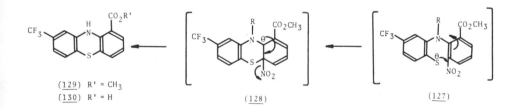

The association between abnormally high levels
of serum lipids and atherosclerosis has been discussed
earlier.  One of the earliest and still most widely
used drugs for normalizing lipid levels and thus
presumably treating atherosclerosis is the phenoxyester
*clofibrate (131).*  The wealth of analogues in this
series has demonstrated that lipid lowering activity
is retained when a second chlorophenoxy group is
substituted onto the beta carbon of the acid moiety.
More recently it was found that the two aromatic
rings can be linked to form an eight-membered heterocycle.  In one example, treatment of potassium di-
chloroacetate with the dipotassium salt of bisphenol
*132* affords the dibenzoxacin *133* directly, after
acidification.  Esterification with methanol gives
the hypolipidemic agent *treloxinate (134).*[24]

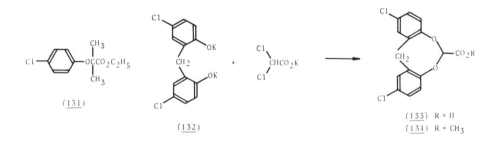

## REFERENCES

1.  B. M. Bloom and J. F. Muren, Belgian Patent
    647,066 (1964); *Chem. Abstr.*, *63:* 11,512a (1965).

2.  J. M. Grisar, U. S. Patent 3,196,150 (1965);
    *Chem. Abstr.*, *63:* 18,116f (1965).

3.  J. Schmutz, U. S. Patent 2,905,590; *Chem. Abstr.*,
    *54:* 5,699n (1959).

4.  D. Lednicer and L. A. Mitscher, Organic Chemistry
    of Drug Synthesis, Vol. I, p. 399, 1977.

5.  E. J. Blanz, Jr., and F. A. French, *J. Med.
    Chem.*, *6*, 185 (1963).

6.  C. L. Zirkle, U. S. Patent 3,131,190 (1964);
    *Chem. Abstr.*, *61:* 4,326a (1964).

7.  J. W. James and R. E. Rodway, British Patent
    1,135,947 (1968); *Chem. Abstr.*, *70:* 87,603r
    (1969).

8.  G. Schilling and T. A. Dobson, German Patent
    2,314,869 (1974); *Chem. Abstr.*, *81:* 25,527n
    (1974).

9.  P. A. J. Janssen, U. S. Patent 3,041,344 (1962);
    *Chem. Abstr.*, *59:* 6,417b (1963).

10. M. Nakanishi, C. Tashiro, T. Munakata, K. Araki,
    T. Tsumagari and H. Imamura, *J. Med. Chem.*, *13*,
    644 (1970).

11. Anon., Belgian Patent 652,938 (1965); *Chem.
    Abstr.*, *64:* 19,575h (1966).

12. Anon., Netherland Appl. 6,411,861 (1965); *Chem.
    Abstr.*, *63:* 16,366a (1965).

13. D. Lednicer and L. A. Mitscher, Organic Chemistry
    of Drug Synthesis, Vol. I, p. 401404, 1977.

14. J.M. Bastian, A. Ebnother, E. Jucker, E. Rissi
    and A. P. Stoll, *Helv. Chim. Acta*, *49*, 214 (1966).

15. E. C. Taylor, Jr., and A. J. Crovetti, *J. Org.
    Chem.*, *19*, 1633 (1954).

16. F. J. Villani, U. S. Patent 3,366,635 (1968); *Chem. Abstr.,69:* 10,372m (1968).

17. D. Lednicer and L. A. Mitscher, Organic Chemistry of Drug Synthesis, Vol. I, p. 405, 1977.

18. D. D. Emrick and W. E. Truce, *J. Org. Chem.,* 26, 1239 (1961).

19. F. Hunziker, F. Kunzle and J. Schmutz, *Helv. Chim. Acta,* 49, 1433 (1966).

20. F. Hunziker, E. Fischer and J. Schmutz, *Helv. Chim. Acta,* 50, 1588 (1967).

21. J. Schmutz, F. Kunzle, F. Hunziker and R. Gauch, *Helv. Chim. Acta,* 50, 245 (1967).

22. C. F. Howell, R. A. Hardy and N. Q. Quinones, French Patent 1,508,536 (1968); *Chem. Abstr.,* 70: 57,923c (1969).

23. B. M. Sutton, U. S. Patent 3,471,482 (1969); *Chem. Abstr.,* 72: 21,701f (1970).

24. J. M. Grisar, R. A. Parker, T. Kariya, T. Blohm, R. W. Fleming, V. Petrow, D. L. Wenstrup and R. G. Johnson, *J. Med. Chem.,* 15, 1273 (1972).

# 15
# β-Lactam Antibiotics

Despite the enormous effort already expended during
the past three decades, the β-lactam antibiotic field
remains one of the most hotly competitive in the
whole field of medicinal chemistry, with new entities
constantly being produced to address one or more the
clinical deficiencies perceived in existing drugs.
Recently, some new basic skeletons have been encoun-
tered in fermentation screening programs, and this
has given the field yet another burst of activity.
*Cefoxitin (31)* is the first fruit of this effort.
Whether the nocardicins, clavulanic acid, thienamycins,
etc., will reach the marketplace is not yet clear.
Meanwhile, intensive work is still being done among
the older ring systems.

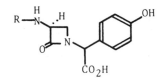

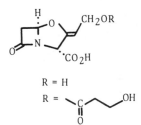

R = H

R =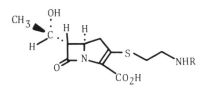

Clavulanic
Acids

R = 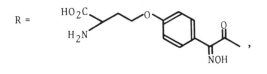,

R = 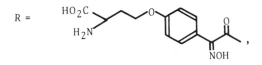,

R = 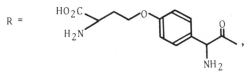,

R = H,

R = $COCH_3$

Thienamycins

R = 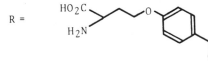,

R =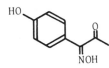

Nocardicins

1. PENICILLINS

The new entries in this section are the result of
manipulation of polar amide side chains to broaden
the antimicrobial spectrum of the penicillins.
*Carbenicillin (1)* is used in the clinic primarily
because of its low toxicity and its utility in treating
urinary tract infections due to susceptible *Pseudomonas*
species.  Its low potency, low oral activity, and
susceptibility to bacterial β-lactamases make it
vulnerable to replacement by agents without these
deficits.  One contender in this race is *ticarcillin*
*(4)*.  Its origin depended on the well-known fact (to
medicinal chemists) that a divalent sulfur is often
roughly equivalent to a vinyl group.  One synthesis
began by making the monobenzyl ester *(2)* of (3-
thienyl)malonic acid, converting this to the acid
chloride with $SOCl_2$, and condensing it with 6-amino-
penicillanic (6APA) acid to give *3*.  Hydrogenolysis
(Pd/C) completed the synthesis of *ticarcillin (4)*.[1]

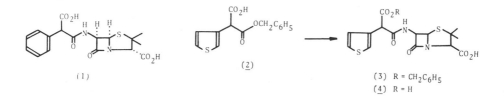

(1)                          (2)                          (3) R = $CH_2C_6H_5$
                                                          (4) R = H

*Ampicillin (5)* remains the penicillin of choice
for many infections because of its oral activity and
good potency against Gram-negative bacteria.  A
number of prodrugs have been examined in attempts to

improve upon its pharmacodynamic characteristics, and
one of these is *talampicillin (8)*.[2]  One synthesis
involved protecting the primary amino group of
*ampicillin (5)* as the enamine with ethyl acetoacetate
*(6)*.  This was then esterified by reaction with 3-
bromophthalide *(7)*, and the enamine was carefully
hydrolyzed with dilute HCl in acetonitrile to produce
*talampicillin (8)*.

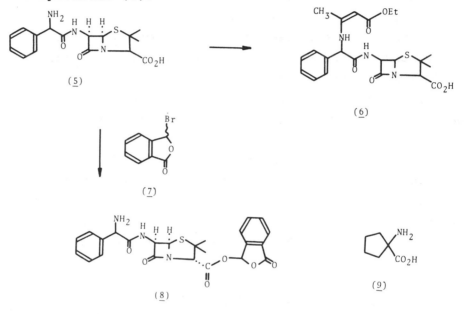

In an attempt to form orally active penicillins
unrelated to ampicillin, use was made of the fact
that certain spiro α-aminoacids, such as *9*, are well
absorbed orally and transported like normal amino
acids.  Reaction of cyclohexanone with ammonium
carbonate and KCN under the conditions of the Bucherer-
Bergs reaction led to hydantoin *10*.  On acid hydrolysis,
α-amino acid *11* resulted.  Treatment with phosgene

both protected the amino group and activated the
carboxyl group toward amide formation (as *12*) and
reaction with 6-aminopenicillanic acid gave
*cyclacillin (13)*.[3]   Interestingly, this artifice

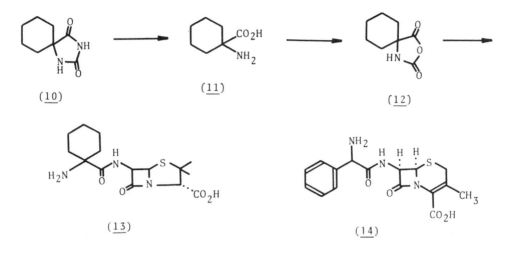

(10)

(11)

(12)

(13)

(14)

seems to have worked, since *cyclacillin* is more
active *in vivo* than its *in vitro* spectrum suggests
would be likely.


2.   CEPHALOSPORINS

The oral activity and clinical acceptance of *cephalexin*
*(14)* has led to the appearance of a spate of similar
molecules.  *Cefadroxyl (16)* is an example.[4]   The
design of this drug would seem to have derived from
the success of *amoxycillin*.   The synthesis of *cefadroxyl*
was accomplished by N-acylation of 7-aminodesacetyl-
cephalosporanic acid (7 ADCA) after blocking the
carboxy group with $(CH_3O)_2CH_3SiCl$ (to *15*).   The

blocking group was removed by solvolysis with butanol
to give *cefadroxyl (16)*.

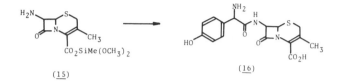

(15)                                                                      (16)

Noting that 1,4-cyclohexadiene rings are nearly
as planar as benzene rings but of greatly different
reactivity, a cephalosporin was synthesized with such
a moiety.  Birch reduction of D-α-phenylglycine *(17)*
led to diene *18*.  This was N-protected using t-
butoxycarbonyl azide and activated for amide formation
via the mixed anhydride method using isobutylchloro-
formate to give *19*.  Mixed anhydride *19* reacted
readily with 2-aminodesacetoxycephalosporanic acid to
give, after deblocking, *cephradine (20)*.[5]

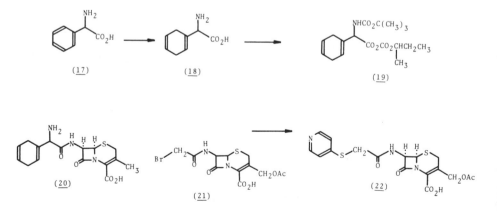

(17)                      (18)                                  (19)

(20)                                      (21)                              (22)

A more traditional cephalosporin analogue is
*cephapirin (22)*. It was made by reacting 7-aminocephalo-
sporanic acid with bromoacetyl chloride to give amide
*21*. The halo group was displaced by 4-thiopyridine
to give *22, cephapirin*.[6]

One of the few successful analogues in the β-
lactam series with an aliphatic side chain is *cephacetrile (23)*. It was made by reacting 7-amino-
cephalosporanic acid with cyanoacetyl chloride in the
presence of tributylamine.[7]

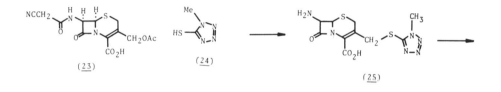

Modifications of the substituent at $C_3$ are
conveniently accomplished using sulfur nucleophiles
to displace the acetoxy moiety which is present in
the fermentation products. *Cefamandole (26)* is such
an agent. Reaction of 7-aminocephalosporanic acid
with thiotetrazole *24* gave displacement product *25*,

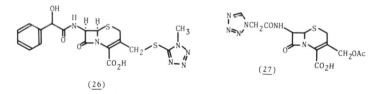

which was subsequently reacted with dichloroacetyl
mandelate to put on the side chain.  Deblocking
during workup produced *cefamandole (26)*.[8]

Reaction of sodio 7-aminocephalosporanic acid
with 1-(1H)-tetrazoylacetic acid gave intermediate
*27*.  Reaction of this last with 2-mercapto-5-methyl-
1,3,4-thiadiazole led to the widely used parenteral
cephalosporin, *cefazolin (28)*.[9]

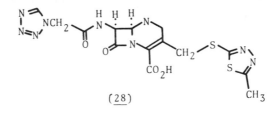

(28)

3.   CEPHAMYCINS

While screening for β-lactam antibiotics stable to
β-lactamases, a strain of *Streptomyces lactamdurans*
was found to contain several such agents which have a
6-α-methoxy group whose electronic and steric properties protect the antibiotic from enzymatic attack.
*Cephamycin C (29a)*, one of these substances, is not
of commercial value, but side chain exchange has led
to much more potent materials.  Of the various ways
of effecting this transformation, one of the more
direct is to react cephamycin C with nitrous acid so
that the aliphatic diazo product *(29b)* decomposes by
secondary amide participation giving cyclic iminoether
*30*.  The imino ether moiety solvolyzes more readily
than the β-lactam to produce 7-aminocephamycinic

acid, which was acylated in the usual way to produce
*cefoxitin (31)* with broad spectrum activity and
excellent resistance to bacterial degradation.[10]

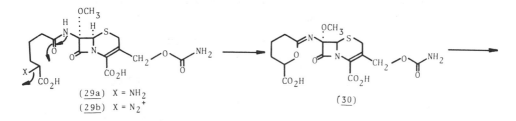

(29a) X = NH$_2$
(29b) X = N$_2^+$

(30)

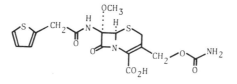

(31)

## REFERENCES

1.  Anon., Belgian Patent 646,991 (1964); *Chem. Abstr.*, *63*: 13,269f (1965).

2.  I. Isaka, K. Nakano, T. Kashiwagi, A. Koda, H. Horiguchi, H. Matsui, K. Takahashi and M. Murakami, *Chem. and Pharm. Bull.*, *24*, 102 (1976); J. P. Clayton, M. Cole, S. W. Elson, H. Ferres, J. C. Hanson, L. W. Mizen and R. Sutherland, *J. Med. Chem.*, *19*, 1385 (1976).

3.  H. E. Alburn, D. E. Clark, H. Fletcher and N. H. Grant, *Antimicrob. Agts. Chemother.*, 586 (1967).

4.  T. Ishimaru and Y. Kodama, German Patent

2,163,514 (1973); *Chem. Abstr.*, *79:* 78,826z
(1973).

5.   J. E. Dolfini, H. E. Applegate, G. Bach, H.
     Basch, J. Bernstein, J. Schwartz and F. L.
     Wiesenborn, *J. Med. Chem.*, *14*, 117 (1971).

6.   L. B. Crast, Jr., R. G. Graham and L. C. Cheney,
     *J. Med. Chem.*, *16*, 1413 (1973).

7.   Anon., Netherlands Patent 6,600,586 (1966);
     *Chem. Abstr.*, *65:* 20,131h (1966).

8.   J. R. Guarini, U. S. Patent, 3,903,278 (1976).

9.   K. Kariyone, H. Harada, M. Kurita and T. Takano,
     *J. Antibiotics*, *23*, 131 (1970).

10.  L. D. Cama, W. J. Leanza, T. R. Beattie and B.
     G. Christensen, *J. Am. Chem. Soc.*, *94*, 1408
     (1972); S. Karady, S. H. Pines, L. M. Weinstock,
     F. E. Roberts, G. S. Brenner, A. M. Hoinowski,
     T. Y. Cheng and M. Sletzinger, *ibid.*, *94*, 1410
     (1972).

# 16

# Miscellaneous Fused Heterocycles

As may be apparent now, compounds in a given structural class are often associated with good biological activity. This means that on the operational level, a good many examples of those structures will be available that have been assigned generic names. In terms of this book, those compounds will merit a chapter or even a section. Thus, for example, although β-lactams represent a relatively narrow structural descriptor, activity in this class is sufficiently promising so that a full chapter is needed to fully cover those compounds. There does, however, exist a sizeable group of compounds that are not so readily categorized, since relatively few examples of each type have been assigned generic names. The medicinal agents discussed below are miscellaneous in that there is no readily apparent unifying thread in terms

of either structure or biological activity by which
to group them, other than in a miscellaneous way.

### 1.   Compounds with Two Fused Rings

Discovery in medicinal chemistry is intimately dependent on available animal test systems.  Except for
certain infectious diseases, it is rare to find a
preexisting animal model for the human disease for
which drugs are being sought.  For example, animals
do not develop atherosclerosis spontaneously.  As a
result, pharmacologists exercise great ingenuity in
devising animal test systems intended to be relevant
to diseases.  Such assays, particularly in the area
of agents acting on the CNS, are often quite indirect
in that the connection to the human disease may be
somewhat circuitous. Those tests are usually validated
as far as possible with test results from drugs known
to be active in the human.  There thus exists the
distinct possibility that an animal test will pre-
ordain the discovery of compounds that act by a
closely similar mechanism, and thus have the same
side effects, as those already on the market. This is
perhaps best illustrated in the field of the centrally
acting analgesics.  The animal tests in this area
have proven very reliable in detecting compounds that
show analgesic activity in man; at the same time, all
drugs discovered by these assays have at least some
of the side effects of the prototype, *morphine*, to a
greater or lesser degree.  For this reason, therapeutic breakthroughs are relatively rare and celebrated
events.

The discovery of an analgesic that acts by a
presumably nonopiate pathway, in fact, resulted from
a clinical trial of the compound in question, *nefopam*
*(4)*, in man.  It might be noted that this trial was
designed to study the drug as a muscle relaxant.  It
should also be noted that *nefopam* fails to show
activity in many of the tests used to detect compounds
with central analgesic activity. At the present time,
there does not seem to exist any solution to that
conundrum, short of the clearly unacceptable alter-
native of using man as the test animal.  The huge
expense and the bureaucratic requirements needed
before embarking on a clinical trial in the late
1970's serve to make this kind of discovery less
common and inclines the field more and more to modest
advances in modulating potency or side effects.  Does
the old saw, "drugs are discovered in the clinic,"
still have relevance?  Time will tell.

Preparation of *nefopam* starts with the acylation
of aminobenzhydrol *1* (obtainable by reduction of the
corresponding benzoylbenzamide) with chloroacetyl
chloride; treatment of the chloroamide *(2)* with
potassium tertiary butoxide results in internal
alkylation to give the eight-membered ring *(3)*.
Reduction of the lactam function with lithium aluminum
hydride gives the amine and, thus, *nefopam (4)*.[1]

Although most nonsteroidal antiinflammatory
agents depend on the presence of an acidic proton for
activity, examples of nonacidic drugs are scattered
among the various structural classes. A furanopyrrole,

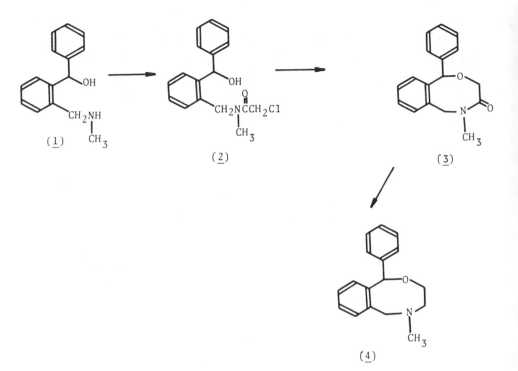

octazamide (11), represents yet another structure
that has been found to act as a peripheral analgesic/
antiinflammatory agent.  Hydrolysis of substituted
furan 5 gives the corresponding diol (6), which is
then reduced catalytically to afford the tetrahydrofuran 7.   Both the method of reduction and the subsequent cyclization suggest that the product has the
cis configuration. Reaction of 7 with tosyl chloride
leads to ditosylate 8; use of that intermediate to
bisalkylate benzylamine affords the bicyclic heterocyclic system (9).  Debenzylation (10) followed by
acylation of the resulting secondary amine with
benzoyl chloride affords finally octazamide (11).[2]

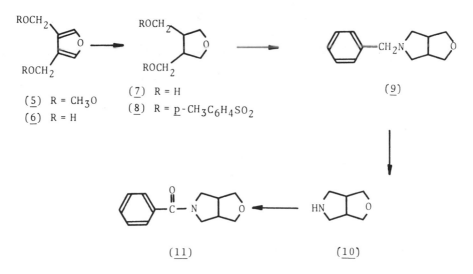

(5)  R = CH₃O
(6)  R = H

(7)  R = H
(8)  R = p-CH₃C₆H₄SO₂

(9)

(11)                    (10)

One of the first pharmacological classes to be
studied by medicinal chemists was local anesthetics.
Many of the guiding principles which are used to this
day, for example, molecular dissection, side chain
substitution and inversion, and the like, were first
developed in the course of those early researches.
The most tangible fruit of that work was the development of a host of local anesthetic drugs; since there
is a limited demand for such agents, the field lay
quiescent for a good many years.  The adventitious
discovery that the local anesthetic agent *lidocaine*
*(12)* showed antiarrhythmic activity in man has lent
impetus to renewed interest in local anesthetics for
new application.  In particular, compounds are being
sought which escape the main shortcoming of *lidocaine*;
that drug is active for clinical purposes by intra-
venous administration only.

Preparation of one of these newer local anesthe-
tic/antiarrhythmic agents, *rodocaine (19)*, starts
with the synthesis of an octahydropyrindene.  Conjugate
addition of the enolate from cyclopentanone to acrylonitrile gives the cyanoketone *13*.  The carbonyl group
is then protected as its ethylene ketal *(14)*, and the
nitrile is reduced to the corresponding primary amine
*(15)*.  Deketalization in dilute acid affords a
transient aminoketone, which spontaneously cyclizes
to the imine *16*.  Dissolving metal reduction (sodium
in ethanol) affords the *trans*-fused bicyclo *17*.[3]
(Catalytic reduction of *16* affords the *cis* isomer.

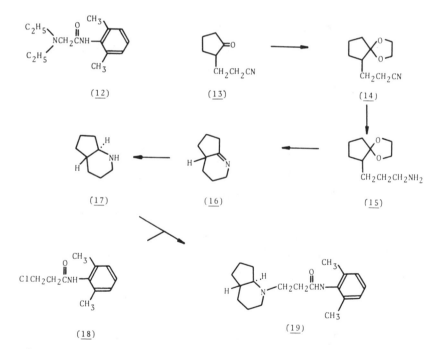

It is unexpected that the presumably thermodynamically controlled metal in alcohol reduction gives the

*trans* compounds; the *cis* isomer is usually the more stable in the analogous all-carbon hydrindane system.) The amide portion of the molecule (*18*) is assembled by acylation of 2,6-dimethylaniline with 3-chloropropionyl chloride. Alkylation of *17* with chloroamide *18* affords *rodocaine* (*19*).[4]

2. Compounds with Three or More Fused Rings

Preparation of rigid analogues of medicinal agents sometimes leads to compounds with greatly increased activity. Briefly, the success of a rigid analogue depends on locking a previously freely rotating side chain or flexible molecule into a conformation that will give a better fit with some putative receptor. Application of this principle to the tricyclic antidepressants does indeed afford a compound, *mianserin* (*26*), which retains the activity of the parent molecule. Preparation of *26* begins with acylation of the benzylaniline *20* (available from the benzophenone) with chloroacetyl chloride to give amide *21*. Treatment with a mixture of phosphorus oxychloride and polyphosphoric acid leads to cyclodehydration of the amide to the corresponding tricyclic intermediate *22*. Displacement of the now allylic chloride by means of methylamine gives the amine *23*; this is then reduced to the diamine *24* with sodium borohydride. Construction of the last ring is accomplished by formation of the cyclic diamide (*25*) from *24* by ester interchange with diethyl oxalate. Reduction of this α-diamide with diborane proceeds with no apparent difficulty to

the diamine, the antidepressant compound *mianserin*
(*26*).[5]

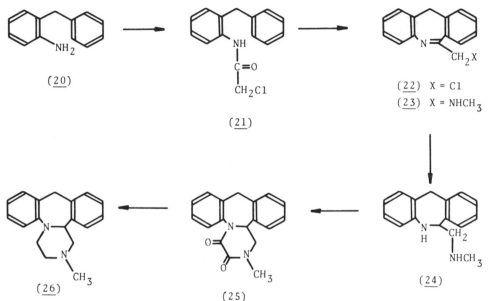

(*20*)

(*21*)

(*22*) X = Cl
(*23*) X = NHCH₃

(*24*)

(*25*)

(*26*)

Application of the same type of reasoning to an
anxiolytic benzodiazepine results in a rigid analogue,
*clazolam (35)*, which also retains the activity of the
parent molecule, *diazepam*.   It should be noted that
in this case it is a benzene ring rather than a side
chain that is conformationally restricted.   Condensation of isatoic anhydride *27* with 2-phenethylamine
(*28*) results in net acylation of the aliphatic amine.
The anhydride is in essence both an activated carboxyl
derivative and a means of protecting the aniline
nitrogen against self-condensation reactions.   The
secondary amine in *29* is then converted to the tosylamide to protect it during subsequent steps.   Treatment
of the amide *30* with phosphorus pentoxide results in

a Bischler-Napieralski cyclization to the dihydroisoquinoline *31*.  The protecting group is then removed
by hydrolysis in strong acid *(32)*, and the double
bond is reduced catalytically.  Alkylation of the
diamine *33* with ethyl bromoacetate proceeds as expected
at the more basic aliphatic amine to give the glycinate
*34*.  Base-catalyzed ring closure of the aminoester
serves to close the diazepine ring; there is thus
obtained the anxiolytic agent *clazolam (35)*.[6]

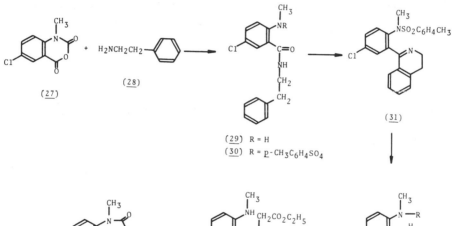

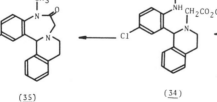

(29) R = H
(30) R = p-CH₃C₆H₄SO₄

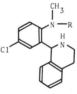

When the pharmacophoric group in a rigid compound is fused in some position remote from that in
the nonrigid compounds, it is likely that the agent
is active by some different biological mechanism.
Thus, although *naranol (40)* is formally related to
the tricyclic compounds, the basic center is in a
quite different position from that in the majority of
tricyclic CNS agents.  Synthesis of *40* is begun by
Mannich reaction of 2-naphthol with formaldehyde and
dimethylamine to afford the adduct *37*.  Reaction of
this aminophenol with the substituted piperidone *38*
affords the tetracyclic product *40* in a single step.

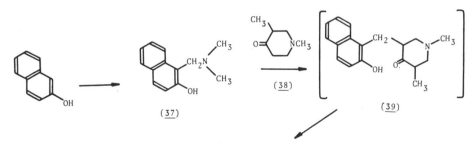

(37)          (38)          (39)

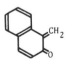

(41)

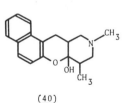

(40)

This seemingly complex transformation can be rationalized by assuming, as the first step, formation of
an enolate of ketone *38*.   Displacement of dimethylamine on *37* by the enolate will give the phenolketone
*39*.   Although both regioisomers of the enolate may in
fact be formed, the observed product is from reaction
of the less hindered enol.   (An alternate sequence
involves loss of dimethylamine from *37* to give
quinonemethide *41*; conjugate addition of the same
enolate will give *39*.)   Simple internal hemiketal
formation gives the product *40*, *naranol*,[7] of unspecified stereochemistry.

Although most available CNS agents are quite
effective, they are not without side effects.   There
is, thus, some impetus for a search for novel structures in the hope that these will be better than
available drugs.   During this search a derivative of
a partly reduced indole, *molindone (48)*, has been
reported to have sedative and tranquilizing activity.
Condensation of oximinoketone *42* (from nitrosation of
3-pentanone), with cyclohexane-1,3-dione in the
presence of zinc and acetic acid leads directly to
the indole derivative *47*.   The transformation may be
rationalized by assuming as the first step, reduction
of *42* to the corresponding α-aminoketone.   Conjugate
addition of the amine to *43* followed by elimination
of hydroxide (as water) would give ene-aminoketone
*44*.   This may be assumed to be in tautomeric equilibrium with intermediate *45*. Aldol condensation of the
side chain carbonyl group with the doubly activated
ring methylene would then result in cyclization to

pyrrole *46;* simple tautomeric transformation would
then give the observed product.  Mannich reaction of
*47* with formaldehyde and morpholine gives the
tranquilizer *molindone (48).*[8]

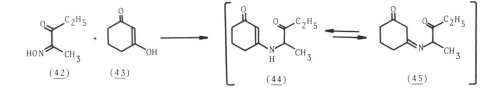

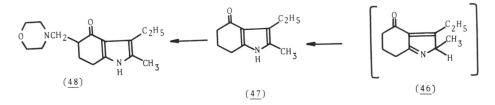

Tricyclic antihistamines as a rule carry aliphatic
nitrogen as a substituent on a side chain attached to
the central ring; the side chain nitrogen may be part
of a heteroaromatic ring.  Conjugate addition of p-
chloroaniline *(49)* to the substituted vinylpyridine
*50* gives the alkylated aniline *51.*  Treatment of that
intermediate with nitrous acid leads to N-nitroso
intermediate *52* which is then reduced to the hydrazine
*(53).*  Reaction of *53* with N-methyl-4-piperidone

under the conditions of the Fischer indole synthesis affords *dorastine (54)*,[9] an antihistamine.

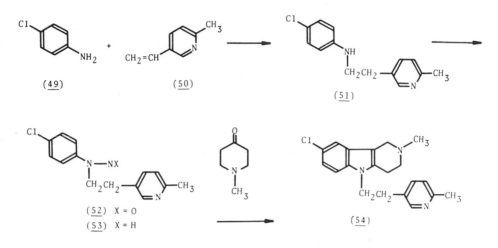

(49)     (50)     (51)

(52) X = O
(53) X = H

(54)

Azanator (59) represents a more classical anti-histaminic structure, since the more basic nitrogen in this case occurs in the side chain.  Preparation

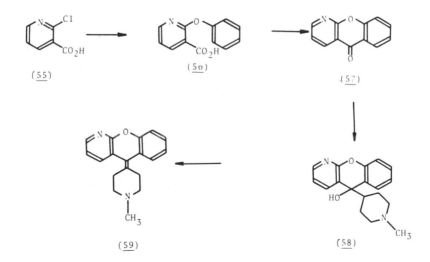

(55)     (56)     (57)

(59)     (58)

of this compound starts with aromatic nucleophilic
displacement on pyridine 55 (see Chapter 14) with
phenoxide anion.  Friedel-Crafts ring closure of the
product (56) by means of polyphosphoric acid leads to
the azaxanthone 57.  This is then converted to the
final product by condensation with the Grignard
reagent from N-methyl-4-chloropiperidine (58), followed
by dehydration to yield 59.[10]

As noted previously, a wide variety of aromatic
systems serve as nuclei for arylacetic acid antiinflammatory agents.  It is thus to be expected that
fused heterocycles can also serve the same function.
Synthesis of one such agent (64) begins with condensation of indole-3-ethanol (60) with ethyl 3-oxo-
caproate (61) in the presence of tosic acid, leading
directly to the pyranoindole 63.  The reaction may be
rationalized by assuming formation of hemiketal 62,
as the first step.  Cyclization of the carbonium ion

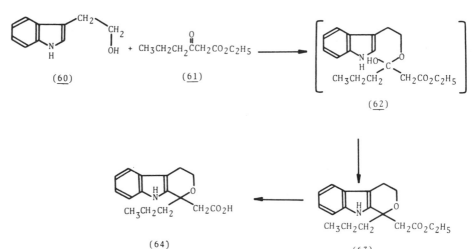

(from loss of hydroxyl) into the nucleophilic indole
2-position will give the observed product (63).
Saponification of the ester gives the antiinflammatory agent *prodolic acid (64).*[11]

A closely related compound, *pirandamine (72),*
bearing a basic rather than an acidic side chain and
having a methylene in place of the indole nitrogen,

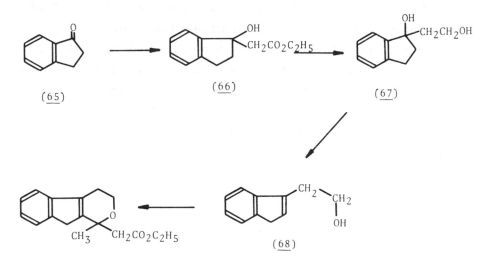

(65)                    (66)                    (67)

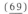

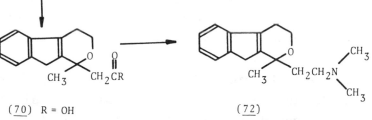

(69)

(70) R = OH
(71) R = N(CH₃)₂

(72)

interestingly exhibits antidepressant activity.
Basically, the same synthetic scheme is used for the
preparation of this analogue as for compound *64*
above.  Condensation of 1-indanone *(65)* with ethyl
bromoacetate and zinc affords Reformatski product *66*;
then, reduction with lithium aluminum hydride gives
diol *67*.  Dehydration with sulfuric acid gives the
indene ethanol *68*.  Acid catalyzed condensation of *68*
with ethyl acetoacetate then gives the fused tetra-
hydropyran derivative *69*, no doubt by a scheme quite
analogous to that above.  The ester is then saponified
to the corresponding acid *(70)*, which is then converted to the dimethylamide *(71)*.  Reduction with
lithium aluminum hydride completes the synthesis of
the antidepressant agent *pirandamine (72)*.[12]

Antidepressant activity is retained in *tandamine*
*(80)*, an analogue in which the indole ring is restored,
the basic side chain is retained, and the oxygen
heterocycle is replaced by the corresponding sulfur-
containing ring.  Acetylation of indole ethanol *60*
affords the corresponding acetate *73*; the indole
nitrogen is then alkylated by means of ethyl iodide
and sodium hydride *(74)*.  Conversion of the side
chain oxygen to sulfur is accomplished by first
treating the alcohol (from hydrolysis of the acetate
*(75)* with phosphorus tribromide to give *76*; displacement of halogen with thiosulfate anion then
affords the covalent thiosulfate *(77)*.  In a departure
from the synthetic scheme used above, the basic side
chain is introduced directly.  Thus, reaction of
thiosulfate *77* with amidoketone *78* in the presence of

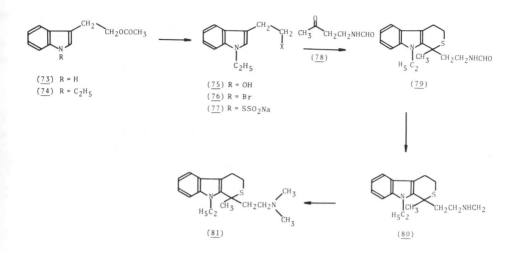

boron trifluoride leads directly to the fused heterocycle *(79)*.  Reduction of the formamide by means of
lithium aluminum hydride then affords monomethyl
derivative *80;* N-methylation of that intermediate
completes the synthesis of the antidepressant agent
*tandamine (81).* [13,14]

  A rather complex fused isoindoline *(87)* has been
found to show good anorectic activity.  This substance
differs from other anorectic agents by not being a
β-phenethylamine analogue.  Preparation of this
compound starts by reaction of a substituted benzoyl-
benzoic acid *(82)* with ethylene diamine.  The product
*(84)* can be rationalized as being the aminal from the
initially obtained monoamide *83.*  This is then subjected to reduction with lithium aluminum hydride

and--without isolation--air oxidation.  Reduction
probably proceeds to the mixed aminal/carbinolamine
*85;* such a product would be expected to be in equilibrium with the alternate aminal *86*.  The latter would
be expected to predominate due to the greater stability
of aldehyde aminals over the corresponding ketone
derivatives.  Air oxidation of the tetrahydroimidazole
to the imidazoline will then remove *86* from the
equilibrium.  There is thus obtained the anorectic
agent *mazindol (87)*.[15]

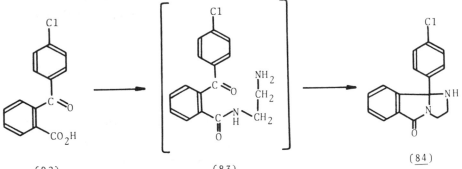

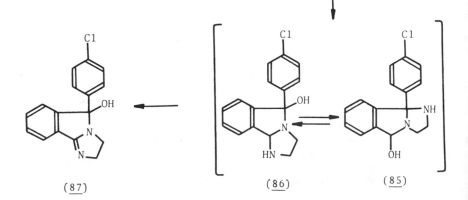

### 3. Purines and Related Heterocycles

Considerable research has been devoted to preparation of modified purines in the expectation that such compounds could act as antagonists to, or possibly false substrates for, those involved in normal metabolic processes. It is surprising to note the relatively small number of such compounds that have found clinical use.

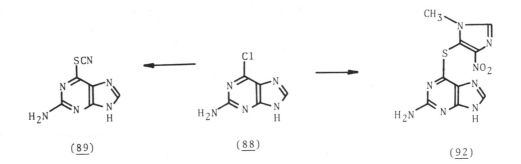

*Thioguanine* is one of the most familiar of the
medicinal purine analogues.  This compound acts as a
false guanine and has found a role as an antineoplastic agent by reason of its resulting activity as
a metabolic inhibitor.  The compound is obtained most
simply by displacement of halogen from 6-chloroguanine
*(88)* with thiocyanate anion.  Hydrolysis of the
product *(89)* yields *thioguanine (90).*[16]

In much the same vein, displacement of chlorine
from *88* with the sodium salt of imididazolethiol 91
affords the antineoplastic agent *thiampirine (92).*[17]
The same reaction starting with purine 93 gives the
immunosupressant agent *azathioprine (94).*[18]

Contraction and relaxation of smooth muscle is
known to be mediated by way of the cyclic nucleotides.
In brief, increase in intracellular levels of cyclic
adenosine monophosphate (cAMP) leads to relaxation of
smooth muscle.  In the normal course of events, cAMP
is hydrolyzed to its inactive form by the enzyme
phosphodiesterase (PDE).  Drugs that inhibit the
action of that enzyme--PDE inhibitors--will tend to
promote smooth muscle relaxation. One such drug,
*theophylline (95)* has found extensive use in treatment
of asthma based on its ability to relax bronchial
smooth muscle.  A search for more lipophilic analogues
of theophylline led to a compound, the hexyl analogue
*96* of theobromine, which seemed to have greater
selectivity for vascular smooth muscle.  Further
biological investigation revealed that the active
agent was in fact the metabolite *101* resulting from
ω-1-oxidation of the aliphatic side chain.

Preparation of the requisite side chain starts by
alkylation of ethyl acetoacetate with 1,3-dibromopen-
tane; the initially formed bromoketone (shown as the
enol *97*) undergoes O-alkylation under the reaction
conditions to give the dihydropyran *98*.  Reaction of
that masked hydroxy ketone derivative with hydrogen

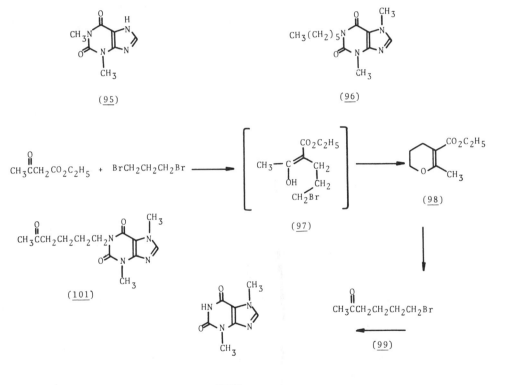

bromide affords the requisite bromoketone (*99*);
reaction conditions are apparently sufficient to

insure decarbethoxylation of the ketoester intermediate.
Alkylation of theobromine (*100*) with *99* affords the
vasodilator, *pentoxifylline (101)*.[18]

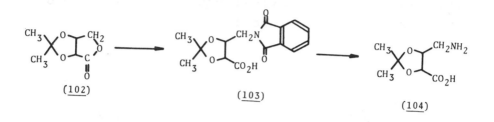

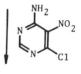

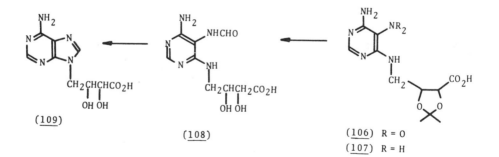

Pharmacognosy, the study of plant products with
medicinal properties, has contributed many structural
leads to drug development.  Although findings have in
recent years been less frequent this discipline

continues to uncover unusual structure-activity
combinations.  In one example, methanol extracts of
the Japanese mushroom *Lentinus edodes* Sing. were
found to have hypolipidemic activity.  The active
compound *eritadenine (109)* proved to be a purine
alkylated with an oxidized sugar fragment; its synthesis can be accomplished as follows.  Ring opening
of the protected lactone *(102)*, derived from erythrose,
with sodium phthalimide gives the acid *103*; hydra-
zinolysis then leads to the amino acid *104*. Displacement of chlorine in pyrimidine *105* by the amine
function on *104* serves to attach the future imidazole
nitrogen and the sugar-derived side chain *106*.  The
nitro group is then reduced by catalytic hydrogenation
*(107)*, the resulting primary amine is the most basic,
and is selectively formylated with formic acid  These
strongly acidic conditions serve to remove the acetonide protecting group as well *(108)*.  Treatment with
sodium hydroxide then serves to close the imidazole
ring, forming *eritadenine (109)*.[19]

The several compounds below *(115, 120, 121)* are
related to purines only in that they contain some
three nitrogen atoms formally distributed among an
indene nucleus.  Despite the varied structures, all
three analogues share activity mediated through the
CNS.  In one of the classical methods for construction
of a pyrimidine ring, synthesis of *115* begins with
condensation of the substituted cyanoacetate *110* with
acetamidine to give the corresponding pyrimidone
*(111)*, shown as the enol.  Treatment with acid probably
results initially in hydrolysis of the acetal function

to give the transient aminoaldehyde *112*.  This then
cyclizes to the corresponding imine under the reaction
conditions, and this interemdiate tautomerizes to the
observed pyrrolopyrimidine *113*.  Reaction with phosphorus oxychloride serves to replace the hydroxyl
group by chlorine *(114)*. Displacement of halogen with
benzylamine gives the muscle relaxant *rolodine (115)*.[20]

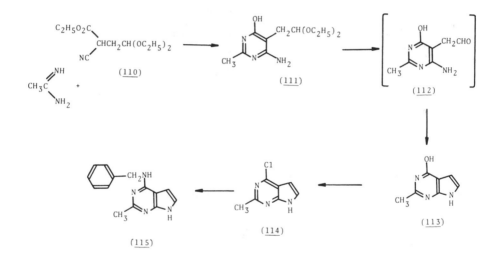

Condensation of aminopyrazole *116* with ethoxymethylene malonic ester gives the product of addition-
elimination *(117)*, which is then cyclized to the
piperidone by heating in diphenyl ether.  The product
tautomerizes spontaneously to the hydroxypyridine
*118*.  The hydroxyl group is then converted to the
chloro derivative by means of phosphorus oxychloride
*(119)*.  Displacement of halogen by n-butylamine gives

the antidepressant compound *cartazolate* (*120*).[21]
Replacement of halogen by the basic nitrogen of
acetone hydrazone affords the antidepressant *etazolate*
(*121*).[21]

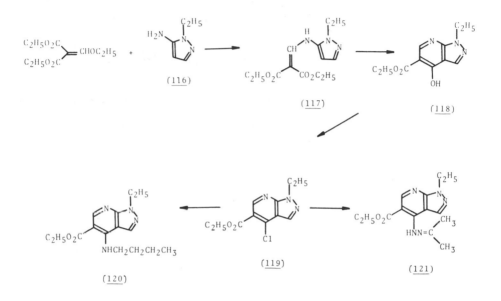

### 4. Polyaza Fused Heterocycles

As noted earlier (see Chapter 12), considerable
latitude exists in the *nalidixic acid* type antibacterial agents as to the exact nature of the two
heterocyclic rings.  The minimum requirement for
activity seems to reside in a fused enaminoketone
carboxylate function.  (Even so, an additional nitrogen
atom may be interposed in that function, viz.
*cinoxacin*.)  Consistent with this, it is interesting
that inclusion of an additional nitrogen atom in the
pyridino ring also gives a molecule (*127*) that shows

antibacterial activity. Synthesis of this agent
begins with successive displacement reactions on
2,6-dichloropyrimidine (122) with pyrrolidine and
then ammonia, leading to the diaminopyrimidine 123.
The rest of the synthesis follows the usual pattern.
Condensation of 123 with ethoxymethylenemalonate
gives the substituted malonate 124. Thermal cyclization serves to form the fused pyridone ring (125);
saponification of the ester with base then gives the
corresponding acid (126). Alkylation of the pyridone
nitrogen with diethyl sulfate completes the synthesis
of piromidic acid (127).[22]

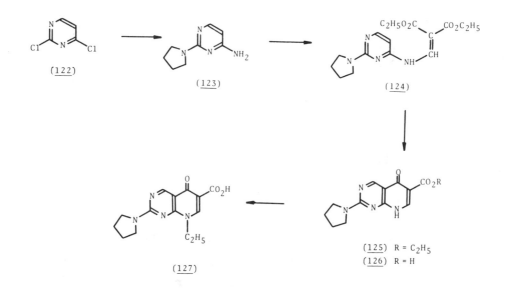

Replacement of methine by nitrogen, i.e.,
replacement of a phenyl moiety by pyridine, is consistent with biological activity in quite a few structural-

biological classes (see Chapter 9).  This retention
of activity in the face of an interchange of aromatic
rings is well illustrated in the case of the acyclic
and tricyclic antihistamines.  It is of note that the
same interchange in at least one tricyclic antidepressant drug (*dibenzepin*, see Chapter 14), affords

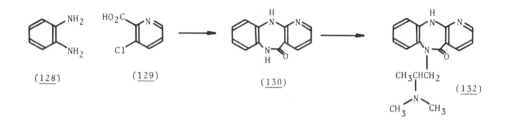

(128)          (129)                      (130)

(132)

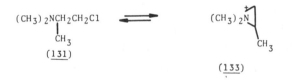

(131)

(133)

an analogue that retains the CNS profile of the parent
compound.  Another centrally acting tricyclic agent
bearing a pyridino moiety (*132*) is prepared as
follows.  Condensation of phenylenediamine (*128*) with
2-chloronicotinic acid (*129*) leads directly to the
tricyclic lactam *130*.  Although the reaction obviously
includes amide formation and nucleophilic aromatic
displacement of chlorine, the order of these steps is

not known. Alkylation of the anion obtained from
treatment of *130* with the chloroethylamine *131* affords
the antidepressant compound *propizepine (132)*.[23] The
last step in this sequence is less straightforward
than it might seem. There is considerable evidence
that such alkylations often proceed by way of the
aziridinium ion *(133)*. It will be appreciated that
attack of the anion at the secondary or tertiary
carbon of the aziridinium ring will lead to different
products. Extensive investigation of this problem[24]
has established that the product from attack at
secondary carbon usually predominates. This is, of
course, the same compound that would be formed by
direct displacement of halogen without involvement of
the aziridnium intermediate *133*.

Two rather broad structural classes account for the
large majority of drugs that have proven useful in
the clinic for treating depression. Each of these
has associated with it some clearly recognized side
effects: the monoamine oxidase inhibitors, most
commonly derivatives of hydrazine, tend to have
undesirable effects on blood pressure; the tricyclic
compounds on the other hand may cause undesirable
changes in the heart. Considerable effort has thus
been expended toward the development of antidepressants that fall outside those structural classes. An
unstated assumption in this work is the belief that
very different structures will be associated with a
novel mechanism of action and a different set of
ancillary activities. One such compound, *trazodone*

(<u>138</u>), has in fact shown clinically useful antidepressant activity without the typical side effects
of the classical drugs. In a convergent synthesis,
reaction of 2-chloropyridine with semicarbazide in
the presence of a catalytic amount of acid affords
the fused triazole *135*. The reaction may be
rationalized by assuming addition of semicarbazide to
the protonated atom of chloropyridine to give intermediate *134*. (Although semicarbazide is a stronger
base, protonation of that compound does not lead to
any reaction.) Elimination of hydrogen chloride

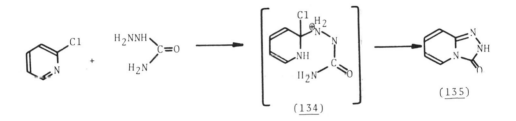

(<u>134</u>)                                            (<u>135</u>)

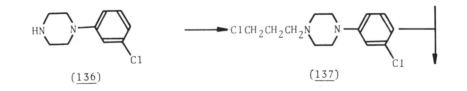

(<u>136</u>)                              (<u>137</u>)

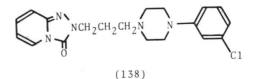

(<u>138</u>)

restores aromaticity, and leads to attack by the
pyridine nitrogen on the semicarbazide carbonyl.
This or the reverse order will give the observed
product *(135)*. Alkylation of piperazine *136* with 1-
bromo-3-chloropropane gives the piperazine derivative
*137*; use of that intermediate to alkylate heterocycle
*135* affords the antidepressant agent *trazodone (138).*[25]

A fused heterocyclic compound *(146)* distantly
related to the antiinflammatory agent *cintazone*
(Chapter 12), which itself can be viewed as a cyclized
derivative of *phenylbutazone*, retains the activity of
the prototype. In the synthesis of *146*, reaction of
the nitroaniline *139* with phosgene gives intermediate
*140*, which is then reacted with ammonia to afford the
substituted urea *(141)*. Cyclization of the <u>ortho</u>
nitrourea function by means of sodium hydroxide leads
to the N-oxide *(142)*; this last reaction represents

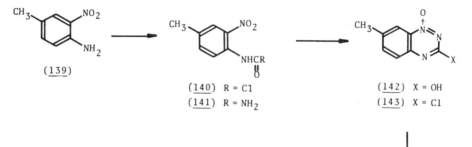

(139)

(140) R = Cl
(141) R = NH₂

(142) X = OH
(143) X = Cl

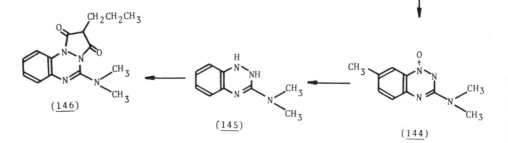

(146)

(145)

(144)

one of a series of transformations in which nitro and
nitroso groups reveal electrophilic character akin to
carbonyl groups.  Reaction of *142* with phosphorous
oxychloride serves to convert the hydroxyl group to
chloride *(143)*, which is then displaced with dimethylamine to give the key intermediate *144*.[27] Catalytic
reduction then converts the azoxide function to the
corresponding cyclic hydrazine derivative *(145)*.
Finally, condensation with diethyl n-propylmalonate
affords the antiinflammatory agent, *apazone (146)*.[28]

   5.  Ergolines
Ergotism, popularly known at the time as "St. Anthony's
Fire," was one of the dread epidemic diseases of the
Middle Ages. Its victims suffered gangrenous degener-
ation, madness, and death. Scientific investigation
eventually revealed that this disease was due to
ingestion of foods prepared from rye which was infected
with a fungus, *Claviceps purpurea*.  These infected
foods were more likely to be ingested in times of
famine, so prevention of ergotism in modern times is
a simple matter.  Chemical investigation of *Claviceps
purpurea* revealed mycotoxins that were amides of
*lysergic acid (147)*, involving a series of unusual
internally cyclized tripeptides.

   Some of these natural products--and drugs made
from them--are known collectively as the ergot alkaloids, and have found use in medicine.  *Ergonovine*,
for example, is a selective stimulant for contraction
of uterine muscle and is used in conjunction with
labor and delivery.  A mixture of hydrogenated ergot
alkaloids--reduced at the 9,10-position--has found

use as a cerebral vasodilator by reason of its α-
adrenergic blocking activity.

Lysergic acid itself has been used as starting
material for a small series of drugs.  This natural
product was until quite recently difficultly accessible
because *Claviceps* molds could only be cultivated on
growing grains and grasses.  Once harvested, the
mixture of ergot alkaloids needed to be subjected to
alkaline hydrolysis to yield the free acid.  The
search for a more efficient method of production led
to the finding of a related mold, *Claviceps paspali*,
which can be grown in submerged culture in
fermentation tanks; this method of culture is addi-
tionally advantageous, as it affords the acid directly,
thus bypassing the hydrolysis step.[28]

The discovery of the potent hallucinogen LSD-25
(*148*), (or in street parlance, "acid"), represents
one of the classics in serendipity.  In the course of
an analogue program on lysergic acid derivatives in
the Sandoz laboratories in Switzerland, Hoffman had
occasion to prepare the simple diethylamide derivative.
On his way home from work that day, he saw the city
of Basle in an entirely new light.  The fantastic
potency of the compound had led him to ingest sufficient drug as dust to experience the hallucinogenic
effect.  Recognizing the probable cause of his "trip,"
he verified the effect by deliberately taking a
second dose.  This is one of those interesting cases
where animal pharmacology and toxicology came after
the human trial.

A number of hallucinogens, including LSD-25,
enjoyed considerable vogue in the counterculture of
the late nineteen sixties.  Since there exists no
legitimate source for the drug (it has no recognized
clinical use), underground laboratories no doubt
broadened their repertoire from acetylation of morphine
(to produce heroin) to include amide formation from
lysergic acid. (The reaction goes particularly well
in dimethylformamide; for some years a major manu-
facturer of this solvent showed this reaction in its
advertisements to illustrate the versatility of their
products!)  Lysergic acid has been prepared by total
synthesis by a group at Lilly[29]; rumor has it that
some of the illicit LSD was racemic, and thus a
product of underground total synthesis. If so, this
reflects a considerable and unexpected degree of
expertise!

Migraine is a particularly virulent form of
headache of which that suffered by the majority of
mankind is but a pale reflection; the common remedies,
such as aspirin, are all but useless against these
attacks.  Although the exact etiology of migraine is
not known, an attack does involve at one stage
dilation of the cerebral vasculature.  The skull is a
bony case that cannot accommodate volume expansion of
any magnitude.  *Methysergide (152)*, a lysergic acid
derivative, which acts as a cerebral vasoconstrictor,
has proven of use in treatment of migraine.  Alkylation of methyl lysergate *(149)* with methyl iodide,
by means of the anion formed with potassium amide,
gives the N-methylated product *(150)*.  This is then

saponified (to *151*) and converted to the amide with
2-amino-1-butanol.  There is thus obtained
*methysergide (152).*[30]

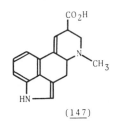

(147)

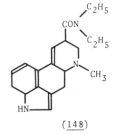

(148)

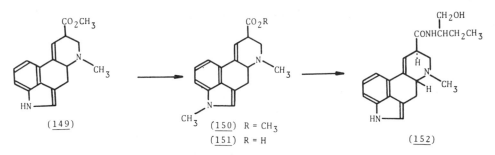

(149)        (150) R = CH₃        (152)
             (151) R = H

A different substitution pattern leads to *157*, a
molecule that exhibits peripheral α-adrenergic
blocking activity.  This is manifested as vasodilating
activity.  Photochemical addition of methanol to the
9,10-double bond of acid *151* affords the methyl ether
with the trans ring fusion *(153)*.[31]  Reduction of the
corresponding ethyl ester *(154)* with lithium aluminum
hydride then gives the carbinol *155*.  Esterification
of that alcohol with substituted nicotinic acid *156*,
gives the vasodilator *nicergoline (157).*[32]

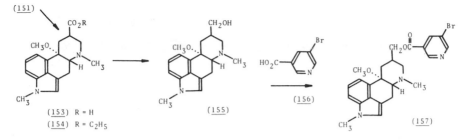

(151)

(153) R = H
(154) R = C$_2$H$_5$

(155)

(156)

(157)

Yet different elaboration of the same molecule affords a compound *(162)* that acts as an inhibitor to the pituitary peptide hormone *prolactin*, the factor responsible for supporting lactation. As such the drug has found use in suppressing lactation and in the treatment of prolactin-dependent breast tumors. In the synthesis of *162*, catalytic hydrogenation of lysergic acid proceeds from the less hindered side of the molecule to afford the derivative with the <u>trans</u> ring junction *(158)*.[30]  As above, reduction of the methyl ester *(159)* gives the corresponding carbinol. This is then converted to the methane sulfonate *(160)*, and that function is displaced with cyanide ion to afford the acetonitrile derivative *161*.

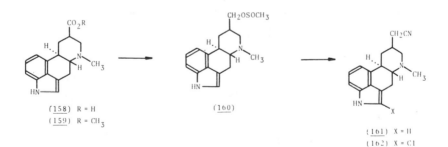

(158) R = H
(159) R = CH$_3$

(160)

(161) X = H
(162) X = Cl

Chlorination with N-chlorosuccinimide at the activated indole 2-position gives the corresponding chloro derivative, the prolactin inhibitor *legotrile (162)*.[33]

# REFERENCES

1.  Anon., Netherlands Application 6,606,390 (1967); *Chem. Abstr.*, *66:* 55535 (1967).

2.  A. D. Miller, U. S. Patent 3,975,532 (1976); *Chem. Abstr.*, *85:* 177393m (1976).

3.  T. Henshall and E. W. Parnell, *J. Chem. Soc.*, 661 (1962).

4.  H. Hermans, K. F. Hubert, G. A. Knaeps and J. J. M. Willems, U. S. Patent 3,679,686 (1972); *Chem. Abstr.*, *78:* 43295 (1972).

5.  W. J. Van Der Burg, I. L. Bouta, J. De Lobelle, C. Ramon and B. V. Vargaftig, *J. Med. Chem.*, *13*, 35 (1970).

6.  H. Otto, British Patent 1,113,754 (1969); *Chem. Abstr.*, *70:* 78031 (1969).

7.  M. Von Strandtmann, M. P. Cohen and J. Shavel, U. S. Patent 3,549,641 (1970); *Chem. Abstr.*, *75:* 91297 (1971).

8.  Anon., Belgian Patent 670,798 (1966); *Chem. Abstr.*, *65:* 7148 (1966).

9.  L. Berger and A. J. Coraz, U. S. Patent 3,409,628 (1968); *Chem. Abstr.*, *71:* 38939 (1969).

10. F. J. Villani, T. A. Mann, A. E. Wefer, J. Hannon, L. L. Carca, M. J. Landon, W. Spivak, D.

Vashi, S. Tuzzi, G. Danks, M. del Prado and R. Lutz, *J. Med. Chem.*, *18*, 1 (1975).

11. C. A. Demerson, L. G. Humber, T. A. Dobson and R. R. Martel, *J. Med. Chem.*, *18*, 189 (1975).

12. I. Jirkovsky, L. G. Humber and R. Noureldin, *Eur. J. Med. Chem.*, *11*, 571 (1976).

13. I. Jirkovsky, L. G. Humber and R. Noureldin, *J. Heterocyclic Chem.*, *12*, 937 (1975).

14. I. Jirkovsky, L. G. Humber, K. Voitw and M. P. Charest, *Arzneimittelforsch.*, *27*, 1642 (1977).

15. P. Aeberli, P. Eden, J. H. Gogerty, W. J. Houlihan and P. Penberthy, *J. Med. Chem.*, *18*, 177 (1975).

16. G. H. Hitchings, G. B. Elison and L. E. Mackay, U. S. Patent 3,019,224 (1962); *Chem. Abstr.*, *58:* 3443a (1963).

17. G. H. Hitchings and G. B. Elison, U. S. Patent 3,056,785 (1962); *Chem. Abstr.*, *58:* 5701 (1963).

18. W. Mohler and A. Soder, *Arzneimittelforsch.*, *21*, 1159 (1971).

19. T. Kamiya, Y. Saito, M. Hashimoto and H. Seki, *Tetrahedron Lett.*, 4729 (1969).

20. R. A. West and L. Beauchamp, *J. Org. Chem.*, *26*, 3809 (1961).

21. H. Hoehn and T. Deuzel, German Patent 2,123,318 (1971); *Chem. Abstr.*, *76:* 59619 (1971).

22. S. Minami, T. Shono and J. Matsumoto, *Chem. Pharm. Bull.*, *19*, 1426 (1971).

23. C. Hoffmann and A. Faure, *Bull. Soc. Chim. Fr.*, 2316 (1966).

24. See for example, D. Lednicer and L. A. Mitscher, Organic Chemistry of Drug Synthesis, Vol. 1, p. 79, 374 (1975).

25. G. Palazzo and B. Silverstrini, U. S. Patent 3,381,009 (1968); *Chem. Abstr.*, *69:* 52144 (1968).

26. F. J. Wolf, R. M. Wilson, K. Pfister and M. Tischler, *J. Amer. Chem. Soc.*, *76*, 4611 (1954).

27. G. Mixich, *Helv. Chim. Acta*, *51*, 532 (1968).

28. A. Stoll and A. Hoffmann, "Chemistry of the Alkaloids," S. W. Pelletier, ed., Von Nostrand, Reinhold and Company, New York, New York, 1970, pp. 267-300.

29. E. D. Kornfeld, E. J. Fornefeld, G. B. Kline, M. J. Mann, R. G. Jones and R. B. Woodward, *J. Amer. Chem. Soc.*, *76*, 5226 (1954); E. C. Kornfeld, E. J. Fornefeld, G. B. Kline, M. J. Mann, D. E. Morrison, R. G. Jones and R. B. Woodward, *J. Amer. Chem. Soc.*, *78*, 3087 (1956).

30. Anon., British Patent 811,964 (1959); *Chem. Abstr.*, *53:* 18969 (1959).

31. W. Barbieri, L. Bernardi, G. Bosiosi and A. Temperilli, *Tetrahedron*, *25*, *2401* (1969).

32. G. Acari, L. Bernardi, G. Bosiosio, S. Coda, G. B. Freguan and A. H. Glaser, *Experientia*, *28*, 819 (1972).

33. J. A. Kornfeld and N. J. Bach, German Patent 2,335,750 (1974); *Chem. Abstr.*, *80:* 146400 (1974).

# Indexes

# Cross Index of Drugs

Adrenal Suppressant

Trilostane

Adrenergic Agents

Adrenalone
Amidephrine
Clorprenaline
Deterenol
Domazoline

Esproquin
Etafedrine
Metizoline
Soterenol

α-Adrenergic Blocking Agents

Fenspiride

β-Adrenergic Blocking Agents

Acebutolol
Atenolol
Bufuralol
Bunitridine
Bunitrolol
Bunolol
Metalol

Metoprolol
Moprolol
Nadolol
Oxprenolol
Phenbutalol
Pindolol
Practolol

485

## β-Adrenergic Blocking Agents (cont.)

Sotalol                          Tiprenolol
Tazolol                          Tolamolol
Timolol

## Aldosterone Antagonists

Canrenoate                       Mexrenoate, Potassium
Canrenone, Potassium             Prorenoate, Potassium

## Anabolic Steroids

Bolandiol Diacetate              Norbolethone
Bolasterone                      Quinbolone
Boldenone                        Stenbolone Acetate
Bolmantalate                     Tibolone
Mibolerone

## Analgesics

Anidoxime                        Molinazone
Anileridine                      Nalbuphine
Anilopam                         Nalmexone
Benzydamine                      Naltrexone
Buprenorphine                    Nefopam
Butacetin                        Nexeridine
Butorphanol                      Noracymethadol
Carbiphene                       Octazamide
Clonixeril                       Oxilorphan
Clonixin                         Proxazole
Dimefadane                       Pyrroliphene
Dipyrone                         Salsalate
Etorphine                        Tetrydamine
Ketazocine                       Tramadol
Letimide                         Volazocine
Methopholine                     Xylazine
Mimbane

## Anesthetics

Etoxadrol                        Tiletamine
Propanidid

### Anorexic Agents

Aminorex
Amphecloral
Clominorex
Fenisorex

Fludorex
Fluminorex
Mazindol
Mefenorex

### Anterior Pituitary Activator

Epimestrol

### Anterior Pituitary Suppressant

Danazol

### Antiadrenal

Trilostane

### Antiadrenergics

Solypertine

Zolterine

### Antiamebics

Bialamicol
Clamoxyquin

Symetine
Teclozan

### Antiandrogens

Benorterone
Cyproterone Acetate

Delmadinone Acetate

### Antianginals

Flunarizine

Nifedipine

### Antiarrhythmic Agents

Amoproxan
Aprindine
Bucainide
Bunaftine
Capobenic Acid
Disopyramide

Pirolazamide
Pranolium Chloride
Pyrinoline
Quindonium Bromide
Rodocaine

## Antibacterials

Acedapsone
Acediasulfone
Acetosulfone Sodium
Biphenamine
Carbadox
Cinoxacin
Diaveridine
Mafenide
Mequidox
Nifuratrone
Nifurdazil
Nifurimide
Nifuroxime
Nifurpirinol

Nifurquinazol
Nifurthiazole
Nitrofuratrone
Ormetoprim
Oxolinic Acid
Phenyl Aminosalicylate
Piromidic Acid
Racephenicol
Sulfabenzamide
Sulfacytine
Sulfanitran
Sulfasalazine
Sulfazamet
Thiamphenicol

## Antibiotics

Amicycline
Cefadroxil
Cefamandole
Cefazolin
Cefoxitin
Cephacetrile
Cephapirin
Cephradine
Cetophenicol
Clavulanic Acid
Cyclacillin

Democycline
Meclocycline
Methacycline
Nitrocycline
Nocarcidins
Sancycline
Talampicillin
Thienamycin
Thiphencillin
Ticarcillin

## Anticholinergic Agents

Alverine
Benapryzine
Benzetimide
Benzilonium Bromide

Butropium
Dexetimide
Domazoline
Elantrine
Elucaine
Glycopyrrolate
Heteronium Bromide

Oxybutynin
Oxyphencyclimine
Parapenzolate Bromide
Pentapiperium Methyl-
   sulfate
Phencarbamide
Poldine Methylsulfate
Proglumide
Propenzolate
Thiphenamil
Tofenacin
Triampyzine

### Anticoagulant

Bromindione

### Anticonvulsants

Albutoin
Atolide
Citenamide
Cyheptamide

Eterobarb
Sulthiame
Tiletamine

### Antidepressants

Aletamine
Amedalin
Amoxapine
Bupropion
Butacetin
Cartazolate
Clodazon
Cotinine
Cypenamine
Cyprolidol
Cyproximide
Daledalin
Dazadrol
Dibenzepin
Dioxadrol
Encyprate
Fantridone
Fenmetozole
Gamfexine
Guanoxyfen
Hepzidine

Intriptyline
Isocarboxazid
Ketipramine
Maprotiline
Melitracin
Mianserin
Modaline
Octriptyline
Oxypertine
Pirandamine
Pizotyline
Propizepine
Quipazine
Rolicyprine
Sulpiride
Tandamine
Thiazesim
Thozalinone
Trazodone
Viloxazine

### Antiemetics

Metopimazine

Trimethobenzamide

### Antiestrogens

Clometherone
Delmadinone Acetate

Tamoxifen

## Antifungals

Biphenamine
Ciclopirox
Econazole
Ethonam

Miconazole
Tolindate
Tolnaftate

## Antihelmintics

Albendazole
Bromoxanide
Bunamidine
Cambedazole
Clioxanide
Cyclobendazole
Flubendazole
Lobendazole

Mebendazole
Niclosamide
Nitramisole
Nitrodan
Oxantel
Oxfendazole
Oxibendazole
Thenium Closylate

## Antihistaminics

Azanator
Azatadine
Clemastine
Closiramine

Dorastine
Mianserin
Rotoxamine
Terfenadine

## Antihypertensives

Aceperone
Alipamide
Amquinsin
Bupicomide
Chlorothiazide
Clopamide
Diapamide
Guanabenz
Guanisoquin
Guanochlor
Guanoxabenz
Guanoxyfen

Hydracarbazine
Indoramine
Leniquinsin
Methyldopa
Metolazone
Mexrenone
Pazoxide
Prazocin
Quinazocin
Trimoxamine
Trimazocin

## Antiinflammatory Steroids

Amcinafal
Amcinafide
Cormethasone Acetate
Cortivazol

Desonide
Difluprednate
Drocinonide
Endrysone

## Antiinflammatory Steroids (cont.)

Flunisolide
Halcinonide
Nivazol

Tralonide
Triclonide

## Antimalarials

Amquinate

Menoctone

## Antimigrane

Methysergide

## Antineoplastics

Azathioprine
Azatepa
BCNU
Benzodepa
Calusterone
CCNU
Dacarbazine
Lomustine
MeCCNU
Melphalan

Oxisuran
Pipobroman
Piposulfan
Procarbazine
Semustine
Tamoxifen
Testolactone
Thiampirine
Thioguanine

## Antiparkinsonism Agents

Carbidopa
Carmantadine

Dopamantine
Lometraline

## Antiperistaltics

Alkofanone
Difenoximide
Difenoxin

Fetoxylate
Fluperamide
Loperamide

## Antiprotozoals

Carnidazole
Flubendazole
Flunidazole
Ipronidazole
Moxnidazole
Nifursemizone

Nimorazole
Nithiazole
Oxamniquine
Ronidazole
Sulnidazole

### Antipyretics

Benzydamine                    Indoxole
Dipyrone

### Antipsychotics

Carpipramine                   Clocapramine

### Antischistosomals

Becanthone                     Oxamniquine
Niridazole                     Teroxalene

### Antispasmodic Agents

Butamirate                     Carmantadine

### Antitrichomonals

Nimorazole

### Antitussives

Amicibone                      Clobutinol
Benproperine                   Codoxime
Butamirate                     Pemerid

### Antivirals

Amantadine                     Methisazone
Famotine                       Rimantadine
Memotine                       Tilorone

### Avian Chemosterilant

Azacosterol

### Bronchodilators

Albuterol*                     Fenspiride
Carbuterol*                    Hoquizil
Clorprenaline*                 Isoetharine*
Doxaprost                      Piquizil
Eprozinol                      Pirbuterol*
Fenoterol*                     Prostalene

Bronchodilators (cont.)

Quazodine
Quinterenol*
Rimiterol*
Soterenol*
   *adrenergic

Sulfontcrol*
Suloxifen
Trimethoquinol*

CNS Stimulants

Amphetaminil
Ampyzine
Azabon
Difluanine
Ethamivan

Flubanilate
Indriline
Mefexamide
Pyrovalerone
Trazodone

Canine Contraceptive

Mibolerone

Cardiotonics

Benfurodil

Dobutamine

Catecholamine Potentiator

Talopram

Cathartics

Bisoxatin Acetate

Oxyphenisatin Acetate

Choleretic

Piprozolin

Cholinergic Agent

Aceclidine

Coccidiostats

Alkomide
Cyproquinate
Decoquinate
Nequinate

Proquinolate
Sulfanitran
Triazuril

### Coronary Vasodilators

Dobutamine
Flunarizine
Medibazine
Mixidine

Nifedipine
Oxprenolol
Oxyfedrine
Terodiline

### Corticoids

Cloprednol
Drocinonide

Flunisolide
Halcinonide

### Cough Suppressant

Amicibone

### Diuretics

Alipamide
Ambuside
Azolimine
Bumetanide
Chlorothiazide
Clazolimine
Clopamide
Clorexalone
Diapamide

Furosemide
Indapamide
Metalazone
Methalthiazide
Prorenone
Ticrynafen
Triflocin
Xipramide

### Estrogens

Epimestrol
Estrazinol
Estrofurate

Fenestrol
Nylestriol

### Estrus Regulators

Cloprostenol
Fluprostenol

Prostalene

### Expectorant

Bromhexine

### Fibrinolytic

Bisobrin

### Gastric Antisecretory

Cimetidine                          Metiamide
Deprostil                           Tiquinamide

### Glucocorticoids

Clocortolone Acetate                Flurandrenolide
Cortivazol                          Formocortal
Descinolone Acetonide               Medrysone
Diflucortolone                      Nivazol
Flucloronide                        Prednival
Fluperolone Acetate

### Hemostatics

Aminomethylbenzoic Acid             Tranexamic Acid

### Hypoglycemic

Isobuzole

### Hypolipidemics

Beloxamide                          Nafenopin
Boxidine                            Pimetine
Clofenpyride                        Probucol
Eritadenine                         Tibric Acid
Halofenate                          Treloxinate
Lifibrate

### Hypotensives

Amquinsin                           Prostalene
Prorenone

### Immunosuppressant

Azathioprine

### Interferon Inducer

Tilerone

## Local Anesthetics

Amoproxan                          Etidocaine
Biphenamine                        Risocaine
Diamocaine                         Rodocaine
Dexivacaine

## Luteolytic Agents

Cloprostenol                       Fluprostenol

## Mucolytic

Bromhexine

## Muscle Relaxants

Baclofen                           Mebeverine
Benzoctamine                       Mesuprine
Cinnamedrine                       Metaxalone
Dantrolene                         Nafomine
Fenalamide                         Pancuronium Bromide
Fenyripol                          Prazepam
Fetoxylate                         Proxazole
Flavoxate                          Ritodrine
Fletazepam                         Rolodine
Flumetramide                       Methixine
Isomylamine                        Xylazine
Lorbamate

## Narcotic Antagonists

Nalbuphine                         Naltrexone
Nalmexone

## Narcotics

Anileridine                        Etorphine
Buprenorphine                      Oxilorphan
Butorphanol

## Non-Steroidal Antiinflammatory Agents

Alclofenac                         Benoxaprofen
Apazone                            Benzydamine
Bendazac                           Cicloprofen

## Non-Steroidal Antiinflammatory Agents (cont.)

Cintazone
Cliprofen
Clonixeril
Clonixin
Clopirac
Diclofenac
Diflumidone
Diflunisal
Etoclofene
Fenamole
Fenbufen
Fenclorac
Fenclozic Acid
Fenoprofen
Fenoterol
Fenpipalone
Flazolone
Flufenamic Acid
Flumizole
Flunisolide
Flunixin
Flutiazin
Furobufen

Indoxole
Intrazole
Isoxicam
Ketoprofen
Meclofenamic Acid
Nimazone
Oxaprozin
Paranyline
Pirprofen
Prodolic Acid
Proquazone
Proxazole
Pyroxicam
Salsalate
Sudoxicam
Sulindac
Suprofen
Tesicam
Tesimide
Tetrydamine
Tolmetin
Triflumidate

## Oral Hypoglycemics

Gliamilide
Glibornuride
Glipizide
Glydanile
Glymidine

Glyoctamide
Glyparamide
Metformin
Tolpyrramide

## Pituitary Suppressant

Danazol

## Progestins

Algestone Acetonide
Algestone Acetophenide
Angesterone Acetate
Cingestol
Clogestone
Clomegestone Acetate

Delmadinone Acetate
Dexnorgestrel Acetime
Ethynerone
Flurogestone Acetate
Gestaclone
Gestonorone

### Progestins (cont.)

| | |
|---|---|
| Haloprogesterone | Norgestomet |
| Medrogestone | Tigestol |
| Methynodiol Diacetate | |

### Prolactin Inhibitor

Lergotrile

### Respiratory Stimulants

| | |
|---|---|
| Dimefline | Doxapram |

### Sedatives

| | |
|---|---|
| Benzoctamine | Nisobamate |
| Clozapine | Tricetamide |
| Midaflur | Trimetozine |
| Alonimid | Perlapine |
| Flunitrazepam | Roletamide |
| Nisobamate | |

### Sedatives - Tranquilizers

| | |
|---|---|
| Acepromazine | Cyprazepam |
| Alpertine | Cyproximide |
| Azaperone | Demoxepam |
| Benperidol | Etazolate |
| Benzindopyrine | Fenimide |
| Bromperidol | Fletazepam |
| Buspirone | Fluspiperone |
| Butaclamol | Fluspiriline |
| Butaperazine | Halazepam |
| Carpipramine | Hydroxyphenamate |
| Cinperene | Imidoline |
| Cintriamide | Lenperone |
| Clazolam | Lometraline |
| Clobazam | Loxapine |
| Clocapramine | Metiapine |
| Clomacran | Milipertine |
| Cloperidone | Molindone |
| Clopimozide | Naranol |
| Clothiapine | Nisobamate |
| Clothixamide | Oxiperomide |
| Cyclophenazine | Penfluridol |

### Sedatives - Tranquilizers (cont.)

Pimozide
Pinoxepin
Pipamperone
Pipotiazine
Prazepam
Spirilene
Sulazepam

Taclamine
Temazepam
Thiothixene
Triflubazam
Tybamate
Uldazepam

### Serotonin Inhibitors

Chlorophenylalanine
Cinanserin
Fenclonine

Fonazine
Mianserin
Xylamidine

### Thyromimetic

Thyromedan

### Uricosurics

Benzobromarone

Halofenate

### Vasoconstrictors

Ciclafrine

Methysergide

### Vasodilators

Aceperone
Bamethan
Benfurodil
Betahistine
Cinepazide
Flunarizine
Hexobendine
Ifenprodil

Isoxsuprine
Mesuprine
Nafronyl
Nicergoline
Oxprenolol
Pentoxifylline
Pindolol
Zolterine

# Index

*Acebutolol*, 109
*Aceclidine*, 295
*Acedapsone*, 112
*Aceperone*, 332
Acetaminophen, 63
*Acetanilide*, 97
Acetylcholine, 71, 93, 97, 294
Acetylenes, hydration, 20
"Acid", 476
Additive effects of substituents, 179
*Adrenalin*, 38
*Adrenalone*, 38
Adrenergic agents, 36, 37
Adrenergic agonists, SAR, 37, 38, 251
Adrenergic antagonists, 105-109
β-Adrenergic antagonists, actions, 107
Adrenergic transmission, 100
Adrenergic transmitters, SAR, 106

*Albendazole*, 353
*Albuterol*, 43
*Albutoin*, 261
*Alclofenac*, 68
Aldosterone, 173
*Aletamine*, 48
*Algestone acetonide*, 171
*Algestone acetophenide*, 171
*Alipamide*, 94
Alonimid, 295
*Alpertine*, 342
*Alphaprodine*, 328
*Alverine*, 55
*Amantadine*, 18
*Ambuside*, 116
Amcinafal, 185
Amcinafide, 185
*Amedalin*, 348
*Amicibone*, 11
*Amicycline*, 228
*Amidephrine*, 41
Aminals, 258, 462
*p-Aminobenzoic acid*, 9
7-Aminocephalosporanic acid (7ACA), 441

501

7-Aminodesacetylcephalo-
  sporanic acid (7ADCA),
  439
α-Aminonitrile, 289
Aminooxazoline synthesis,
  264
6-Aminopenicillanic acid
  (6APA), 437
Aminopyrine, 262
Aminorex, 265
Amiquinsin, 363
Amoproxan, 91
Amoxapine, 428
Amphecloral, 48
Amphetamine, 47
Amphetaminil, 48
Ampicillin, 437, 438
Ampyzine, 298
Amquinate, 370
Anagram, 235
Anesthetic, injectable, 15
Angesterone acetate, 165
Anidoxime, 125
Antagonists,
  β-adrenergic, 41
  to histamine, 251
Anticholinergic activity,
  71, 221
Antidepressant, 31
Antidepressant activity, 7
Antipyrine, 63, 261
Antisecretory, gastric, 3,
  4
Antisecretory activity, 2
Antitussive, 11
Antiulcer activity, 2
Apazone, 475
Aphrodisiac, reputed, 347
Appetite depressants, 47
Aprindine, 208
Arbuzov reaction, 420
Aromatization, by loss of
  methyl group, 147, 149
Arrhythmias, cardiac, 33
Aspirin, 63, 89
Atenolol, 109

Atropine, 71
Autonomic nervous system,
  36
Azabon, 115
Azacosterol, 161
Azanator, 457
Azaperone, 300
Azaphilone, 282, 296
Azatadine, 424
Azathioprine, 464
Aziridinium ion, 11, 208,
  219, 325, 472
  regiochemistry, 59
Aziridinium salt, 72
Azolimine, 260

Baclofen, 121
Bamethan, 39
BAS, 96
BCNU, 12
Becanthone, 413
Beckett-Casey rule, 328
Beloxamide, 56
Benapryzine, 74
Bendazac, 351
Benfurodil, 355, 356
Benorterone, 156
Benoxaprofen, 356
Benperidol, 290
Benproperine, 100
Benzbromarone, 354
Benzetimide, 293
Benzilate esters, 74
Benzilonium bromide, 72
Benzindopyrine, 343
Benzoctamine, 220
Benzodepa, 122
Benzothiadiazines, 383
Benztriamide, 290
Benzydamine, 350
Betahistine, 279
Bioisosterism (see also
  biological isosterism),
  278
Biological isosterism, 233
Birch reduction, 145, 147,

152, 440
1,3-Biscarbamates, 21
Bischler-Napieralski
  cyclodehydration, 140,
  377, 404, 427, 453
  reaction, 224
Bismethylenedioxy protect-
  ing group, 190
β-Blockers, 41
Blood-brain barrier, 52,
  213
Bolandiol diacetate, 143
Bolasterone, 154
Boldenone 10-undecylenate,
  153
Bolmantalate, 143
Boxidine, 99
Breakthroughs, therapeutic,
  446
Bromindione, 210
Bromperidol, 331
Bromhexine, 96
Bromoxanide, 94
Bronchodilator, 3, 5, 38,
  45, 108
Bucainide, 125
Bucloxic acid, 126
Buformin, 21
Bufuralol, 110
Bumetanide, 87
Bunaftine, 211
Bunamidine, 212
Bunitridine, 215
Bunitrolol, 106, 110
Bunolol, 110, 215
Bupicomide, 280
Buprenorphine, 321
Bupropion, 124
Burimamide, 251
Buspirone, 300
Butacetin, 95
Butamirate, 76
Butaclamol, 226
Butorphanol, 325
Butropium bromide, 308

Calusterone, 154
Cambendazole, 353
c-AMP, 464
Canrenone, 174
Carpipramine, 416
Capobenic acid, 94
Carbadox, 390
Carbencillin, 437
Carbidopa, 119
Carbinoxamine, 32
Carbiphene, 78
Carboxylation of phenols,
  86
Carbuterol, 41
Cardiotonic agent, 53
Carisoprodol, 21
Carmantadine, 20
Carmustine, 12
Carnidazole, 245
Cartazolate, 469
CCNU, 12
Cefadroxil, 440
Cefamandole, 441
Cefazolin, 442
Cefoxitin, 435, 443
Cephalexin, 439
Cephamycin C, 442
Cephradine, 440
Cephapirin, 441
Cetophenicol, 46
Chloramphenicol, 28, 45
Chlordiazepoxide, 401
Chlormadinone acetate, 165
p-Chlorophenylalanine, 52
Chlorothiazide, 395
Chlorpromazine, 409
Cholinergic transmission,
  71
Cholinesterase, 294
Chromone synthesis, 391
Ciclafrine, 266
Ciclopirox, 282
Cicloprofen, 217
Cimetidine, 253
Cinanserin, 96
Cinepazide, 301

*Cingestol*, 145
*Cinnamedrine*, 39
Cinnoline synthesis, 387, 394
*Cinoxacin*, 388
*Cintazone*, 388, 474
*Cintriamide*, 121
*Citenamide*, 221
*Clamoxyquin*, 362
Clavulanic acid, 435
*Clazolam*, 452, 453
*Clazolimine*, 260
*Clemastine*, 32
*Clioxanide*, 94
*Cliprofen*, 65
*Clobazam*, 406
*Clobutinol*, 121
*Clocapramine*, 416
*Clocortolone*, 193
*Clodazon*, 354
*Clofenpyride*, 101
*Clofibrate*, 79, 101, 432
*Clogestone*, 166
*Clomacran*, 414
*Clomegestone acetate*, 170
*Clometherone*, 170
*Clomifene*, 127
*Clominorex*, 265
*Clonixeril*, 281
*Clonixin*, 281
*Clopamide*, 93
*Cloperidone*, 387
*Clopimozide*, 300
Clopirac, 235
*Cloprednol*, 182
Cloprostenol, 6
*Clorprenaline*, 39
*Closiramine*, 424
*Clothiapine*, 429
*Clothixamide*, 412
*Codeine*, 317
*Codoxime*, 318
Conjugate addition, 2, 72, 123, 140, 144, 147, 154, 175, 220, 237, 343, 412, 450, 455, 456

Corey lactol, 4
Cormethasone acetate, 194
Cormethasone acetate, 196
Cortisone, 176, 179
*Cortivazol*, 191
Cotinine, 235
*Curare*, 162
*Cyclacillin*, 439
*Cyclazocine*, 327
Cyclic adenosine mono-phosphate, see cAMP
*Cyclobendazole*, 353
Cyclopropanation, 32, 166, 168, 174. 223, 297
*Cyheptamide*, 222
Cypenamine, 7
*Cyprazepam*, 402
*Cyprolidol*, 31
*Cyproquinate*, 368
*Cyproterone acetate*, 166
*Cyproximide*, 293

*Dacarbazine*, 254
*Daledalin*, 348
*Danazol*, 157
*Dantrolene*, 242
*Dapsone*, 112
Darzens condensation, 374
*Dazadrol*, 257
Debrisoquin, 374
*Decoquinate*, 368
Dehydrogenation,
  with chloranil, 144, 147, 170, 182, 190
  with DDQ, 147, 191
  microbiological, 189, 192, 196
  with selenium dioxide, 160, 166, 179
*Demoxepam*, 401
*Deprostil*, 3
*Descinolone*, 187
*Descinolone acetonide*, 187, 189
*Desonide*, 179
*Deternol*, 39

Dexivacaine, 95
Dexnorgestrel acetime, 152
Diabetes, 116
Diamocaine, 336
Diapamide, 93
Diaveridine, 302
Diazepam, 452
Diazoxide, 395
Dibenzepin, 424, 471
Dichloroisoproterenol, 106
Diclofenac, 70
Dicyanamide, 21
Dieckmann cyclization, 72
Difenoximide, 331
Difenoxin, 331
Diflucortolone, 192
Diflumidone, 98
Diflunisal, 85, 86
Difluoromethylene groups,
  from ketones, 196
Difluprednate, 191
Dihydrocodeinone, 318
Dihydropyridine synthesis,
  283
Dihydroxyphenylalanine,
  see DOPA
Dimefadane, 210
Dimefline, 391
Dioxadrol, 285
Diphenoxylate, 331
1,3-Dipolar addition, 301
Dipyrone, 262
Disopyramide, 81
DNA, 12
Dobutamine, 53
Doisynolic acid, 9
Domazoline, 256
DOPA, 52, 119
Dopamantine, 52
Dopamine, 51
Dorastine, 457
Doxapram, 236, 237
Doxaprost, 3
Drocinonide, 186

Econazole, 249

Elantrine, 418
Elucaine, 44
Encyprate, 27
Endorphins, 317
Endrysone, 200
Enkephalins, 316
Ephedrine, 39
Epimestrol, 13
Epinephrine, 38, 105
Eprozinol, 44
Ergonovine, 475
Ergotism, 475
Eritadenine, 467
Eschweiler-Clark methyla-
  tion, 29, 162, 210, 28(
Esproquin, 373
Estradiol, 136
Estrazinol, 142
Estriols, 138
Estrofurate, 137
Estrogenic activity, 9
Estrogens, 137
Estrone, 137
Estrus synchronization,
  6, 183
Etafedrine, 39
Etazolate, 469
Eterobarb, 304
Ethacrynic acid, 103
Ethamivan, 94
Ethonam, 249
Ethynerone, 146
Etidocaine, 95
Etoclofene, 89
Etorphine, 321
Etoxadrol, 285

False substrates, 161
Famotine, 37
Fantridone, 421
Fenalamide, 81
Fenbufen, 126
Fenclorac, 66
Fenclozic acid, 269
Fenestrel, 9
Fenimide, 237

Fenisorex, 391
Fenmetozole, 257
Fenoprofen, 67
Fenpipalone, 293
Fenoterol, 38
Fenspiride, 291
Fenyripol, 40
Fetoxylate, 331
Fibrinolysis, 8
Fire, St. Anthony's, 475
Fischer indole synthesis, 340, 457
Flavoxate, 392
Flazalone, 337
Fletazepam, 403
Flubanilate, 98
Flubendazole, 354
Flucloronide, 198
Fludorex, 44
Flufenamic acid, 69
Fludrocortide, 198
Flumetramide, 306
Fluminorex, 265
Flumizole, 254
Flunarizine, 31
Flunidazole, 246
Flunisolide, 181
Flunitrazepam, 406
Flunixin, 281
Fluperamide, 334
Fluperolone acetate, 185
Fluprostenol, 6
Flurandrenolide, 180
Flurogestone acetate, 183
Fluspiperone, 292
Fluspirilene, 292
Flutiazin, 431
Food and Drug Administration, 447
Formocortal, 189
Friedel-Crafts cyanation, 212
Furobufen, 416
Furosemide, 87
Fusaric acid, 279

Gamfexine, 56
Ganglion blocking agent, 287
Gestaclone, 169
Gestonorone caproate, 152
Gliamilide, 286
Glibornuride, 117
Glipizide, 117
Glucocorticoids, 177
Glyoctamide, 117
Glyoxals, from methyl-ketones, 42
Glyparamide, 117
Grewe synthesis, 327
Guanabenz, 123
Guanethidine, 100
Guanisoquin, 375
Guanochlor, 101
Guanoxabenz, 123
Guanoxyfen, 101

Halcinonide, 187
Halofenate, 80, 102
Haloform reaction, 88
Haloprogesterone, 173
Hepzidine, 222
Heroin, 315
Heteronium bromide, 72
Heterosteroids, 139-142
Hexobendine, 92
Histamine,
    antagonists, 250
    $H_1$ and $H_2$ receptors, 251
    in ulcer formation, 251
Hoquizil, 381
Hycanthone, 413
Hydantoin synthesis, 261
Hydracarbazine, 305
Hydroxylamine-o-sulfonic acid, 7
Hydroxylation, osmium tetroxide, 138
Hypoglycemics, oral, 20
Hypotensive agent, 5

Ibuprofen, 218, 356

Ifenprodil, 39
Imidazole,
  synthesis, 246, 249, 254
  tautomerism, 243
Imidazoline synthesis, 256
Imidazolinone synthesis,
  260
Imidazolone synthesis, 291
Imidoline, 259
Imipramine, 420
Indapamide, 349
Indazole synthesis, 350
Indoles, as starting
  material for benzo-
  diazepines, 405
Indomethacin, 345
Indoramin, 344
Indoxole, 254, 340
Inflammation, 63
Influenza A, 18
Inhibition,
  of cholinesterase, 294
  of DNA gyrase, 370
  of DNA synthesis, 12
  of dopamine β-
    hydroxylase, 279
  of MAO, 266
  of monoamine oxidase, 7,
    27
  of phosphodiesterases,
    379, 464
  of prolactin, 479
  of sympathetic trans-
    mission, 100
Insertion reaction, 27
Interferon, inducer, 219
Intrazole, 345
Intriptyline, 223
Ipronidazole, 244
Isobuzole, 272
Isocarboxazid, 266
Isoetharine, 9
Isolectronic groups, 253
Isomylamine, 11
Isoniazid, 266
Isoproterenol, 37, 107

Isoxicam, 394
Ivanov salt, 68

Ketamine, 16
Ketazocine, 328
Ketoprofen, 64

β-Lactamases, 442
Leniquinsin, 363
Lenperone, 286
Leprosy, 111
Lergotrile, 480
Letimide, 393
Leucine enkephalin, 317
Lidocaine, 95, 449
Lifibrate, 103
β-Lipotropin, 317
Lithium dimethyl cuprate,
  4
Lobendazole, 353
Lometraline, 214
Lomustine, 12, 15
Loperamide, 334
Lorbamate, 21
Loxapine, 427
LSD-25, 476
Lucanthone, 413
Luteolytic activity, 6
Lysergic acid, 475

Mafenide, 114
Mannich reaction, 17, 40,
  45, 57, 155, 223, 233,
  234, 261, 336, 362, 410,
  454, 456
MAO, see monoamine oxidase
Maprotiline, 220, 221
Mazindol, 462
Mebendazole, 353
Mebeverine, 54
MeCCNU, 12
Meclocycline, 227
Meclofenamic acid, 88
Medibazine, 30
Mediquox, 390
Medroxyprogesterone

acetate, 165
Medrysone, 200
Mefenamic acid, 280
Mefenorex, 47
Mefexamide, 103
Melitracin, 220
Melphalan, 120
Memotine, 378
Menoctone, 217
Meperidines, 328
  reversed, 331
Meprobamate, 21
Mesuprine, 41
Metabolic activation, 464
Metabolism, of steroids,
  138
Metalol, 41
Metformin, 20
Methacycline, 227
Methadone, 328
Methionine enkephalin, 317
Methisazone, 350
Methixene, 413
17-Methyltestosterone, 156
Methynodiol diacetate, 149
Methysergide, 477
Metiamide, 252
Metiapine, 429
Metizoline, 256
Metolazone, 384
Metoprolol, 109
Mexenone, 175
Mianserin, 451
Mibolerone, 144
Miconazole, 249
Midaflur, 259
Migraine, 477
Milipertine, 341
Mimbane, 347
Mineralocorticoids, 177
Minocycline, 228
Mixed agonists-antagonists,
  318
Mixidine, 54
Modaline, 299
Molecular dissection, 9,

17, 96, 237, 315, 325,
  449
Molinazone, 395
Molindone, 455
Monoamine oxidase, 7, 49
Moprolol, 109
Morazone, 261
Morphine, 314
Morphine rule, 17, 328
Moxnidazole, 246

Nadolol, 110
Nafenopin, 214
Nafomine, 212
Nafronyl, 213
Nalbuphine, 319
Nalidixic acid, 370, 469
Nalmexone, 319
Nalorphine, 318
Naloxone, 318, 323
Naltrexone, 319
Naranol, 454
Nef reaction, 2
Nefopam, 447
Nequinate, 369
Nexeridine, 17
Nicergoline, 478
Niclosamide, 94
Nifedipine, 283
Nifuratrone, 238
Nifurdazil, 239
Nifurimide, 239
Nifuroxime, 238
Nifurpirinol, 240
Nifurquinazol, 383
Nifursemizone, 238
Nifurthiazole, 241
Nimazone, 260
Nimorazole, 244
Niridazole, 269
Nisobamate, 22
Nithiazole, 268
Nitronic acid, 2
Nivazol, 159
Nocardicins, 435
Noracymethadol, 58

Norbolethone, 151
Norepinephrine, biological
   effects, 38
Norethindrone, 145
Norgestrel, 151
19-Nortestosterone, 142
Nucleophilic aromatic
   substitution, 64, 65,
   79, 89, 95, 281, 282,
   406, 410, 413, 425

Octazamide, 448
Octriptyline, 223
Opium, 314
Organoboranes, amination,
   7
Ormetoprim, 302
Oxamniquine, 372
Oxantel, 303
Oxaprozin, 263
Oxazepam, 402
Oxazole synthesis, 263
Oxazolinone synthesis,
   246, 265
Oxfendazole, 353
Oxibendazole, 352
Oxidation,
   metabolic, 464
   microbiological, 160,
   180, 183, 196, 373
   by nitroalkanes, 28
   with ruthenium tetroxide,
   404
Oxilorphan, 325
Oxiperomide, 290
Oxisuran, 280
Oxolinic acid, 370, 387
Oxprenolol, 109
Oxyfedrine, 40
Oxymorphone, 319
Oxypertine, 343
Oxyphencyclimine, 75
Oxyphenisatin, 350
Oxytetracycline, 226

Pancuronium bromide, 163

Papaver bracteatum, 319
Papaver somniferum, 314,
   318
Paraaminosalicylic acid,
   89
Paranyline, 218
Parapenzolate bromide, 75
Parasympathetic nervous
   system, 71
Pargyline, 27
Parkinson's disease, 52,
   119
Pazoxide, 395
Pemerid, 288
Penfluridol, 334
Pentapiperium methyl-
   sulfate, 76
Pentazocine, 325
Pentoxifylline, 466
Perhydropyrindene synthesis,
   450
Perlapine, 425
Pharmacophore, 233, 237,
   242, 255, 278, 361
Pharmacognosy, 466
Phenbutalol, 110
Phencarbamide, 97
Phenmetrazine, 261
Phenyl aminosalicylate,
   89
Phenylbutazone, 388, 474
Phenylephrine, 265
Phenylpiperidinols, 334
Physical dependence, 314
Pill, the, 137, 164
   for canines, 144
Pimetine, 286
Pimozide, 290
Pindolol, 342
Pinoxepin, 419
Pipamperone, 288
Pipobroman, 299
Piposulfan, 299
Piprozolin, 270
Piquizil, 381
Pirandamine, 459

*Pirbuterol*, 280
*Piromidic acid*, 470
*Pirprofen*, 69
*Pizotyline*, 420
*Poldine*, 74
Poldine methylsulfate, 74
Polonovski reaction, 240,
  402
Potassium canrenoate, 174
Potassium mexrenoate, 175
Potassium prorenoate, 175
Poultry, epidemics in, 366
*Practolol*, 106, 108
*Pranolium chloride*, 212
*Prazepam*, 405
*Prazosin*, 382
*Prednisolone*, 178
*Prednival*, 179
*Probucol*, 126
*Procarbazine*, 27
*Prodolic acid*, 459
Prodrug, 48, 50, 89, 198,
  363
*Progesterone*, 164
*Proglumide*, 93
*Propanidid*, 79
Propenzolate, 75
*Propizepine*, 472
*Propoxyphene*, 57
*Propranolol*, 105, 107, 212
*Proquazone*, 386
*Proquinolate*, 368
*Prorenone*, 175
*Prostalene*, 5
*Proxazole*, 271
Purine synthesis, 467
Psilocybine, 342
Psychotomimetic activity,
  71
*Pyrantel*, 303
Pyrazine synthesis, 298
Pyridazine synthesis, 304
Pyrimidine synthesis, 302,
  467
*Pyrinoline*, 34
*Pyrovalerone*, 124

*Pyroxicam*, 394
*Pyrroliphene*, 57

*Quazodine*, 379
Quinate coccidiostats,
  366-370
*Quinazosin*, 382
*Quinbolone*, 154
*Quindonium bromide*, 139
Quinolone synthesis, 363
Quinoxaline synthesis, 388
*Quinterenol*, 366

Reaction, time honored, 92
Rearrangement,
  Beckmann, 419
  of benzisothiazoles, 393
  Chapman, 89
  cyclopropylcarbinyl, 223
  Fries, 42, 43, 355
  glycidic ester, 374
  Hofmann, 49, 117, 279
  isoxazole to cyano-
    ketone, 159
  lactone-amide, 282
  ring exchange, 236
  Smiles, 430
  Stevens, 124
  Wagner-Meerwein, 323,
    347
Receptors,
  α-, 105
  α-adrenergic, 37
  β-, 105
  β-adrenergic, 37
  as drug targets, 50
  for opioids, 316
Reductive alkylation, 47,
  55
Reformatsky reaction, 209,
  355, 424, 460
Retro-Claisen reaction, 49
Rigid analogues, 50, 223,
  284, 296, 451
*Rimantadine*, 19
*Rimiterol*, 278

*Risocaine*, 91
*Ritodrine*, 39
Ritter reaction, 19
Robinson annulation, 224
*Rodocaine*, 450
*Roletamide*, 103
*Rolicyprine*, 50
*Rolodine*, 468
*Ronidazole*, 245
*Rotoxamine*, 32

*Salbutamol*, 280
*Salsalate*, 90
*Sapiens, homo*, 316
*Semustine*, 12, 15
Serotonin, 96, 343
Serum cholesterol, 56, 78, 161
Slow release drugs, 143
*Solypertine*, 342
*Sotalol*, 41
*Soterenol*, 40
*Spirilene*, 292
*Spironolactone*, 172
*Stenbolone acetate*, 155
Strecker reaction, 119
*Streptokinase*, 377
*Sudoxicam*, 394
*Sulazepam*, 403
*Sulfabenzamide*, 112
*Sulfacytine*, 113
*Sulfanilamide*, 112
*Sulfanitran*, 115
*Sulfapyridine*, 114
*Sulfasalazine*, 114
*Sulfazamet*, 113
Sulfonamide diuretics, SAR, 87
*Sulfonterol*, 42, 43
*Sulindac*, 210
*Sulnidazole*, 245
*Sulpiride*, 94
*Sulthiame*, 306
*Suprofen*, 65
*Symetine*, 29
Sympathetic blocker, 363

Sympathetic nervous system, 36
Sympathomimetic, 47
  agents, 36, 365
  α- agents, 255

*Taclamine*, 224
*Talampicillin*, 438
*Talopram*, 357
*Tamoxifen*, 127
*Tandamine*, 347, 460
*Tazolol*, 110, 268
*Teclozan*, 28
*Temazepam*, 402
*Terodiline*, 56
*Tesicam*, 379
*Tesimide*, 296
*Testolactone*, 160
Tetrahydropyrimidine synthesis, 303
Tetrahydroquinoline synthesis, 371
Tetrazole synthesis, 301, 345
*Tetrydamine*, 352
*Thalidomide*, 296
Thebaine, 318
*Thenium closylate*, 99
Theobromine, 456
*Theophylline*, 464
*Thiabendazole*, 352, 353
1,2,5-Thiadiazole synthesis, 271
1,3,4-Thiadiazole synthesis, 272
*Thiamphenicol*, 45
*Thiampirine*, 464
Thiazole synthesis, 240, 269
Thiazolinone synthesis, 270
Thienamycin, 435
*Thioguanine*, 464
*Thiothixene*, 412
Thioxanthone synthesis, 400

*Thozalinone*, 265
*Thyromedan*, 79
*Thyroxine*, 78
*Tibolone*, 147
*Tibric acid*, 87
*Ticarcillin*, 437
*Ticrynafen*, 104
*Tienilic acid*, see
  ticryanfen
*Tigestol*, 145
*Tiletamine*, 15, 16
*Tilorone*, 219
*Timolol*, 272
*Tiquinamide*, 372
*Tofenacin*, 32
*Tolamolol*, 110
*Tolazoline*, 106
*Tolindate*, 208
*Tolmetin*, 234
*Tolnaftate*, 211
*Tolpyrramide*, 116
Torgov-Smith synthesis, 140
*Tralonide*, 198
*Tramalol*, 17
*Tranexamic acid*, 9
*Tranylcypromine*, 7, 50
*Trazodone*, 472
*Treloxinate*, 432
Triacetone amine, 288
*Triamcinolone*, 185
*Triampyzine*, 298
Triazinedione synthesis,
  305
*Triazuril*, 305
*Tricetamide*, 94
*Triclonide*, 198
*Triflocin*, 282
*Triflubazam*, 406
*Triflumidate*, 98
*Trilostane*, 158, 159
*Trimazosin*, 382
*Trimethoprim*, 302
*Trimethoquinol*, 374
*Trimetozine*, 94
*Trimoxamine*, 49
Trip, 476

Tryptamine, 343
*Tybamate*, 22

Ulcerogenic potential, 64
Ullman reaction, 413, 425,
  428, 429
*Urokinase*, 376

Vasodilator, 30
*Viloxazine*, 306
Vilsmeir reaction, 189
*Volazocine*, 327
von Braun demethylation,
  321

Whipworm, 303
Willgerodt reaction, 68
Wittig condensation, 3, 6
Wittig reaction, 420
Woodward hydroxylation,
  215

*Xipamide*, 93
*Xylamidine*, 54
*Xylazine*, 307

Yohimbine, 347

*Zolterine*, 301

# Errata for Volume One

In a work of this magnitude it is an unfortunate
fact of life that errors will creep in. We are
grateful to our friends and students who have enabled
us to compare their lists with ours. Fortunately,
the majority are typos and other grammatical mistakes
that are embarassing but do not obscure the meaning
nor the veracity of what we were conveying. These
have been corrected in subsequent printings of the
work and are not reproduced here. Those mistakes that
are less obvious and/or which we feel might mislead
those not familiar with the particular subject matter
involved are listed here. The interested reader can
annotate volume 1 accordingly. Every effort has
been made to ensure that the number of mistakes that
creep into volume 2 have been held to a minimum. It
is hoped that the authors have the reader's understanding if not forebearance for those which remain.

| Page | Line | Old Entry | New Entry |
|------|------|-----------|-----------|
| 6 | 19 | tropane. | tropane.[13] |
| 8 | 9 | Hydrogenation | Cyanohydrin reaction |
| 8 | 11 | ester, 19. | ester, 20. |
| 11 | Tab. | (X and Y for ambucaine are reversed.) | |
| 16 | 3 | (64) | (64a) |
| 16 | 4 | (65) | (65a) |
| 16 | | Formula 64 | 64a |
| 16 | | Formula 65 | 65a |
| 17 | | Formula 74 | $(CH_2)_2$ |
| 17 | 6 | butylamine | propylamine |
| 18 | 21 | (85) via | (88) via |
| 32 | 6 | ,36, | ,39, |
| 33 | 1 | 43, | 42, |
| 33 | 5 | 43, | 42, |
| 33 | 29 | 41 | 47 |
| 34 | 2 | (7). | (7).[14] |
| 36 | 8 | (8). | (8).[14] |
| 36 | 7 | dicyclonime | dicyclomine |
| 36 | 13 | dihexyrevine | dihexyverine |
| 38 | last | clocental (25) | clocental (75) |
| 42 | 14 | -1-methylpyrro-diline | -1-methylpyrrolidine |
| 47 | 2 | azacyclonol | pipradol |
| 47 | 4 | pipradol | azacyclonol |
| 54 | | Formula 76 | |

| | | | |
|---|---|---|---|
| 66 | 2 | pronethanol | pronethalol |
| 66 | 4 | soltalol | sotalol |
| 67 | | Formula 6 | (remove "6") |
| 68 | | Formulas 37 and 38 | (numbers are reversed) |
| 70 | | Formula 51 | (remove "51") |
| 70 | 15 | $(54).^{12}$ | $(54).^{13}$ |
| 70 | 23 | (58) | (59) |
| 70 | 26 | phenylbutanone-2 | phenylpentanone-2 |
| 72 | 17 | oxoethazine | oxoethazaine |
| 74 | 7 | fencamfine | fencamfamine |
| 78 | 3 | p-chloroaceto-phenone | p-methylacetophenone |
| 78 | | Formulae 109, 110, 111 | $(p-CH_3)$ |
| 86 | 2 | isopropylbenzene | isobutylbenzene |
| 86 | 15 | alkylation of | alkylation with ethyl iodide of |
| 86 | 16 | base with ethyl iodide affords | base affords |
| 86 | 23 | monoethyl | monomethyl |
| 86 | | Formulas 1-5 | $CH_3-CHCH_2-$ with $CH_3$ |
| 90 | 5 | dimethylamine | diethylamine |
| 90 | 6 | carbetapentane (39) | (38) |
| 90 | | Formula 38 | 38, $X=N(C_2H_5)_2$ |
| 91 | | Formula 44 | |

| | | | |
|---|---|---|---|
| 92 | 6 | cyclopyrazolate | cyclopyrazate |
| 93 | 11 | benactizine | benactyzine |
| 96 | 10 | phenol, 77. | phenol, 77a. |
| 96 | 13 | of 77 | of 78a |
| 96 | 15 | ether (79). | ether (79a). |
| 96 | 19 | of 79 | of 79a |
| 97 | 4 | (80) to afford | to afford |
| 97 | | Formula 77 | 77a |
| 97 | | Formula 78 | 78a |
| 97 | | Formula 79 | 79a |
| 97 | | (Unnumbered formula should be 80) | |
| 100 | 15 | ,2,$^2$ | ,2,$^1$ |
| 102 | | (Formula 7 is superfluous and should be removed.) | |
| 111 | | Formula 16 | X=Z=CH$_3$; Y=H |
| 111 | 17 | of 21 | of 20 |
| 111 | 18 | hydrazone (24) | hydrazone (23) |
| 115 | 5 | (42).[9,10] | (43).[9,10] |
| 116 | 2 | moxysylyte | moxisylyte |
| 117 | last | (66).[19] | (66).[18] |
| 119 | | Formulas 76 and 75 | (convert Cl to CH$_3$) |
| 120 | | Formula 81 | |

$$R - \langle\bigcirc\rangle\ \text{(Cl, Cl)} - OCH_2CO_2H$$

| | | | |
|---|---|---|---|
| 123 | | (Compound 94 should be spelled sulfaproxyline.) | |
| 136 | 4 | 1930s | 1920s |
| 137 | 3 | piperidine | azepine |
| 137 | 7 | tolazemide | tolazamide |

| 137 |    | Formulas 190, 191, 193 | |
|-----|----|------------------------|---|
| 138 | 3  | carbutemide | carbutamide |
| 138 | 5  | 1-butyl-3-metanyl-urea | 1-butyl-3-meta-nilylurea |
| 141 | 9  | thiazosulfone | thiazolsulfone |
| 150 |    | Formula 29 | |
| 151 | 17 | amytriptylene | amitriptyline |
| 151 | 23 | methylpipyridine | methylpiperidine |
| 152 | 6  | tylene | tyline |
| 153 |    | Formulas 45/46 | |
| 172 |    | Formula 78b | (Replace angular Me group by H but leave formulae 78a and 78c alone.) |
| 173 |    | Formula 80 | |
| 174 | 7  | eneone (91) | eneone (95) |
| 175 |    | Formula 92 | (Also remove arrow from 91.) |

| | | | |
|---|---|---|---|
| 176 | 39 | (109), | (107), |
| 180 | | Formula 124 | 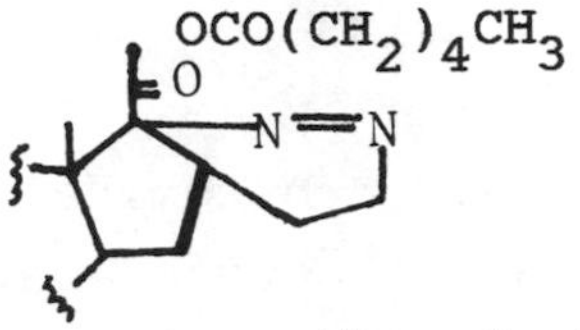 OCO(CH2)4CH3 O N N |
| 183 | | Formula 145 | |
| 186 | Tab. | norethinodrel | norethynodrel |
| 193 | | Formulas 174 and 175 | (Renumber to 174a and 175c) |
| 196 | 21 | N-bromosuccinide | N-bromosuccinimide |
| 196-7 | | Formulae 192-198 | 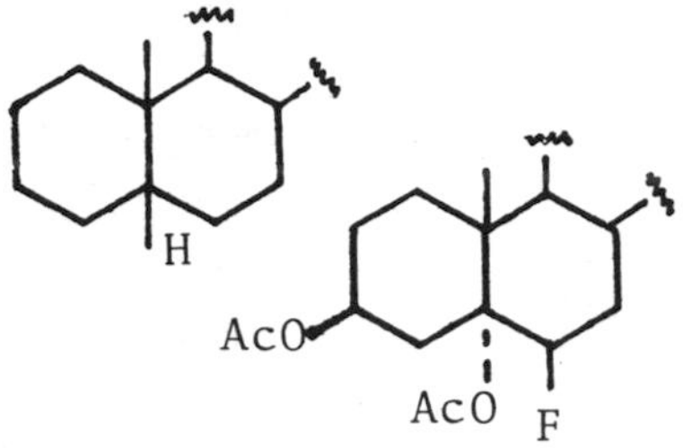 H AcO AcO F |
| 198 | | Formulae 205-207 | |
| 199 | | Formulae 211-212 | |
| 200 | | Formula 219 | |
| 203 | | Formula 240 | OH instead of OAc |
| 213 | | Formulae 1-3 | 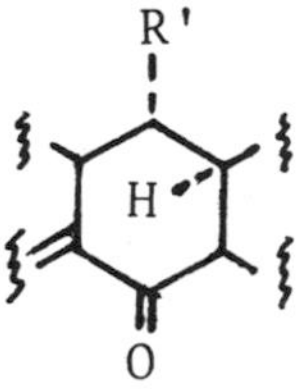 R' H O |
| 213 | | Formulas 9 and 10 | 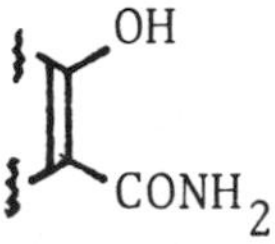 OH CONH2 |
| 219 | | Formulas 3 and 4 | 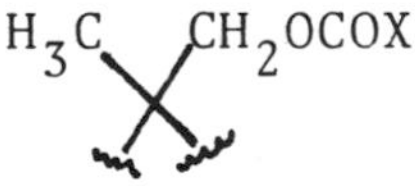 H3C CH2OCOX |
| 225 | | Formula 47 | 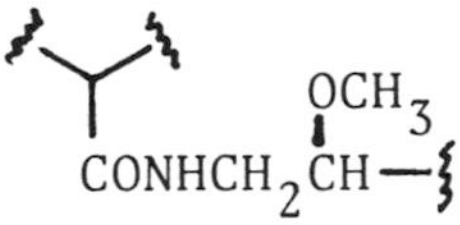 OCH3 CONHCH2CH |

| | | | |
|---|---|---|---|
| 224 | | (Unnumbered formula is 41.) | |
| 231 | last | gives nifurprazine (46).[13] | gives the thiadiazole analogue (46) of nifurprazine (46a).[13] |

232     Add formula 46a

$$O_2N - \underset{O}{\bigcirc} - CH= CH - \underset{N=N}{\bigcirc} - NH_2$$

| | | | |
|---|---|---|---|
| 233 | 8 | isocarboxazine | isocarboxazid |
| 233 | | Formula 50 | (Reverse the methyl and allyl groups.) |
| 234 | 18 | reduction affords | reduction and methylation affords |
| 234 | 19 | (61), | (61a). |
| 235 | | Formula 68 | $CH_3(CH_2)_3CH(CO_2C_2H_5)_2$ |
| 235 | | Formula 61 | |

$$\underset{R_2N}{\phantom{x}} \underset{CH_3}{\phantom{x}} \quad 61, \ R=H$$
$$61a, \ R=CH_3$$

241     Formula 95

$$\underset{N}{\overset{CH_3}{\bigcirc}} - SH$$

242     Formula 101

$$- CH_2 - \underset{NH}{\overset{C}{\underset{\|}{C}}} OCH_3$$

242     Formula 102

$$- CH_2 - \underset{N}{\overset{H}{\underset{N}{\bigcirc}}}$$

| | | | |
|---|---|---|---|
| 246 | 4 | (132); | (130); |
| 246 | 2 | acetophenone | propiophenone |
| 246 | last | tetratoin | tetrantoin |

| 246 |      | Formulae 130–133 | $C_2H_5-C$ |
| 247 | 10   | aminitrazole | aminitrozole |
| 249 | 27   | ambient | ambident |
| 257 | 9    | glutethemide | glutethimide |
| 257 | 12   | aminogluthemide | aminoglutethimide |
| 260 | 6    | guancycline | guanacline |
| 263 | 6    | (71). | (71a). |
| 263 | 8    | (72). | (72a). |

263    (Renumber formulas 71 and 72 to 71a and 72a.)

263    (An arrow should connect formulas 73 and 74.)

264    Formula

264    Formulas 75–79

| 265 | 8    | uracyl | uracil |
| 265 | 12   | uracycls | uracils |
| 266 | 15   | (92).[28] (94),[29] | (94).[28] (95),[29] |
| 266 | 1    | amisotetradine | amisometradine |
| 265 | last | aminotetradine | aminometridine |
| 269 | 1    | 105 | 105a |
| 269 |      | entry 110 | $CH_3CHCH_2CH_2CH_3$ |
| 270 | 6    | allilic | allylic |
| 262 | 2    | phenylacetonitrile | p-chlorophenylaceto-nitrile |
| 262 |      | Formulas 63–65 | (add a p-chloro group) |
| 272 |      | Formula 124 | |

278   19   171.                    171a.

279        Formula 171             171a.

281        Formula 182             $\{\!-\!NHCNH_2$ with NH above and double bond

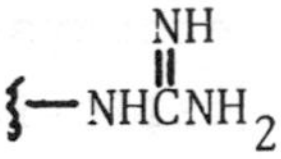

287   last  (4).                   (4).[2]

295        Formula 30              40 (also remove +)

301   1    furfuryl               tetrahydrofurfuryl

301        Formulae 82-85          $-CO_2C_2H_5$

301        Formulae 85-87

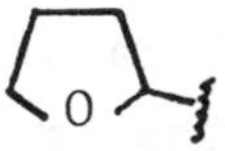

305   7    prolidine              prodilidine

308   20   pirintramide          piritramide

315        Formula 14

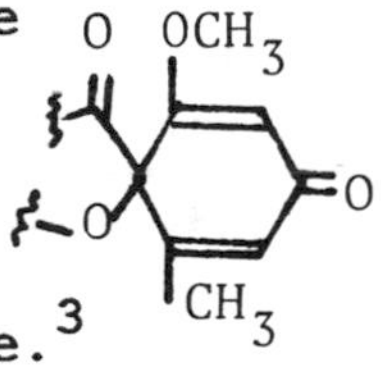

316   15   predominate            predominate.[3]

318   last  scision                scision.[7]

319   5    Rawaulfia              Rauwolfia

320   13   fused to               fused α to

320   17   potassium per-         potassium chlorate
           chlorate

320        Formulas 30-32

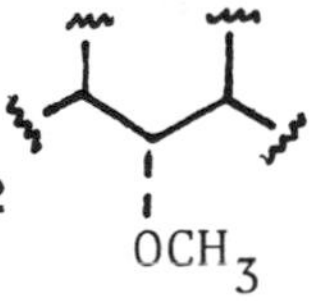

321   7    synthesis.            synthesis.[12]

322        Formulas 47-49

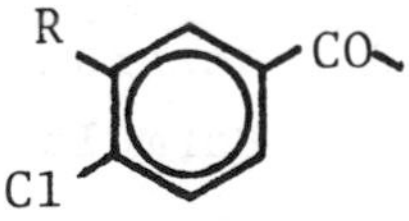

| | | | |
|---|---|---|---|
| 325 | 13 | clonitazine | clonitazene |
| 325 | 14 | etonitazine | etonitazene |
| 327 | 3 | ethoxysolamide | ethoxazolamide |
| 333 | last | salicylaldehyde | acetophenone |
| 334 | | Formulae 21-30 should have a $CH_3$ group | |

instead of H as 30 is

| | | | |
|---|---|---|---|
| 335 | 13 | ,35, | ,35a, |
| 336 | | Formula 35 | 35a |
| 336 | 8 | the bronchodilator | the antiasthmatic |
| 336 | 9 | its extremely insoluble disodium | its disodium |
| 337 | | Formulas 46 and 47 | -CHOH- |
| 338 | 23 | cincona | cinchona |
| 340 | 10 | 59. | 59.[13] |
| 343 | | Formula 76 | 76a |
| 346 | 15 | ,101. | ,103. |
| 346 | 19 | (103) affords | (101) affords |
| 348 | 13 | same | name |
| 352 | 8 | diethylamine | piperidine |
| 352 | | Formula 138 | |

| | | | |
|---|---|---|---|
| 355 | 29 | anthralic | anthranilic |
| 355 | 30 | anthranillic | acetic anhydride |
| 356 | | Formula 163 | |

| | | | |
|---|---|---|---|
| 358 | | Formula 182 | |
| 358 | | Compound 179 | ethiazide |
| 359 | 1 | trichlomethiazide | trichlormethiazide |
| 359 | 7 | cyclopentadiene.[49] | cyclopentadiene.[44] |
| 359 | 2 | althizide | althiazide |
| 359 | 16 | altizide | althiazide |
| 365 | 13 | the oxime | the N-methyl analogue of the oxime |
| 365 | | Formula 14 | $N-CH_3$ |
| 366 | 7 | of diazepam | of desmethyldiazepam |
| 368 | 22 | amide (37). | amide (36). |
| 368 | 25 | The N-methylated analog of inter- mediate, 15, contains | Intermediate 15 contains |
| 370 | 1 | cloxazepam | cloxazolam |
| 373 | 28 | of 3, | of 1, |
| 376 | | Formula 22 | |
| 379 | 1 | (30) | (31) |
| 380 | | Formulas should all have $CH_2CH(CH_3)N(CH_3)_2$ as the side chain. | |
| 386 | 6 | piperactizine | piperacetazine |
| 389 | 8 | of the methylthio- substituted | of substituted |
| 389 | 8 | phenothiazine with | phenothiazine 113 with |
| 389 | 10 | (115).[19] | (114).[19] |

| 389 | 14 | (114) | (115) |
| 389 |    | Formulae 112, 113 and 115 | $-SCH_3$ |
| 390 | 5  | pyrrolidyl | piperazinyl |
| 390 | 9  | at the expense of | in favor of |
| 390 |    | Formulas 118 and 120 | $\{-N\bigcirc$ |
| 390 |    | Formulas 117 and 119 | $-N(CH_3)_2$ |
| 394 | 5  | propanthe- | pronanthe- |
| 394 | 34 | catalyst. | catalyst.[3] |
| 400 | 7  | thiothixine | thiothixene |
| 401 |    | Formula 42 | $-N\bigcirc N-CH_3$ |
| 404 | 10 | amytriptyline | amitriptyline |
| 405 |    | (The unnumbered formula should be 76) | |
| 405 | 10 | dibenzepine | dibenzepin |
| 410 | 32 | 4, a | 4,[1] a |
| 410 | 36 | phenbencillin | phenbenicillin |
| 414 | 21 | carbencillin | carbenicillin |
| 414 | 17 | amoxycillin (35) | amoxycillin (28a) |
| 414 |    | Formula 27, $R=CO_2CH_2C_6H_5$, X=H | $X-\bigcirc-\overset{NHR}{\underset{}{CH}}-\{$ |
| 414 |    | Formula 28, R=X=H | |
| 414 |    | Formula 28a, R=H, X=OH | |
| 417 | 11 | 43. | 43.[24] |
| 426 | 10 | oncolyltic | oncolytic |

| 426 | 12 | oxidate | oxidase |
| 429 | 9 | (39). | (39).[8] |
| 430 | 2 | (47);[10] | (47);[11] |

Changes To Be Made In The Index:

Althiazide

Aminitrozole

Aminoglutethimide

Aminometradine

Amisometradine

Amitriptyline, 151, 404

Benactyzine

Benzphetamine

Betamethasone

Biperiden

Butallonal

1-Butyl-3-metanilyl urea

Caramiphen

Carbenicillin

Carbetidine

Carbutamide

Carisoprodol

Chlorimpiphenine

Chloropyramine

Chlorotrianisene

Cromoglycic acid

Clonitazene

Cloxazolam

Ethoxzolamide

Etonitazene

Fencamfamine

Flumethiazide

Glutethimide

Guanacline

Gaunochlor

Guanoxan

Hydroflumethiazide

Iodothiouracil

Isocarboxazid

Isoproterenol

Levarterinol

Levalorphanol

Mebhydroline

Mephenoxalone

Metaproterenol

Metaxalone

Methaphenilene

Methdilazine

Methyclothiazide, 360

Methylthiouracil

Methyridine, 256

Cyclopyrazate
Debrisoquine
Desipramine
Dexamethasone
Dicyclomine
Dihexyverine
Dimetacrine
Dipiproverine
Dithiazanine
Etriptamine
Ethacrynic acid
Ethiazide
Prolintane
Pronethalol
Propylthiouracil
Prontosil
Protriptyline
PTU, see propylthiouracil
Rescinnamine
Sotalol
(delete Sulfadiazene, 128)
Sulfaproxyline
Tetrantoin
Thiomestrone
Thiazolsulfone
Trichlormethiazide
Trifluperidol
Trihexyphenidyl
Tripelennamine
Uracils

Moxisylyte
Nikethamide
Norethynodrel
Nortriptyline
Oxoethazaine
Paraethoxycaine
Pargyline
Phenbenicillin
Pholcodine
Piperacetazine
Piritramide
Prodilidine